SUPERBUG

Previous books by Geoffrey Cannon:

Dieting Makes You Fat (co-author, 1983, 1984)
The Food Scandal (co-author, 1984, 1985)
Fat To Fit (1986)
The Politics of Food (1987, 1988)
The Good Fight (1989)
Food and Health: the Experts Agree (1992)

SUPERBUG

Nature's revenge

Why antibiotics can breed disease

Geoffrey Cannon

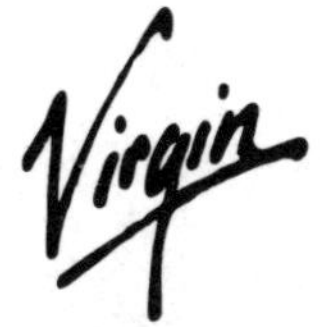

To Ben, Matt and Lou–
with love always

First published in Great Britain in 1995 by
Virgin Publishing Ltd
332 Ladbroke Grove
London W10 5AH

Research: Angela Henderson
Appendix: Kirsten Rowley

A catalogue record for this book is available from the British Library

ISBN 1 85227 364 X

Type design by Roger Kohn
Typeset by Phoenix Photosetting, Chatham, Kent
Printed and bound in Great Britain by
Mackays of Chatham PLC, Chatham, Kent

If you try to eradicate Nature, she will in time rise up silently and confound your foolish arrogance.

Horace
Epistles; 1st century BC

Drugs are much too serious a thing to be left to the medical profession and to the pharmaceutical industry.

D. Laurence and P. Bennett
Clinical Pharmacology; 1992

Contents

Acknowledgements

Superbug has been five years in the making, and my first and foremost thanks are to my collaborators Angela Henderson, who did much of the initial research for the book, and to Kirsten Rowley, who compiled the Appendix. Interviews with scientists in the USA and in Scandinavia were made possible by a Winston Churchill Travelling Fellowship, and I am grateful to the Winston Churchill Memorial Trust and in particular to Brigadier-General Sir Richard Vickers and to Anne Knocker, for their support and kindness.

The idea of *Superbug* was guided by the writings of many scientists on infection, medicine and public health. I am especially indebted to the late Professor René Dubos, the late Professor Thomas McKeown, Professor Nevin Scrimshaw and Professor Lewis Thomas.

To my mind a mark of a great scientist is an interest not just in research, but also in its social implications. I owe a special debt to five leading scientists who very generously gave me much of their time to explain the meaning of their work. These are Professor Graham Dukes, lately head of the World Health Organisation's European office pharmaceutical programme in Copenhagen who has written the Preface of this book; Professor Richard Lacey, head of the department of Medical Microbiology at Leeds University, who has written the Foreword and Afterword; Professor Tore Midtvedt, head of the department of Medical Microbial Ecology at the Karolinska Institute in Stockholm; Dr Richard Novick of the Public Health Research Institute in New York City; and Professor Thomas O'Brien, Medical Director of the department of Microbiology at Brigham and Women's Hospital, Boston.

A large number of scientists and workers in the field were interviewed for *Superbug* or guided me to relevant research; or else read and commented on the book or relevant chapters or sections in draft. Thanks to Professor Jerry Avorn, Dr Peter Borriello, Andrew Chetley, Dr Mariam Claeson, Dr Peter Davey, Dr Richard Dickinson, Dr

Georgia Duckworth, James Erlichman, Professor Stanley Falkow, Professor Sydney Finegold, Professor Rolf Freter, Dr Leo Galland, Kevin Gopal, Professor Sherwood Gorbach, Dr Jeremy Hamilton-Miller, Professor Tony Hart, Professor Ken Harvey, Professor David Hentges, Dr Scott Holmberg, Dr John Hunter, the late Brian Inglis, Professor Calvin Kunin, Professor Harold Lambert, Professor Marc Lappé, Professor Philip Lee, Professor Stuart Levy, Professor Alan Linton, Dr Frank Loew, Dr Alan Long, Dr Rosalind Maskell, Charles Medawar, Dianna Melrose, Professor Robert Metcalf, Professor Alan Percival, Professor Sandy Raeburn, Dr Anita Rampling, Professor Michael Rawlings, Professor David Reeves, Professor Donald Rucker, Philippa Saunders, Dr Mildred Seelig, Dr Robert Tauxe, Dr John Threlfall, Professor Dirk van der Waaij, Joy Wingfield and Professor Steven Witkin.

Last and special thanks to my publisher, Rob Shreeve, whose suggestions and support as the book progressed were vital; my editors Lorna Russell and Nancy Duin; my advisors Gerrard Tyrell and Sophia Roper; my agent Deborah Rogers, whose legendary kindness has been put to the test; and to Imogen Sharp, with love. I have spent more time writing books and less time with my family than I care to remember; thus the dedication of this book to my sons Ben and Matt and my daughter Lou.

Preface

by Professor Graham Dukes

During the last quarter of a century, we have become acutely aware of a series of problems caused by our social and economic development; although not always so painfully aware that we have been goaded to find solutions. Sometimes we may be too clever for our own good. More often, we have been much more clever at making discoveries than in making good use of these discoveries. The essence of our foolishness is that we solve one problem, but in so doing create a much bigger problem. Too much knowledge, not enough wisdom, perhaps.

For men, aerosol shaving cream with a Freon propellant is, early in the morning, a minor convenience; but the hole in the ozone layer that it helps to create threatens to be a global disaster. For women of a certain age, hormones in beauty creams may just possibly smooth out wrinkles, but may be rather more likely to promote cancer. Lead in petrol? The slow poisoning of life around every roadway, not to mention the effect of the increased burden of lead on the intelligence of children, is too high a price to pay for a smoother-running engine.

COLLUSION WITH OUR FOOLISHNESS

Manufacturers of such commodities make profits by colluding with us in our foolishness. In such cases, and many more like them, the idealists who seek to alert us to the damage done, and the officials who, as in such cases, make regulations in the public interest, are opposed by an unholy alliance of those who supply and those who demand. Restriction, let alone prohibition of any daily habit, is condemned as outrageous intrusion into both commercial enterprise and personal freedom.

Besides – we are so often told in such cases – evidence of risk is just anecdotal, and not based on data from randomised double-blind scientific trials. The weight of effort, ingenuity, pressure and equivocation that society is capable of bringing to bear in order to defend its most unwise habits, is staggering. Common sense sometimes wins in the end, but usually only after much harm, sometimes irreparable, has been done.

The antibiotic story, as Geoffrey Cannon tells it in this book, is blacker than most other stories of human failing. With antibiotics, the risks are so great, and society's understanding of these risks is so meagre.

For a generation that has come to live with the appalling horror of AIDS, it should be easy to realise just how devastating an unstoppable disease epidemic may be. Why then are we so apathetic about the dangers of antibiotic overuse and abuse? One partial explanation is that penicillin and other early antibacterial drugs were originally hailed with awe as miracle cures, and ever since then it has been assumed that the flood of new antibiotics, and the vast increase in antibiotic use, is an unmixed blessing.

THE GLOBAL MENACE

Even physicians sometimes seem to think that antibiotic overuse is not a problem; after all, the frivolous prescription of antibiotics for a patient is not very likely to expose that individual to immediate risk. The menace is to fellow-patients – across the ward, across the city, across the world – who blur into a faceless anonymity about which it is hard to generate concern. Even if the individual boomerang returns, in the form of a new drug-resistant and perhaps virulent or invasive infection that is hard to treat, both the patient and the physician may not understand that such a superbug has been created by previous use of antibiotics.

For many years now, specialist professionals have expressed more and more concern about the ill-effects of antibiotics, in the dry language of science in learned journals. Recently, appalling phenomena like drug-resistant tuberculosis in the community, and virtually untreatable potentially deadly multi-resistant hospital pathogens like *Staphylococcus aureus*, have made sensational headlines and baffling mass media stories. But the basic issues are straightforward, as well as bleak and stark. If we go on abusing antibiotics as we now do, we are faced with a return to a medical dark age, in which antibiotics no longer work against a vast range of infections, some created by antibiotics, some perhaps epidemic and deadly. It is good that Geoffrey Cannon has now presented these issues in simple terms, in the hope that we shall at last understand, and act.

But who should act? *Superbug* very properly starts with the people most concerned: patients themselves. You are less likely to be offered an antibiotic unnecessarily if you question what is prescribed for you. Many doctors, fortunately, do listen to well-informed, determined patients.

DOCTORS, INDUSTRY AND GOVERNMENTS

The medical profession has a key responsibility, guided by microbiologists and pharmacists, and also by impartial sources that emphasise the need for drugs to be prescribed rationally. In some countries, and in some areas even within countries like the UK and the USA where market forces are so strong, many doctors are using antibiotics more cautiously. But nowadays nobody can be completely protected against the ill-effects of irresponsible antibiotic use: with infections carried across the world on every jetliner, we are all vulnerable to superbugs.

In some developing countries, within East Africa for example, a combination of prudence and poverty has resulted in excellent 'essential drugs' programmes, so that most people are prescribed only a few well-selected antibiotics. But these nations could at any time be overwhelmed by drug-resistant epidemics bred in their affluent cities, where antibiotics are grossly overused and abused.

What of industry? The pharmaceutical industry is sensitive to criticisms, and we can be grateful for its research successes and appreciative of its attempts to maintain ethical standards. The fact remains, though, that in a great part of the world reckless use of antibiotics is made worse by aggressive marketing and promotion of drugs. It is also true that when the US National Institutes of Health attempted a global initiative in the mid 1980s designed to stop antibiotic misuse, their work was thwarted by a number of major pharmaceutical companies able to put pressure on the White House. And even when one company sets proper standards for drug promotion and sales, another company will jump in to grab more market share.

What of governments, and ministries of health? History shows that national drug policies are an unhappy confusion, with restrictive measures occasionally imposed, but usually only after a disaster has already occurred. Neither individual nations nor international bodies such as the European Union have so far developed any broad policy to ensure that drugs serve the community properly. Governments like that of the UK whose drug regulations are designed to ensure the quality, efficacy and relative immediate safety of each individual product entering the market, seem to believe they are doing enough.

There is little inclination to tackle issues like the overuse, abuse, proliferation and redundancy of permitted drugs, let alone ignorance and misunderstanding of their benefits, risks and longer-term ill-effects on public health, except when a government's hand is forced by media scandal or soaring costs. Policy-makers must be pressed relentlessly to think and act in the public interest.

But it is too easy to point the finger of blame at patients, doctors, drug companies or health authorities. Like most major social problems, the overuse and abuse of antibiotics is a tangled web.

PUTTING THE CITIZEN FIRST

Recently I was discussing these issues with a group of medical students who first blamed industry advertising. I asked them to think again. What emerged on the blackboard was literally, a series of vicious circles and spirals. Aggressive advertising of third-generation cephalosporins did indeed seem to push doctors to prescribe these new and very expensive drugs in situations where an older, simpler, safer, antibiotic would be the rational choice. So why the advertising? Because patents on the old antibiotics had expired, prices had fallen, and they were too cheap to generate enough profits to finance the research that would produce even more sophisticated fourth-generation cephalosporins. And why was that research, costing altogether maybe hundreds of millions of dollars and pounds, needed? Because energetic advertising and promotion campaigns had led to overuse and abuse, which in turn inevitably bred new generations of drug-resistant bacteria, effectively and profitably treated only by ever-new drugs. And so on, and on.

The final analysis was complex, and led to questioning of patent law, national and local drug purchasing policies, the training of medical students, the financing of research, and many other interrelated issues. The fearful problem of antibiotic resistance outlined in *Superbug* must now become a national and international priority, to be resolved not just in private by policy-makers, but also by means of informed public debate.

In his book, Geoffrey Cannon starts at the right point. However many vicious circles and spirals we identify, they all have a common centre, and that is the patient, which is to say the citizen – you, and me. This is the place to start, and start now, rather than continuing just to discuss disaster until it overwhelms us.

Graham Dukes MD MA LLM
Professor of Drug Policy Studies,
University of Groningen, the Netherlands
Formerly Head of Pharmaceuticals Programme,
World Health Organisation, European Region

Foreword

by Professor Richard Lacey

We all know that antibiotics save lives; but they probably do not do so as often as is generally believed. Antibiotics are the second favourite drug prescribed by doctors throughout the world. Indeed, patients come to expect them for all sorts of minor symptoms, from sore throats to colds, coughs, earache, diarrhoea and cystitis. Sometimes the writing of a prescription for an antibiotic provides the speediest means for ending a medical consultation. Patients have come to expect these 'wonder' drugs for almost every complaint.

A few years ago I had just completed a lecture in a Middle Eastern country, when a doctor asked: 'What antibiotics should I recommend for headache?' After some discussion, it transpired that the issue was that meningitis could cause headaches, and that patients could not afford tests to see if they had meningitis: so antibiotics were given – just in case.

But there is a down side to reflex or compulsive antibiotic prescribing. The human body needs its own harmless bacteria for full health. The bacteria in the intestines are particularly valuable, for preventing dangerous germs getting a foothold, for making vitamins, for developing the immune system, and for digesting some of our food.

REASONS TO BE CAREFUL

The use of antibiotics is often associated with side-effects, either directly caused by the drug, such as allergies to penicillins, or growth defects in the developing body from tetracycline, or else as a result of their destruction of our beneficial bacteria. Furthermore, antibiotics are bound to select resistant bacteria that might spread and cause problems in other patients who might really need them. It follows that if the patient did not require antibiotics in the first place, then these drugs are only doing harm.

I am writing these comments with some considerable experience of research and use of antibiotics, both as microbiologist and as a medical doctor. In this highly recommended book, Geoffrey Cannon presents a meticulous analysis of such issues as seen from the view of the patient. There is of course implied criticism of the over-prescription of antibiotics by doctors, and their over-promotion by the massive multinational pharmaceutical companies. These criticisms are fully justified.

But the overriding message is to you, the reader and potential patient. When you have a condition for which antibiotics are of no benefit and therefore are only harmful, do not pester your doctor for a prescription. If in the surgery you are told that your sore throat is due to a virus and therefore untreatable with antibiotics, please accept this advice.

In his analysis, Geoffrey Cannon explores both the reasonable and the unreasonable uses of antibiotics. The particular details of each available product are to the best of my knowledge, correct.

This book has been incubating for some years. Like Geoffrey Cannon's other major works, it contains a wonderfully detached analysis of the issues involved. Of course there are some ideas, even speculation, that a trigger-happy prescriber might question; but I hope that most doctors will be sympathetic with the message, which is that we should reduce our expectation of benefit from antibiotics, except in cases of really serious bacterial infections such as meningitis, enteric fever, tuberculosis, or infections of the heart, kidneys or blood where they really are needed.

Currently, most people on average take a course of antibiotics once or twice a year. If this book has the effect of reducing this average to once every five or ten years, then Geoffrey Cannon's energy and enthusiasm will have been worthwhile.

Richard W Lacey MA MD PhD FRCPath DCH
Professor of Medical Microbiology, University of Leeds

Introduction

In effect, antibiotics are pesticides used on people. Farmers and gardeners who use chemicals do so to destroy bugs they think are a nuisance to their crops, flowers or vegetables. Likewise, people who accept antibiotic chemotherapy do so to check or kill bugs they or their doctors believe will harm them. The general word for pesticide, including herbicides, insecticides and the rest, is biocide. This has much the same literal meaning as antibiotic: killer of life (-cide as in homicide, bio- as in biology); or against (anti-) life.

The life in question is of course that of bugs, visible or invisible. Pesticides, used carefully, are vital for modern agriculture and horticulture. But they have a bad reputation, because we sense that the world needs visible bugs and that most of them have a purpose on the planet. To use an old-fashioned phrase, they are links in the great chain of being. Pesticides do indeed kill living things that attack plants, but it is now common knowledge that they also kill beneficial or beautiful creatures, create a devastation in which previously harmless bugs become virulent pests, and breed mutant superpests immune to chemical bombardment.

Farmers thus risk being put on a treadmill, dependent on ever greater and possibly futile use of increasingly expensive agrichemicals. Many insects now are biocide-resistant, the result of the use of insecticides. Mutant strains of insects that carry human disease also multiply as a result of treatment with pesticides: the malaria mosquito is now commonly a superpest, immune to insecticides. We are all used to the idea that the ecological havoc caused by pesticides is vast and incalculable.

BENEFITS OF ANTIBIOTICS

Antibiotics have a good reputation; but they do to the natural world and to us what pesticides do to smaller creatures. The good news about antibiotics is well known. They can indeed be wonderfully effective, and are vital treatment for dangerous invasive bacterial infections of the vital organs.

Virtually all farmers and gardeners use pesticides of some type or another on occasion. Quite right too. Similarly, you would be mad to refuse antibiotic treatment for reliably diagnosed bacterial infections of the blood (septicaemia), lining of the brain (meningitis) or heart (endocarditis), the lungs (pneumonia), kidneys (nephritis), or sexual organs (gonorrhoea, syphilis).

It is quite likely that at some time in your life you or a member of your family will be infected by a really dangerous bacterial disease that should be cured by an appropriate antibiotic. Never forget this. Take care to find a general practitioner who is interested in positive health, who likes to discuss treatment, who prefers to avoid drugs, who respects antibiotics as a precious resource, and who normally will prescribe them only when reasonably sure that your illness is caused by an invasive bacterial infection. Such a doctor is a real friend in need, and might even save your life.

RISKS: TOXICITY

The bad news about antibiotics is less well known. Everybody knows – or should know – that there is no such thing as a completely safe drug. Any antibiotic may cause acute illness. But this is not a reason to panic. Most common acute ill-effects of antibiotics are trivial or transient: these include rashes, dizziness, headaches, cramps and diarrhoea. Many antibiotics commonly used in general practice are relatively safe, notably penicillins. Most relatively dangerous anti-bacterials, such as all sulphonamides, streptomycin and chloramphenicol, are now not often used in developed countries like the UK (with the exception of co-trimoxazole, a sulphonamide combined with trimethoprim, still often prescribed for cystitis, bronchitis and other infections).

Doctors should warn their patients of possible ill-effects of any course of antibiotics they prescribe, and it is normally bad practice to go on prescribing courses of antibiotics for obstinate infections, unless the patient is closely observed. Most relatively serious acute illnesses caused by antibiotics are ill-effects of heavy doses and/or long courses not referred to or overlooked by doctors.

Carefully prescribed, antibiotics are uncommon causes of severe illness, and their immediate toxicity is usually problematic only when they are used on vulnerable people such as babies, young children, pregnant women, the elderly, and on surgical, immunodeficient or otherwise very ill hospital patients. But on rare occasions even just one course can kill otherwise generally healthy people. These calamities, including severe anaphylactic shock and pseudomembranous colitis, both of which can be caused by a number of commonly prescribed antibiotics, are reason enough to avoid them for simple infections that normally will clear up without drug treatment. But for invasive bacterial infections of vital organs, the balance of risk and benefit is overwhelmingly in favour of taking the antibiotic as prescribed.

PESTICIDES USED ON PEOPLE

Toxicity is the least of the risks of antibiotics. As now used, their main ill-effects, which they have in common with pesticides, are insidious and invisible, and a menace not just to the individual, but to public health.

Curiously, nowadays we tend to think green about everything except ourselves. The last ecological frontier is not thousands of miles away, in the Antarctic ozone layer or the Brazilian rain forest, but on us and a few inches inside us: the bacteria and other microbes that have evolved with us. We have been brought up to believe that bacteria are generally harmful, and to confuse hygiene with sterility. This is a mistake.

We need the bugs that live on and in us; almost all of them have evolved to be harmless or positively health-giving to their hosts, whether human, animal or plant. Among other functions, harmless bacteria protect us against invasive infection simply by being there. The bacteria in our guts, sometimes known as friendly flora, amount to a vital organ of the body.

There is also no such thing as a magic bullet, meaning a drug whose one and only effect is to destroy disease. Exactly like pesticides, antibiotics make waves in the ecosphere. The more they are used, and the more broad-spectrum in their effect, the more bacterial species they devastate, creating a microbiological wasteland. This is liable to be invaded and colonised by other bacterial species, some originally harmless, others essentially harmful, and also by moulds, viruses and other microbes, which may cause what is known as superinfectious disease. Two superinfections, of the gut caused by *Clostridium difficile* bacteria, and the vagina caused by *Candida albicans* mould, are now common as a result of antibiotic use.

Genetically, humans have not changed much since the beginning of history. But the smaller and simpler any species, the faster it can evolve in response to environmental change. Insects are small; bacteria are microscopic one-cell organisms. Pesticides and antibiotics put what is called 'selective pressure' on bugs, pushing them to develop and share defence mechanisms, genes that give immunity to chemical attack. Constant use of pesticides inevitably creates plagues of disease caused by mutant visible bugs, immune to many or even all available chemicals. Likewise, constant use of antibiotics inevitably creates epidemics of disease caused by mutant invisible bugs, immune to many or even all available drugs. These multi drug-resistant bacteria and other microbes are known as superbugs.

Most antibiotics now in use have been devised and marketed for treatment of bacterial and other infections caused by previous use of antibiotics. Most hospital infections are now caused by species or strains of bacteria harmless or trivial in their ill-effects half a century ago. Like farmers, doctors and their patients are now on a chemical treadmill. And superbugs spread their resistance round the world on a microbiological genetic information superhighway. The bacteria that next infect you with disease are unlikely to be exactly the same in their genetic coding as the original pre-antibiotic species.

MUTANT STRAINS

When I started to research *Superbug* in 1989, the greatest fear of microbiologists was that one day a 'doomsday superbug' would evolve: a mutant strain of some bacterial species liable to cause epidemics of deadly disease, immune to every drug known to modern medical science. The most likely candidate was *Staphylococcus aureus* in the form known as MRSA (methicillin-resistant *S. aureus*). This is a dreadful pathogen that occurs in hospital wards in the UK, the USA, Australia and many other countries, bred as a result of constant overuse of antibiotics over the years by surgeons and doctors, and now often immune to every drug except the very expensive and unusually toxic vancomycin. One day, it was feared, MRSA would mutate to become everything-resistant, effectively putting hospital doctors back in a pre-antibiotic dark age, helplessly watching their patients die.

In 1991 I went to New York to see Dr Richard Novick, a world authority on drug resistance. He told me that outside the laboratory, MRSA was still vulnerable to vancomycin. But he also told me that the doomsday superbug had arrived. The second most common cause of hospital infections in the USA now, are enterococci, bacteria that originally were relatively harmless, but now commonly cause infections of wounds, blood and vulnerable vital organs, that may kill weak or old patients. Certain species and strains of enterococci had evolved in the late 1980s to become immune to all known antibiotics, including vancomycin, and in Dr Novick's opinion were likely in time to become epidemic and also to transfer total drug resistance to staphylococci. The result could be a global epidemic, perhaps the greatest disaster ever created by modern medical practice.

This dark thought aside, though, it could be said that superbugs are just a glitch, a negative aspect of a success story. Even though the pharmaceutical industry and the medical profession have to run faster round the treadmill to develop new antibiotics and to find ones that work, some drug will usually be successful treatment against bacterial infections that were epidemic killers up to half a century ago, before the age of antibiotics.

This is true, for generally healthy people in rich countries like the UK and USA. The prospect is not so rosy, though, for debilitated patients, nor for people in poor countries subject to uncontrolled epidemics now often in new forms resistant to available drugs – which may then travel around the world. The malaria mosquito is now commonly immune to insecticides. The malaria microbe is also now commonly immune to antibiotics.

To my mind though, what is most worrying about antibiotics is not just that they breed drug-resistant superbugs, but that they create conditions in which all sorts of mutant strains of bacteria and other micro-organisms thrive and multiply. A religious person could sincerely say that only God knows what drugs have done and will do to bugs. In nature, species of butterflies and other insects can be seen over a few generations to evolve subtle variations in response to change in climate. So do microbes, very much faster; and the selective pressure of antibiotics pushes bacteria to develop mechanisms of protection in a new environment.

Such mutations may, if only by chance, transform a species originally harmless to humans, or a cause only of trivial infection, into variants, sub-species or what are in effect new species, causing new or virulent and even deadly diseases. Such mutant strains, monster superbugs, may or may not be vulnerable to drugs. Does this really happen? Oh yes, here and now.

THE SCALE OF THE PROBLEM

Wisely used, antibiotics are a blessing. But antibiotics are now vastly overused and abused.

The US National Institutes of Health has estimated that by the year 2000, a total of 50,000 tons of antibiotics will be used every year throughout the world on humans, animals and plants, amounting to a vast unplanned, unchecked and uncontrollable exercise in genetic manipulation. This scale of use makes mass microbial mutation, and with it new diseases, inevitable.

The threat of new epidemics caused by mutant bacteria and other microbes is not just theoretical. Leading scientists, worried in the 1980s, are now appalled. Professor Michael Levin is head of the department of the infectious diseases of children at St Mary's Hospital, London, the place where in 1928 Alexander Fleming identified the antibiotic properties of a penicillium mould. In the autumn of 1993, 65 years later, Dr Levin gave the Darwin Lecture for the British Association for the Advancement of Science. With special reference to children, he said, 'So great is the number of new or re-emerging infectious diseases that it would be impossible even to mention a small proportion of them.' He instanced septicaemia, meningitis, pneumonia, nephritis, bacterial infections of the bones and joints and of wounds, and gonorrhoea, tuberculosis, cholera and typhoid fever, all increasing, often in new or drug-resistant forms.

He also mentioned previously unknown diseases of children, such as staphylococcal toxic shock syndrome, Kawasaki disease, and Brazilian purperic fever, 'not even dreamed of ten to fifteen years ago'. This last horrible infection, first identified in the 1980s in Sao Paulo, is now known to be caused by the bacterium *Haemophilus Aegypticus*, previously known to be almost harmless. Professor

Levin said: 'It now seems that a subtle mutation in the genetic make-up of this innocent bacterium has transformed it into a rampant killer.'

In March 1994 *Newsweek* magazine published a cover feature with the title 'The End of Antibiotics'. Quoting the federal Centers for Disease Control and Prevention (CDC), this stated that in the US in 1992, a total of '13,300 hospital patients died of bacterial infections that resisted the antibiotics doctors fired at them . . . It was not that they had infections immune to every single drug but rather that, by the time the doctors found an antibiotic that worked, the rampaging bacteria had poisoned the patient's blood, scarred the lungs or crippled some other vital organ.'

Some American scientists interviewed for this book, Professor Thomas O'Brien of Harvard University, Professor Stuart Levy of Tufts University in Boston, and Professor Stanley Falkow of Stanford University in California, were quoted. Drug resistance is 'unparalleled in recorded biologic history', said Dr Levy. He too cited septicaemia, meningitis, pneumonia, wound infections and tuberculosis; and also dysentery and other bacterial infections, all now increasing in new or multi drug-resistant forms.

In 1993 and 1994 a number of special meetings were held throughout the world in which scientists wondered what to do about the new plagues among us, caused by superbugs. One of these was held at Rockefeller University, New York. Its organiser, Professor Alexander Tomasz, stated in his report in the *New England Journal of Medicine* in April 1994 that 'the 1990s have brought a worldwide resurgence of bacterial and viral diseases. An important factor in this phenomenon is the acquisition of antibiotic-resistance genes by virtually all major bacterial pathogens.' His list included epidemic blood and wound infections caused by MRSA; multi drug-resistant tuberculosis, now out of control in New York; and mutant strains of pneumococci that are now a global menace, causing severe ear infections as well as meningitis and pneumonia.

He also stated that the doomsday superbugs, the everything-resistant enterococci Dr Richard Novick mentioned to me in 1991, had by 1993 killed 323 hospital patients throughout the USA: not yet an epidemic, but cause for concern. In 1994 medical journals recorded that some mutant enterococci were not just immune to vancomycin but actually fed off it. The ultimate drug-eating everything-resistant monster superbug has been created, and is beginning to live and breed in hospitals now.

Professor Tomasz went further than the CDC, citing evidence that every year in the USA, 60,000–70,000 people now die from hospital infections, half or more of which are caused by drug-resistant superbugs; and he reckoned that hospital infections altogether cost the US healthcare system $4.5 billion a year, or more. What about the UK? Statistics like these are easier to find from US sources, and British doctors may say that American colleagues spray antibiotics and extrapolations around enthusiastically. Also, very often it is a matter of opinion whether very ill patients die from a hospital infection or from underlying disease. But it is probably safe to say that superbugs contribute to the deaths of many thousands of hospital patients in the UK, at a cost to the NHS of tens if not hundreds of millions of pounds every year.

In the summer of 1994 the *British Medical Journal* published an interview by its editor Dr Richard Smith with Sir Dai Rees, chief executive of the UK Medical Research Council, responsible for allocating public money to medical science. The first question concerned the greatest challenges facing modern medicine. Sir Dai said: 'We know that we will have an ageing population; and we fear the development of more micro-organisms resistant to antibiotics.' Later in 1994 the UK Parliamentary Office of Science and Technology published a report, 'Diseases Fighting Back'. This said, 'Drug resistance is a problem potentially affecting many thousands of UK patients. The consequences to patients vary widely; for some, contracting a drug-resistant infection may be no more than a minor inconvenience necessitating a slightly prolonged course of treatment. For others however, failure to respond to the initial course of treatment may have more serious implications (e.g. extended hospital stay) or even make the difference between life and death, particularly if the patients are vulnerable (e.g. very young, old, or ill).' You have been warned.

WHO IS RESPONSIBLE?

I am sometimes asked, 'Are you a doctor?' No, I am not. If this question implies that only people with medical qualifications should write about health and disease, I do not agree. Legal definitions of wrongdoing are technical, but this does not mean that only lawyers can understand right and wrong. Key decisions on peace and war are complex, but it does not follow that modern states are best governed by generals. Indeed, the doctrine of 'leave it to the experts' is unwise. Democracy depends on the supremacy of the laity: and if lay people, whether politicians or citizens, are ill-informed, the fabric of society disintegrates.

Certainly, anybody whose views on medicine may be influential should be well-advised. The thesis of *Superbug* depends on modern medical and microbiological science. The main text of the book is fully referenced to the specialist literature. Much of the most powerful testimony cited is that of leading research scientists. And *Superbug* is not an argument for homoeopathy or complementary therapies (although some readers may prefer these to allopathic treatments depending on drugs) or for a return to an imaginary pre-antibiotic arcadia. Antibiotics are a precious resource. We should make the best of them.

As individuals, this responsibility is ours to share with our medical advisors. We should be less inclined to blame doctors for our illnesses, when treatments don't work or go wrong. Disease is too important to be left just to doctors. We should be impatient with science's ignorance about what makes us ill and what keeps us well, and be prepared to have well-informed opinions of our own. Indeed, it would be good if the word 'patient', suggesting that when we go to the doctor we are receptacles, fell into disuse, to be replaced by a sturdier word like 'client'.

SCIENCE AND SPECULATION

Most of *Superbug* simply gathers together information published in textbooks and leading medical journals, and testimonies of leading research scientists, some specially interviewed for the book, presenting this evidence in plain language. There is I think good reason based on reasonably solid science to believe that as now used, antibiotics do more harm than good.

Sometimes *Superbug* goes beyond standard textbooks, but not beyond science: many research findings on ill-effects of antibiotics are new. Occasionally I have been more speculative, basing arguments not on the results of controlled trials, but on biologically plausible reasoning and consultation with specialists in the field.

For example, it seems to me that heavy or regular use of some antibiotics, liable to damage the mucosal lining of the gut wall and thus our immune defences, is for this and other reasons possibly one cause (please note, *possibly one* cause, not *the* cause) of a number of diseases that baffle modern medical science, some much more common in the last half-century. These include gut diseases such as irritable bowel syndrome, Crohn's Disease and even colon cancer; some forms of arthritis; and the debilitating illness known as chronic fatigue syndrome or ME.

I might have omitted hypotheses not yet supported by substantial and consistent research. But I have included some in the book, clearly identified as relatively speculative. Just as medical practice is based on cases, hypotheses are the starting point for investigation, and I hope *Superbug* will encourage the funding of more scientific research into the risks, and the benefits, of antibiotics.

WIDER MEANINGS

Superbug is about antibiotics, bacteria and human disease, and that perhaps is a broad enough theme. But in the time I have been researching and writing the book, it seems to me that the antibiotic story is a parable, resonant with meaning. What does it mean to be ill, and to be well? When is it wise and when foolish, to fight disease? How should we relate not only to doctors, but to other professional people on whom we depend? Are diseases essential to evolution? Do drugs mask the human condition? What are the proper limits of science and technology? Should we see nature as Gaia, a vast intelligence besides which we are children? How can we best respect our place in the world? These and other questions are here for you to consider.

Meanwhile, I hope that *Superbug* will help you to protect your own health, and that of your friends and family, by treating antibiotics with respect and using them carefully. As a citizen, you may also wish to take action.

Geoffrey Cannon
London
and Copenhagen, Stockholm, Oslo,
Boston, Chicago, Palo Alto, New York
January 1995

Part One

Blind Faith:
Doctors and Patients

The aspects of things that are most important for us are hidden, because of their simplicity and familiarity. One is unable to notice something – because it is always before one's eyes. We fail to be struck by what, once seen, is most striking and most powerful.

Ludwig Wittgenstein
Philosophical Investigations; 1953

I continue to listen in astonishment when politicians compete among themselves to prove that their care and concern for the National Health Service is greater than that of any of their opponents. The one guaranteed way of proving how much you care is to demonstrate that, during your time of office, more patients had operations, more outpatients had more treatments, and more doctors issued more prescriptions! If people continue to see health in terms of the provision and consumption of illness services, and a spiralling increase in these illness services year after year, then there is no solution to the problems of the National Health Service.

Jonathon Porritt
Former director, Friends of the Earth; 1989

1 The New Priesthood

KEEP ON TAKING THE PILLS

Antibiotics have a wonderful reputation. We are brought up to believe in them, as a great blessing. And so they can be. In the last half-century, antibiotics and other antimicrobial drugs have saved the lives and restored the health of countless people. They have indeed been effective against the bacterial infections that ravaged Europe and America in the nineteenth century.

The fabulous reputation that antibiotics still enjoy is not just a folk memory. Most readers of this book have probably at some time been successfully treated with antibiotics for trivial or serious bacterial infections. To the best of my knowledge I personally have never had a bad experience with antibiotics; they seem to work, for me. Without antibiotics many people alive today would have died as children or earlier in adult life: two, who as distinguished biological scientists should know what they are talking about, are friends of mine.

But there is a worm in this rose. Like all effective drugs, antibiotics can be toxic, in the sense that they can have acute ill-effects. They should never be taken lightly. Those now available on prescription in the UK, the USA and other countries where the use of drugs is carefully regulated, have between them very many immediate ill-effects, most trivial, some serious.[1,2,3] On rare occasions, antibiotics kill generally healthy people.

As with the contraceptive pill, the benefits of antibiotics are evidently so obvious that it may seem ungrateful to question their effects as now used. Certainly, books on antibiotics written for the general reader usually maintain a somewhat uncritical tone. In his introduction to *Antibiotics: the Comprehensive Guide*,[4] pharmacologist Dr John Halliday correctly writes: 'The development of a wide range of antibiotics means that many previously life-threatening conditions can now be successfully treated.' He concludes: 'There is much reason for optimism, and these are no less exciting times than those of the early pioneers in the field of antibiotics.'

While his book, published in 1990, includes formidable lists of 'side-effects and warnings', Dr Halliday's approach remains resolutely enthusiastic. 'Might frequent use of antibiotics be a bad thing?' is a question asked in the introduction. His answer suggests that we can't do without these drugs.

> It is often said that taking antibiotics hinders the development of one's immunity and that it is better to fight off infections without recourse to drugs. However, there is no strong scientific evidence to support this belief, and it should never deter anyone from justifiable treatment.

Moreover:

> Serious or chronic infections can develop if a condition is not treated, and these can be much more of a problem than any, quite probably imagined, harm caused by antibiotics.

However, in contrast, some books and papers written for a scientific readership are not so enthusiastic about antibiotics. Here, for example, is Professor Calvin Kunin of the Department of Internal Medicine at Ohio State University, writing in the standard textbook *Principles and Practice of Infectious Diseases*.[5]

> Untoward toxic effects of antibiotics are well known; they range from death from anaphylaxis [allergic shock] or aplastic anemia [irreversible damage to bone marrow and thus to blood cells] with penicillin and chloramphenicol, respectively, to severe diarrhoea from lincosamides, rash from ampicillin, nephrotoxicity [kidney damage] and ototoxicity [hearing damage] from the aminoglycosides, and bleeding disorders with some of the new betalactam antibiotics.

These are just a few of the very many acute ill-effects of antibiotics now on the market.[2] Take just one of these, anaphylaxis (also known as anaphylactic shock), in a little more detail. People who are said to be 'allergic' to certain antibiotics have actually become sensitised by past courses of the drug, which, although previously tolerated, then effectively becomes a poison. The antibiotics that have this effect are the betalactams (penicillins and cephalosporins) and also the sulphonamides. Wasp stings and many other substances can cause anaphylaxis but, with radiographic contrast agents, antibiotics are the most common single cause.[6]

It is reckoned that one in five to ten people in the USA is now sensitised in this way to penicillin and other antibiotics, of which around one in every 5000 will react very badly. Such severe anaphylaxis, which can disrupt vital organs and the nervous system, is fatal in up to one in ten cases of the one in 5000 who react this way. Anaphylactic shock is reckoned to kill 500 people a year in the USA; scaled down, this amounts to around 100 deaths a year in the UK, with antibiotics one important cause. This is why doctors are likely to ask new patients whether they are sensitive to penicillin before making out a prescription.

'Systemic anaphylaxis represents the most dramatic and potentially catastrophic manifestation of immediate sensitivity' began a review published in the leading US medical periodical, the *New England Journal of Medicine*.[6] 'The typically explosive and unforeseen nature of severe reactions often hampers treatment . . . It is imperative that an anaphylactic event be recognized quickly, since it may swiftly become life-threatening.'

But such disasters should be put in proportion. When bacterial infections invade vital organs, antibiotics are vital treatment. In the early days of antibacterial drugs, sulphonamides and penicillin were and still can be spectacularly successful treatment against dangerous infections that previously had left doctors and patients helpless. Examples are bacterial infections of the lungs (pneumonia), the lining of the brain (meningitis), and the blood (septicaemia), infections originating in wounds, and in the sexual organs (gonorrhoea, syphilis). Antibiotics have been formulated that make open-body surgery a routine procedure. So-called 'heroic' surgery that involves massive multi-organ and/or transplant high-tech procedures, that may save lives, at least for a while, often cannot be risked without systematic antibiotic 'cover' designed to check bacteria, otherwise liable to waft in from a hospital's infected atmosphere and invade patients' exposed anatomy.

Cases of death known to be directly caused by antibiotics prescribed to generally healthy people by qualified practitioners in countries such as the UK and the USA, are fairly rare. Antibiotics are indeed, rational treatment for serious invasive bacterial infections.

However, less fearful immediate ill-effects of antibiotics are common, and all the more so when patients are generally debilitated. Quoting an American hospital survey, Dr Kunin states: 'Approximately 5 percent of the hospitalized patients who are given an antibiotic will experience some adverse reaction to the drug and about 20 percent of patients requiring medical care have a history of adverse reaction(s) to an antibiotic.' That's a lot of people.

THE DOCTOR AS MAGICIAN

Antibiotics have a potent effect on our bodies. They also have a potent effect on our minds. Our understanding of the meaning of health and disease, and of how we get well after being ill, is profoundly affected by our belief in antibiotics, which reinforces our faith in doctors, and doctors' confidence in drug therapy.

More and more thinking people are now taking responsibility for their own health, and are encouraged to do so by thoughtful health professionals, together with a growing number of practitioners who preach prevention. Various classes of prescription drugs, notably barbiturates and tranquillisers, are now notorious for their insidious ill-effects. Women are understandably uneasy about ill-effects of the contraceptive pill. And for a while, public confidence in the pharmaceutical industry was rocked by the catastrophes of thalidomide and Opren – prescription drugs that, on occasion, caused fearful ill-effects.

Yet we still tend to believe that drugs prescribed by doctors must be good for us. The alternative is to take responsibility for our own health, which most people living in countries where medicine seems cheap (because of insurance or subsidy from taxpayers) are not prepared to do.

Medical students are told not to overuse or abuse antibiotics, and doctors working in hospitals are now trained to be more careful in their use of antibiotics, compared with, say, fifteen or twenty-five years ago. Many general practitioners now don't go along with the routine prescription of antibiotics for trivial infections. That said, though, microbiology, the science of microscopic living things like bacteria and fungi, no longer has an important place in the curriculum of medical students, and the use of antibiotics in general practice and in hospitals continues to increase.

There is a curious dissonance in the attitude of the medical profession to antibiotics. On the one hand, doctors are well aware that these potent drugs have very many 'side-effects' (as ill-effects are often called). On the other, the reputation of antibiotics – evidently shared by both doctors and patients, indeed by almost everybody – is as wonderful savers of life and givers of health: miracle cures.

The special place of antibiotics in our hearts has deep foundations in history. Everybody alive in the world today in reach of a radio, television or doctor is brought up to believe in antibiotics. Technology has displaced religion in the minds of most people living in industrialised countries, and antibiotics are seen as the characteristic gift of modern medicine – more generously given than any gift of God, for 'the Lord giveth and He taketh away' whereas the mysterious drug in the pill or the needle offered to us as a scientific sacrament transforms illness into health, fear into hope, grief into joy, even the threat of death into the promise of life. It is no wonder that our attitude to antibiotics may be reverential.

Fanciful? Perhaps to those of us who live in the West. But this is certainly how antibiotics are so often advertised by the pharmaceutical industry to impoverished people throughout the developing world, who are led to believe that their health and welfare, and that of their children, depends on antibiotics and other drugs.

And for us in the West, the legend of antibiotics goes far beyond science. Sir Alexander Fleming, the British microbiologist who shared a Nobel prize for identifying the antimicrobial power of penicillin, has his own unique place in the public imagination. Like the story of King Alfred's cakes and Sir Isaac Newton's apple, every British schoolchild knows the story of Fleming's plate, the laboratory culture dish he had colonised with staphylococcus bacteria that, by chance, were killed by penicillin spores that filtered up from another laboratory one day in September 1928 while he was away on holiday. The plaque marking Fleming's discovery, on St Mary's Hospital in Praed Street, London, near Paddington station, is a short walk from my house; passing by as I often do, I feel the thrill of being by a place where the history of the world was changed.

Fleming's place in history is based on an accident. Yet he is universally seen as one of the titans who shaped the twentieth century and, like Albert Einstein and Robert Oppenheimer, demonstrated the power of science to give a new definition to our lives. In the past, explorers such as Christopher Columbus and James Cook discovered the shape of the exterior world. In the twentieth century, the new maps have been of the interior world, of our minds and our bodies; and scientists such as Sigmund Freud and Alexander Fleming displaced soldiers and explorers as our models of greatness.

DRUGS AS ELIXIRS

At first, antibiotics were thought to be miracle drugs. Just as alchemists searched for the 'philosopher's stone', the means to turn base metal into gold, chemists still search for the 'magic bullet', the drug that always cures and never does harm. And the power of antimicrobial drugs to kill invisible organisms that cause deadly diseases obviously is marvellous. Early stories about the effect of penicillin on the lives of individual people have become modern gospels. Here, for example, is the story told by Louise Carter, a midwife, as quoted in *Miracle Cure: The Story of Antibiotics* by Dr Milton Wainwright, published in 1990.[7] In 1943, she was attending Mrs Phyllis Andrews, who had given birth to a healthy baby but was suffering from puerperal (or childbed) fever, a bacterial infection of the womb and birth passage that had spread through her bloodstream and was liable to kill her.

> Nurse Carter recalls how one evening she heard hurried footsteps outside her ward, and the consultant, a Mr Verwood, entered already gowned and masked and obviously ready for action. He asked her for a 10cc syringe of water and then began to scrub up. Taking the syringe, he injected the contents into one of two vials containing a yellow powder. The powder dissolved and immediately gave off a pungent smell, which somewhat shocked Nurse Carter. The solution was then injected into a bottle of dextrosaline which was given as a drip into the woman's veins.
>
> Incredibly, after only half an hour the patient's blood pressure had begun to rise, her temperature had dropped two degrees, and her pulse had fallen to a reasonable level of 90. The second bottle of the new drug was given, and by 5.40 in the morning, Mrs Andrews opened her eyes and with some bewilderment asked for a cup of tea. Nurse Carter summed up her account in the following words: 'And so I left that happy little family, a proud relieved father, a beautiful contented baby, and a happy young mother snatched from the very brink of death by a miracle drug.'

This simple story has the power of elemental myth. Notice its language and its symbols. The sense of wonder Louise Carter felt is much like that of Christ's disciples as described in the New Testament. Her story is that of an alchemist's dream come true, and its images – of the masked man whose potion, poured into the veins of a woman near death, restores her to smiling and innocent life – are those of a fairy story.

With antibiotics, we have become accustomed to perceive the modern doctor not just as a healer, but as more of a magician, with a hypodermic wand. We, too, have seen what Nurse Carter saw, if not in real life, then in the movies and on television, in the fables that give doctors unique status as benefactors. The picture of the clear-eyed, firm-jawed, white-suited actor, whose bedside manner consists of focusing his gaze on the point of a syringe containing a life-saving drug, is one of the icons of our age.

In such scenes, there is typically no dialogue between the doctor, who knows and gives, and the patient, who is ignorant and receives, and who is transfixed in wonder and transformed by the doctor's gift, with no doubt or question. This image works best when the doctor is a man and the patient is a woman. In the transaction, the man is indeed godlike, whereas the patient (as we all know) loses identity as a person.

And it is our belief in the drug that gives the doctors their power.

Much of my own work in public health is done with doctors, and many of these friends and colleagues of mine are admirable men and women, hard-working, thoughtful and conscientious. My local general practitioner works in a group practice; she and her partners are efficient and friendly, and don't pretend to know everything. When my late wife Caroline was very ill for a long time in the late 1980s, she was given extraordinary care by doctors working in the community. And physicians have often taken time out to give me excellent treatment and advice. Generally speaking, I have a lot of respect for the doctors I know.

Doctors are of course fallible and often suffer a great deal of stress. The rates of divorce, alcoholism, drug addiction and suicide are high in the medical profession, and doctors on average do not live longer than other people of their social class.[8] They are human. Yet so often we persist in elevating physicians and surgeons to a superhuman status in our minds, which is unhelpful to us and also to them. Noting the awe in which surgeons are typically held, compared with the public healthy disrespect for politicians, the veteran Labour politician Denis Healey once pointed out, half in jest, that surgeons' dissatisfied customers are often not in a position to complain, being either unconscious or dead!

When we sign a legal contract, we know we should read the small print so that we will know what we are letting ourselves in for. Taking care with such transactions does not mean we think that lawyers are fools or crooks, but that we choose to make a conscious decision, and to share responsibility with the people with whom we are dealing. We question our advisers when making financial decisions, not because we think that accountants and bank managers are incompetent, but because we know that the best deals do not come 'off the peg' but are designed for us personally, for our individual requirements and circumstances, and also because any kind of real, sustained relationship requires mutual respect.

Typically, this is not how things are between us and doctors. We expect the doctor to 'make us better' but how, we don't know. In his book *The Wound and the Doctor*[8], Dr Glin Bennet writes:

> Ignorant patients are easier to deal with than those who are well informed, and the medical machine runs more smoothly if people do not ask questions but place themselves, childlike and docile, into the hands of their doctors . . . Doctors may not deliberately keep their patients in ignorance but they certainly want to maintain strict control over the clinical relationship. They are in an almost unassailable position since they possess all the information about the patients who, in turn, know practically nothing, yet are highly anxious; and that increases the doctors' power still further.

But it takes two to turn a person into a patient. We tend to assume not only that 'the doctor knows best' but also that the doctor knows all there is to know about drugs. When criticised for an air of aloof mystery, doctors often say that patients don't want to know, but just want drugs as a means to get rid of their symptoms and get on with life. No doubt this is often true.

Doctors sometimes give drugs an added mystique by referring to their ill-effects as 'idiosyncratic' or to patients' illness caused by drugs as 'hypersensitivity'. While it is indeed true that some people are more vulnerable than others, these words do rather suggest that the harm done is somehow the fault of the patient, not of the drug (nor of the doctor).

Thus, our trust in doctors is so often a blind faith. The contract we accept from the doctor without scrutiny or question, the emblem of medical authority, is the prescription: the slip of paper which, in the familiar wry joke, is written in a code that can only be deciphered by a fellow professional, the pharmacist. We know practically nothing about the meaning of this transaction.

Exaggerated? Well, here are some questions about you and antibiotics. When did you last take a course of antibiotics? What are the generic and the trade names of the drug you took? What was the dose, and for how many days did you take it? What bacterial infection was diagnosed, and what bacterial species was the microbiological cause of the infection? How many courses of antibiotics have you taken, say, in the last five years? And what were the infections for which they were prescribed?[9]

If you can answer those questions, here are two more. What are the most common ill-effects of all the antibiotics you have taken? Have you suffered illness as a result of taking antibiotics and, if so, what did you do to protect yourself then or for the future? Try asking all these questions of yourself, or your partner, or your family.

THE DARK SIDE

We may not want to know about the ill-effects of prescription drugs, but I think we need to know, not only for ourselves but also for the sake of those who are close to us. I have never met a doctor who says that patients should be kept in the dark about drugs. At the same time, I don't know many non-medical people who are knowledgeable about the acute illnesses that can be caused by antibiotics, with the notable exception of those who believe that in their cases, the treatment was worse than their diseases, some of whom have formed mutual-help groups.

Writing about the acute ill-effects of antibiotics is problematic, for a number of reasons. First, it is worth repeating that properly prescribed for a serious invasive bacterial infection, the likely benefit to the individual of any antibiotic far outweighs any possible risk of acute illness caused by the drug.

Second, it is likely that most serious illnesses directly caused by antibiotics outside hospital are a result of heavy and/or prolonged use of drugs, particularly the 'broad-spectrum' types, with inadequate medical supervision: this is not really the fault of the drug, and may well not be the fault of the doctor either, especially in the many countries where antibiotics are available over the counter. Third, perhaps with the exceptions of allergic reactions and gut disorders, most serious acute ill-effects of antibiotics are complications of hospital treatment, which in developed countries like the UK and USA can usually be checked by doctors unless the patient is very vulnerable or debilitated.

Fourth, most relatively toxic older antibacterial drugs such as the sulphonamides, streptomycin, chloramphenicol and the tetracyclines, on the market for up to half a century or more, which may have been taken regularly by middle-aged and elderly readers of this book earlier in their lives, are now mostly reserved for severe or relatively uncommon bacterial infections in countries like the UK and the USA where drugs are carefully regulated. Penicillins in their many forms remain the antibiotics most commonly prescribed in general practice because they are effective and also remarkably safe in use compared with other drugs.

Fifth, singling out individual antibiotics for comment can be invidious. While manufacturers understandably advertise the benefits of their own branded drugs to the medical profession, and while patients may know any antibiotics they take or have taken by their trade names, health benefits and risks are normally of the drug generically, not specifically of any branded product. Indeed, whole families of antibiotics, such as the cephalosporins, the glycopeptides and the quinolones (to name three others)[2] tend to have their own character, and comments on any individual or generic drug in a family tend at least to some extent to be true for the others. Yes, it is all rather complicated.

Sixth, discussion of any kind of risk is diffuse without numbers and definitions. When it is said that a specific ill-effect of a drug is 'common', what does 'common' mean? One in five? Or one in five hundred? What does 'rare' mean? One in a thousand? Or one in ten million? And what about 'very rare'? One in a million, or one case noted in the literature? Terms like these are often used in the scientific literature without quantification. I think they should be given a precise meaning; meanwhile, I have given numbers when I can find them.

Also, when is an illness trivial and when is it serious? To my mind, an illness is trivial when recovery without damage takes only up to a few days, even though it may cause acute distress at the time. A serious illness is either prolonged or liable to get worse or cause lasting damage, and for any of these reasons a suitable case for medical treatment. That's my opinion; again, such terms are usually not defined in the literature. Until there is universal agreement on numbers and definitions, which must surely come as part of the on-line databases that should in time be available to all physicians and all interested citizens, anybody trying to assess the benefits and risks of drugs is involved in some tiresome guesswork.

And seventh, the fundamental problem with antibiotics is not their direct acute ill-effects, serious though these can be, but their indirect ill-effects on the individual, and the general consequences of their overuse and abuse on public health – more of this later in the book.

All this said though, and bearing in mind that I am giving just some examples of the immediate problems that can be caused by antibiotics simply so that you can see they should be used with care, a look at the standard pharmacological textbooks used by physicians and microbiologists[1,3] together with reference books compiled for the general reader[2,10] does show that with all their value, antibiotics are not magic bullets.

Co-trimoxazole, for example. This is a combination drug, being made up from sulphamethoxazole, a sulphonamide, and an antibiotic from another family, trimethoprim. It is the only sulphonamide drug still commonly prescribed in the UK. The adverse effects of co-trimoxazole as listed in the pharmacists' bible, *Martindale: the Extra Pharmacopeia*[1] fill four triple-column small-print pages in this 2000 page tome. They include headache, giddiness, weakness, inability to sleep and anaemia. A handbook for the general reader compiled by Professor Peter Parish[2] states that the adverse effects of co-trimoxazole include those of the sulphonamides as a group of drugs, also mentioning diarrhoea, nausea, confusion and hallucinations.

One of the most troublesome aspects of many ill-effects of antibiotics is that they mimic illnesses that have other causes. A physician, however alert and well guided by textbooks and manuals, may not always spot the difference.

Uncommon but more serious ill-effects of co-trimoxazole include disorders of the blood, kidneys and liver. Most ill-effects though, according to *Martindale*, are to the skin and the digestive system, and the drug has been known to cause immunosuppression – weakening of the means whereby the body protects itself against infection.[11,12]

As another example, streptomycin is effective against a number of infections and was a popular drug until the 1960s. In common with the other drugs in its group, the aminoglycosides, it can however damage a nerve in the inner ear that controls the sense of balance; on rare occasions this damage can be irreversible.[1] As already mentioned, hearing can also be affected: another ill-effect is tinnitus, a constant noise in the ears that sometimes sounds like bells ringing.[2,3] For these and other reasons streptomycin is reserved in the UK only for a few serious bacterial infections, although it remains commonly available in developing countries.

One rare but severe ill-effect of nitrofurantoin, an antibiotic used for urinary tract infections, is peripheral neuritis – inflammation of the nervous system at the body's extremities, such as the hands and feet.[1] First signs include tingling and numbness. This is also an ill-effect of sulphonamides.

The toxicity of antibiotics is not a dark secret known only to specialists such as microbiologists and pharmacologists. Every general practitioner is given detailed information about the risks as well as the benefits of antibiotics, and such data is updated regularly in reference manuals issued or available to doctors, by medical bodies, the pharmaceutical industry itself or in the UK by the Consumers' Association.[13] As another example, erythromycin is an antibiotic in the macrolide group, commonly used as an alternative for people known to be allergic to penicillin. It is available in generic form (sold under its own name) and also in a number of branded versions. In general it is regarded as a relatively safe drug: a review written for specialists says: 'One of the major advantages of erythromycin is its low incidence of serious side-effects and its excellent safety record.'[14]

However, the 1993–4 edition of the ABPI Data Sheets, issued regularly to general practitioners in the UK by industry and made up into an annual book,[13] says of one formulation of erythromycin that: 'It may be accompanied by malaise, nausea, vomiting, abdominal colic and fever. In some instances, severe abdominal pain may simulate the pain of biliary colic, pancreatitis, perforated ulcer, or an acute abdominal surgical problem ... Initial symptoms have developed in some cases after a few days of treatment, but generally have followed one or two weeks of continuous therapy.' More generally, *Martindale*[1] says: 'Gastrointestinal disturbances are fairly common with erythromycin, especially with large doses', adding however, that 'serious side-effects are rare'.

Any antibiotic can cause gut disorders. One specific ill-effect of tetracyclines, effective against many bacterial infections including facial acne, is that they penetrate teeth and can eventually cause staining and destruction of tooth enamel. 'Many unfortunate children have teeth yellowed by this drug, given to them when they were babies or young children, or to their mothers when they were in the womb,' states Professor Parish.[10] Tetracyclines also penetrate into bone, and can cause stunting in young children.[1] For these reasons, in Britain and most developed countries they are now not normally recommended for pregnant women or for children under the age of twelve. These are just a few of the very many examples of the toxicity of antibiotics. Again, readers who want a comprehensive guide are referred to the medical and general literature.[1,2,3,10]

Before I started work on this book I had no idea just how many immediate and acute ill-effects antibiotics may have. It would be comforting to believe that ill-effects of antibiotics are always either trivial or rare. But that's not what the textbooks say. It would also be comforting to believe that antibiotics cause acute ill-effects only when they are overused and abused. But that's not true either. What proportion of people who take antibiotics suffer as a result? Nobody knows: probably, the majority of victims never connect cause and effect, never realise that drugs prescribed by doctors are making them ill; or else suffer in silence.

2 Imperfect Medicine

OVERUSE AND ABUSE

Antibiotics are overused and abused: there's no doubt about that. A series of surveys summarised in a World Health Organisation report, published in 1983[15], estimated that physicians use antibiotics irrationally or inappropriately on anything between two fifths and two thirds of all occasions. Dr Peter Parish comments:[2]

> Antibiotic misuse covers the whole spectrum of medical practice – from the unnecessary use of antibiotics to treat viral infections (for example, viral sore throats) by some family doctors, to the blunderbuss use of antibiotics by some surgeons in the hope of preventing post-operation infections.

When both doctors and their patients believe that antibiotics (perhaps with rare exceptions) do no harm, overprescription is inevitable. A common reason is 'insurance' against the possibility of future bacterial infection. A general practitioner explained:[16] 'It's not just rubbish that one gives in most cases. For example, if they complain of a sore throat, I generally give penicillin. It's unnecessary in most cases, but one could turn out to be a streptococcal infection, which could have serious consequences.' However, a survey of prescribing in Scottish hospitals published in 1979, concluded that in two thirds of cases there was no good evidence that antibiotics were needed: 'Since 11 percent of all antibiotic exposures were associated with undesirable side-effects, it was concluded that the risks of therapy were greater than the benefits to be expected, at least in a substantial proportion of the patients studied.'

Professor David Reeves is a leading British consultant microbiologist. Interviewed for this book in his laboratory at Southmeads Hospital, Bristol, he indicated that little has changed since the late

1970s. Why do general practitioners overprescribe antibiotics? I asked. 'Patient expectation first,' he said. 'It's very difficult to convince patients who have what they perceive as an infection not to have an antibiotic. Like a sore throat, for example, which is usually caused by a virus.[17] It actually takes more time to explain to them that they don't need an antibiotic than it does to write out a prescription.

'Next the natural concern of the GP about a patient who will be at home and not under direct supervision, as they would be in hospital. And third, the desire on the GP's part for the patient not to return unnecessarily. If they have got some therapy, they are less likely to come back. If they have got no therapy, and are no better the next day, they are more likely to come back. If they have taken antibiotics – even if they are no better than they would have been if they hadn't taken the antibiotics – they are less likely to come back. So time pressure is an important factor for GPs. And I don't blame them.'

The 1983 WHO report came to much the same conclusion. In Western countries, where most antibiotics are administered by medically (or dentally) qualified practitioners, the health professional

> may find it difficult to resist pressure from the patient or his family. He [or she] is also motivated to do the best for the patient; unless he has a good knowledge of the management of microbial infections, of antibiotic action, and of the current local state of susceptibility of pathogens [disease-causing microbes] to antibiotics, he may be tempted to give unnecessary treatment. He may feel that, even if an antibiotic is unlikely to do good, it will do no harm, or he may attempt to ensure the efficacy of treatment by giving larger doses or more prolonged treatment than is necessary.

Doctors often overuse and abuse antibiotics both in general practice and in hospitals. In 1983 Dr Reeves and colleagues published a paper in the *British Medical Journal*[18] giving the results of a survey of antibiotic prescription at Southmeads Hospital. Despite the 'generally high quality of its medical staff and the presence of an active microbiology department, between a quarter and a third of all antibiotic prescriptions were reckoned to be unnecessary.' The conclusion was:

> Most prescriptions were written by junior staff who, in the absence of guidance from their seniors and because of their frequent moves,

> would require a widespread and continual education programme. Published concern about the quality of antibiotic prescription appears to be justified.

Overuse of antibiotics is at best a waste of money. It can be a disaster if only because antibiotics are toxic and may cause allergic reactions as well as many other ill-effects. Reviewing Dr Reeves' paper later in the year, the *Lancet* commented[19]: 'Informed antibiotic prescription is essential to limit the emergence of resistant bacteria and to avoid unnecessary toxicity and expense.'

OVERPRESCRIPTION

Earlier, in 1981, the *Lancet* published another editorial on overuse and abuse of antibiotics by doctors.[20] It began:

> Antibiotics, apparently, continue to be prescribed rather indiscriminately . . . Surveys in North America suggest that the use of antibiotics is increasing; often they are prescribed when there is no evidence of bacterial infection, or in the wrong dose, or by the wrong route.

Later the same year, the *Lancet* published the results of another hospital survey, this time carried out at the Central Middlesex Hospital in London.[21] The use of antibiotics therapeutically (to treat infection) and prophylactically (to protect against possible future infection, notably during surgery) was assessed.

Most of the patients were treated before the infectious agent was identified, and in half of these cases the physicians were unable to say what bacterial species might be causing the infection. Thus, in a major London teaching hospital, where resources are as good as can be, some of the time doctors are guessing. In the case of 'preventive' treatment: 'Only 7 percent of antibiotics prescribed for surgical prophylaxis fulfilled all the criteria used to assess the suitability of choice of drug and the method and timing of its administration.' In other words, surgeons are liable to order antibiotic 'cover' without thinking through the consequences both for the patient and for the hospital environment. Careful use of antibiotics in hospital is vital 'not only because of their cost but also because the price of their misuse, especially in hospital, may be unnecessary morbidity and mortality, high hospital infection rates and rapid obsolescence of the most valuable drugs'.

This study was followed by two more: on the use of antibiotics in hospital for lower respiratory tract infections such as bronchitis and pneumonia; and on their use for urinary tract infections, notably cystitis. In the first study, it turned out that use of antibiotics was wrong or questionable more often than it was right, one reason being that junior doctors were not much good at interpreting X-rays. In most other cases,

> the diagnosis appeared to have been made on very tenuous clinical evidence, probably influenced by the view that to omit to prescribe antibiotics is a more serious sin than to prescribe them unnecessarily. The fact that only one of these prescriptions was subsequently altered by the consultant staff suggests that such a view may be widely shared.

The second study, of urinary tract infections, produced a similar result: 'It was considered that both initiation and continuation of antibiotic treatment was justified for 28 out of 55 patients and that either initiation or continuation of treatment was unjustified for 27 out of 55 patients.' Bluntly, the doctors were wrong just about as often as they were right.

The general conclusion from both these studies of antibiotic use in hospitals was 'There is a lot of overprescribing'.[17] These British studies are evidently typical. Professor Calvin Kunin of Ohio State University, an authority on infectious diseases, wrote in 1985[22]: 'There are now numerous studies in representative hospital populations that document that antimicrobial agents are used for unjustifiable reasons, or that the wrong drug, dose or duration of therapy is selected, about half the time.'

So if antibiotic prescriptions in hospitals, with all their microbiological laboratory backing, are somewhat of a toss-up, what of antibiotic prescriptions in general practice, with doctors working under pressure both from patients and from salesmen? No wonder so many doctors are defensive about their use of antibiotics.

In the 1970s, Dr Milton Silverman and Professor Philip Lee, in their book *Pills, Profits and Politics*[23], stated:

> The growing use of antibiotics to prevent infection has apparently been the principal reason for the rapid and indeed alarming increase

> in the prescribing of these drugs during the last few years. Some physicians justify this use on the basis that the risk is slight, the cost to the patient is usually not great, and the patient is pleased to see that his physician is doing something for him.

But use of antibiotics 'just in case' infection develops is usually 'not clinically justifiable. It presents needless risks and causes unnecessary expense. At the worst, it may be fatal for the patient.'

Since Drs Silverman and Lee wrote this, nothing has changed for the better. 'Antimicrobial drugs are often prescribed inappropriately, irrationally, and inefficiently,' writes Dr David Greenwood in the introduction to his textbook *Antimicrobial Therapy*, published in 1989.[24] 'The cost of such wasteful prescribing in terms of unnecessary adverse reactions in the patient, or simply in terms of cash, can only be guessed at.'

A 'guesstimate' of the cash loss can be made. The worldwide market value of antibiotics for the year 1990 has been reckoned at US$18,000,000,000 (US$18 billion).[25] If half of all antibiotics are wrongly used, this amounts to a waste of $9 billion a year. What about the cost to the UK National Health Service? The UK market for antibiotics is roughly one-fortieth of the world market. So on these estimates, and given an exchange rate of say US$1.50 to the pound, in 1990 the total amount wasted on antibiotics in the UK, almost all of it at taxpayers' expense, was around £150 million a year. How much suffering is caused by wrong use of antibiotics is, of course, incalculable.

POPGUN PHARMACY

In developed countries such as the UK and USA the market for potent drugs is restricted by making them subject to prescription by doctors. Nevertheless, in such countries the administration of antibiotics is sometimes thoughtless or irresponsible. Doctors are, after all, human, and they are usually conscientious. The main reason why antibiotics are overprescribed or wrongly prescribed is that we all, doctors included, have a lot of wrong ideas about antibiotics.

In a review published in 1989[26], Dr Jerome Kim of the division of infectious diseases at Duke University Medical Center, North Carolina, identifies a system of beliefs held by physicians that explains why they – and we – tend to overuse and abuse antibiotics. Most of these beliefs are based on the idea that antibiotics are weapons in a war against an invisible enemy army, and so could be called the nine commandments of the germ theory of disease:

1 '*Broader is better*' – always prefer the drug with the broadest spectrum of activity against the widest range of bacterial species (most of which will be either harmless or beneficial).
2 '*Failure to respond is failure to cover*' – the body is unprotected unless and until drugs are used.
3 '*When in doubt, change drugs, or add another*' – the more complex and potent the drug cocktail, the better.
4 '*More diseases, more drugs*' – ill-effects can be confused with illnesses.
5 '*Sickness requires immediate treatment*' – the body cannot be trusted or allowed to defend itself.
6 '*Response implies diagnosis*' – if the drug seems to work, the disease has been identified.
7 '*Bigger diseases, bigger drugs*'
8 '*Bigger diseases, newer drugs*' } a medical man's versions of the war leader's slogan: 'Blitz 'em with our best!'
9 '*Antibiotics are non-toxic*' – self-explanatory

These beliefs are wrong, says Dr Kim, and he is right. 'The immediacy of suffering, the desire to alleviate distress, the desire for action, the fears of errors of omission, and [he adds, as an American] the fear of litigation, all favor impulsive therapeutic activity over accurate diagnosis and specific therapy.' He warns against what he calls a spiralling 'escalation of treatment of suspected but undocumented infectious diseases', which is often futile, sometimes damaging or even deadly in its effect on the individual, and (as we shall see) can be immeasurably dangerous in its effects on the community.

Professor Richard Lacey agrees. Dr Lacey of Leeds University, who has written the foreword and afterword of this book, is well known in Britain for his radical views on the safety of food, notably its contamination with salmonella, listeria and other micro-organisms. However, his main scientific work has been concerned with antibiotics and their safety. Head of the department of medical microbiology at Leeds University, he is also responsible for drug prescription policy in the hospitals governed by the Leeds Health Authority.

Dr Lacey describes beliefs like those listed by Dr Kim as 'antibiotic folklore'. In a critical review published in 1988[27], he says that a broad-spectrum antibiotic 'has the superficial appeal that it can be used for many different types of infection without the need to make an exact diagnosis [but] is usually a second-rate option for many indications'. He confirms that the broader the spectrum of the drug, the more damage it is likely to do inside the gut. Also, he believes that the policy that 'the more severe the infection, the more powerful the dose' is potentially disastrous. Generally the ones who suffer most from infections are infants, the elderly and people who are already weak or vulnerable for other reasons; for them, powerful doses of antibiotics can be dangerous. And it is not necessarily true that virulent bacteria are killed more effectively when a drug dose is increased; indeed, penicillins and some other antibiotics may be less effective in higher doses.

In Dr Lacey's opinion, a tenth 'commandment' of antibiotic folklore is: 'Complete the course.' This is a standard instruction that physicians give when prescribing antibiotics and means that patients should keep on taking the drugs until they are finished, even if, in the meanwhile, all symptoms of infection have vanished. But is it true that bugs continue to lurk in the body, ready to multiply again and flare into illness, even after the patient has apparently recovered?[28] Common sense suggests no – and Dr Lacey says that common sense is usually correct. The more antibiotics you take, the greater the risk of ill-effects; they 'should be prescribed only for as long as there is clinical need'. As a rule, he says, when you feel better, stop taking the drugs, and return the remainder to the pharmacist.

From time to time, while researching this book, I found standard medical practice for antibiotics contradicted by microbiologists, the scientists best placed to know the facts about microbes and antibiotics. Microbiologists are usually research scientists who do not treat patients, but medical microbiologists such as Dr Lacey also care for patients in hospital, and many believe that antibiotics are overused and abused by physicians looking for a quick result.

'Complete the course' remains a standard doctor's order. But Dr Lacey is not the only eminent microbiologist who believes that patients should trust their own sense of well-being. Professor Tore Midtvedt is head of the department of medical microbial ecology at the Karolinska Institute in Sweden. I went to Stockholm to see him. He said: 'Patients are usually very wise. They may stop a little bit ahead of what the doctors have told them to do.' In the case of some serious infections carried by bacteria that become embedded in the body, such as osteomyelitis, endocarditis, brucellosis or tuberculosis, 'feeling better' is not a reliable sign that the bacteria are dead. But, Dr Midtvedt said, 'In most acute infections, by far the most common infections for which antibacterials are used, "feeling better" does indicate that you have had enough of the drug.'

In Dr Midtvedt's experience, physicians have always tended to overprescribe antibiotics. Take urinary tract infections such as cystitis in women, he said. A generation ago, 'when I started to study medicine, all patients had to receive a ten-day course for a urinary tract infection. As a microbiologist, I couldn't understand that. The microbes were dead long before the end of the course. So I said so, in one of the medical journals. My old teacher, he went crazy. "You should complete, you should complete! When it is stated, it should be done!" he told me.' Recalling this confrontation, Dr Midtvedt smiled. 'Just follow the master,' he said.

In Richard Lacey's view, antibiotics are prescribed far too often. He finds that of all the people who have had their infections identified in his laboratory, less than one in a hundred has been treated with appropriate antibiotics. And most of these infections are self-limiting – that is, they will eventually clear up by themselves without any use of drugs.[29]

The great Canadian physician Sir William Osler, writing over half a century ago, before the antibiotic era, worried about the way doctors use drugs. They must understand the disease and also the patient, he said, or else they will 'flounder along in an aimless fashion, practising a sort of popgun pharmacy, hitting now the malady and again the patient, he himself not knowing which'. We are all, doctors included, brought up to have faith in antibiotics, and all too often, our faith is blind.

We in the West are in thrall to a theory of health and disease which is wrong. Our good health is largely our own responsibility. But antibiotics, more than any other drugs, block this insight, because they delude us into thinking that we need not care about our health until we are ill, when the doctor will cure us. We are drawn to antibiotics like moths to a flame.

3 Unconquered Epidemics

MIRACLE DRUGS: THE LEGEND

Typically, doctors are conscientious, but may be blind to the dangers of antibiotics because of their legendary status. We are enthralled by these drugs. Among all others, they have a unique reputation as safe and good, notwithstanding evidence to the contrary.

Indeed, one of the pillars that hold up the edifice of modern medicine is the belief that almost everybody shares: that antibiotics and other antimicrobial drugs, administered by suitably qualified doctors, conquered the rampant epidemics of infectious diseases that destroyed the health and the lives of countless millions of people in industrialised countries until well into the twentieth century.

Thus, an American authority, cited by Milton Wainwright in his book *Miracle Cure*[7], said in the 1950s:

> Thanks to antibiotics, a million and a half lives were saved in the first fifteen years of the sulfonamide and antibiotic era . . . Of the lives saved from 1938 to 1952 inclusive, 1,000,000 would have died of pneumonia and influenza, 76,000 mothers would have died of puerperal fever, 136,000 of syphilis, and 90,000 of appendicitis.

Dr Wainwright himself is even more enthusiastic:

> The impact of antibiotics on medicine can perhaps be appreciated from the fact that in 1920 the life expectancy of the average American was around 54 years, while a baby born today can expect to live until he or she is nearly 75. It has been calculated that ten years of this improvement in life expectancy has resulted directly from the introduction of antibiotics.

Claims like these, based on comparisons of death statistics at different times, are obviously questionable. Why influenza is mentioned is unclear; its microbiological cause is viral, not bacterial, and antibiotics generally have no effect on viruses. Appendicitis should not be a killer disease in any society with adequate hospitals (as there were in the US in the 1950s), and is included presumably to allow for complications caused by bacterial infection before or after surgery. Puerperal fever results from foreign bacteria passing into the vagina and sometimes the womb during childbirth, especially after complications involving forceps or surgery, but this potentially deadly disease is now uncommon in industrialised countries, not solely because of treatment with antibiotics, but principally because of prevention due to better maternal health and better ward hygiene.

Generally, there is no way to tell how many lives in a population have been lengthened or saved by antibiotics as compared with, say, improved infant nutrition, slum clearance and/or clean air legislation. But the general drift of such claims seems plausible because, of course, it is true that antibiotics are effective treatment against bacterial infections.

And this is why we see Alexander Fleming as one of the great heroes of our era. We believe that antibiotics are the key that doctors use to unlock the door beyond which are the open fields in which we can enjoy good health and long life, free from disease. Hence our deference to doctors: for they hold the key – the drug. If antibiotics had never been developed, or if we doubted their value, we would not be so dependent on doctors.

I say 'free from disease' rather than 'free from infection' because antibiotics have such a grip on our imagination that we tend to confuse disease with infection. 'Disease', according to one dictionary definition, is 'a condition of the body, or of some organ or part of the body, in which its functions are disturbed or deranged.' Thus (in alphabetical order) angina, bronchitis, cancers, diabetes, eczema, familial hypercholesterolaemia, gallstones and high blood pressure are all diseases but only one of these, bronchitis, is an infection (and only sometimes a bacterial one). But we are less inclined to think of non-infectious conditions as real diseases. A survey on 'The Concept of Disease', the results of which were published in the *British Medical Journal*[30], concluded: 'To the layman a disease seems to be a living agency that causes illness.' In other words, diseases somehow have an existence separate from the diseased person, and a germ is not so much the carrier as, somehow, the disease itself. So diseases are something we 'catch', 'out of the blue', and we refer to the 'dreaded lurgi' as if disease is an alien from space.

Another conclusion of this survey, in which the views of lay and medical people were compared, was:

> The importance of the role of the doctor bore a strong relation to disease connotation. Conditions in which the doctor had a definite role to play were regarded as diseases by 69 per cent of laymen and over 80 per cent of the doctors, while those in which the doctor is unlikely to be important rated as diseases in about 16 per cent of cases by laymen and 32 per cent by the doctors.

Thus, the quintessential disease seems to be an infection that we believe a doctor can cure with drugs. By contrast, we are inclined to doubt whether non-infectious conditions not much affected by medical interventions – such as obesity or depression or senile dementia – are 'real' diseases. To qualify as a disease, an illness could be said to need a micro-organism, a pharmaceutical and a physician – or, as a wag might put it, a bug, a drug and a quack. No wonder antibiotics are so important to the medical profession. This is the context in which people often say something like 'I feel terrible, but the doctor hasn't given me anything, so I suppose I must be all right.' Or 'The doc said I had a few problems, so he's fixed me up with some pills.'

If all diseases were infections, attitudes such as these might make some sense. But the fact is that most of the major diseases suffered in industrialised countries today are not infections. Drugs often ease the symptoms of non-infectious diseases, and may slow or even stop the disease process, but they usually cannot give a full cure. By the time people start to suffer symptoms of arthritis, cancers, coronary heart disease, diabetes, multiple sclerosis, osteoporosis and many other debilitating or deadly conditions, the disease process is likely to be advanced and ineradicable. The effective approach to non-infectious diseases is prevention rather than treatment, and they are therefore primarily the responsibility of all of us as informed citizens, rather than that of the medical profession.

But as long as we do not see the difference between infections and non-infectious diseases, and as long as we also believe that antibiotics are a sure-fire cure for infections, we will always tend to neglect ourselves and – thinking, for example, of heart disease as if it is somehow like syphilis – rely on doctors for a quick fix of drugs 'to make us better'.

MIRACLE DRUGS: THE REALITY

Antibiotics are not cure-alls. They are also not miracle drugs, for the legend that antibacterials and antibiotics conquered the great epidemic infections of our recent past is not true.

In 1976, the British Department of Health published an official report, *Prevention and Health: Everybody's Business*[31], a remarkable document that redefined the role of doctors and drugs in the conquest of disease. Referring to the infectious plagues of Victorian Britain, it states:

> The decline was well under way before the discovery of specific curative and preventive measures, and therefore to a considerable extent must have been due to non-specific causes like a reduction in overcrowding, safer food, better nutrition, improved personal hygiene, and the educative activities of doctors and district nurses.

Three years later, the distinguished epidemiologist Professor Thomas McKeown published his masterpiece *The Role of Medicine*[32], which includes his careful and unchallenged analysis of the decline of infectious epidemics in Britain since the eighteenth century. What effect did immunisation and drug therapy have on these scourges?

> These measures had little effect on the death-rate before 1935 [when sulphonamides, the first widely used antibacterials, were introduced] and since that time have been less important than other influences. Diphtheria was the only common infection in which a specific measure, immunisation, may have been the main reason for its decline; in the other common ones (tuberculosis, pneumonia, measles, whooping cough and scarlet fever), mortality had fallen to a relatively low level before effective medical intervention was possible.

Professor McKeown proves his point by means of graphs tracking the decline, over the decades, in the rates of death from the infections that became major epidemics during the Industrial Revolution. On these graphs, he charts the points in time when medical treatments such as vaccination and antibiotics became generally available. If these marvels of modern medicine (which indeed they are) actually had conquered epidemic infections, this should have been evident on the graphs. Typically, though, there is little or no change in the drop in the death rates. He concludes: 'The modern improvement in health was initiated and carried quite a long way with little contribution from science and technology . . . The therapeutic advances of the last few decades have had little effect on death rates.'

The incidence of certain invasive, potentially deadly bacterial infections has certainly been reduced by antibiotics in the last 50 years. Such diseases include meningitis, endocarditis and bacterial infections of the bones (osteomyelitis) and other invasive infections to which accident victims and surgical patients are exposed, or which can follow complications of other infections. Penicillin accelerated the decline of syphilis, and together with other antibiotics checked the spread of gonorrhoea, notably among soldiers in wartime. And while bacterial pneumonia – a common threat to old people who are already ill – and puerperal fever were in decline before the introduction of the sulphonamides in the 1930s, analysis of statistical records indicates that antibiotics accelerated the reduction in incidence of these two diseases. Both were once epidemic killers in hospitals, so antibiotics have to that extent made hospitals safer places for the elderly and for women in childbirth.

Generally speaking, though, the evidence from public health records supports Professor McKeown's conclusion that while in some cases antibiotics accelerated the decline of epidemic bacterial infections, neither they nor any other medical therapy are the main reasons why Western society is now relatively free from the great nineteenth-century scourges. The rise and fall of epidemic disease is usually not greatly affected one way or another by drugs.

It may seem strange that treatment that is effective for individuals may have little or no effect on public health. But consider an analogy: death on the roads. The police and ambulance service, together with hospital casualty units and highly trained surgical staff, save the lives of countless people who otherwise would die in traffic accidents. But the overall rate of death on the roads in any country is mainly determined by policy on traffic signalling, speed limits, seatbelts, drink-driving, the standard and attitude of motorists, and the quality of policing and of the roads themselves. A remote island where everybody drives slowly and carefully might have no medical services and no road accidents. A stretch of trunk road subject to ice and fog and with badly signalled junctions might have medical crash units always on call and be an accident black spot. As with road accidents, so with infectious disease: the key factors are not medical or surgical intervention, but environmental conditions, social policy and individual behaviour.

The most authoritative writer on the rise and fall of infectious epidemics is Professor René Dubos, who had a unique knowledge of antibiotics. As a young man, he emigrated from France to the United States at the invitation of Professor Selman Waksman, the scientist who identified streptomycin as an effective treatment for tuberculosis. Dubos himself went on to discover tyrothricin, an antibacterial that was in medical use before penicillin, and also gramicidin, a variant of which was the antibiotic most commonly used by the Soviets to treat wounds in their war of national survival against Nazi Germany.

Professor Dubos comes to the same conclusion as Professor McKeown. In his book *The White Plague*[33], first published in 1952, he writes:

> With the decrease in mortality from tuberculosis, there has taken place in the Western world a similar or in some cases an even greater fall in the mortality caused by other infections. This is true not only of intestinal diseases like typhoid fever or the diarrhoeas, which are transmitted mainly by contaminated food and water, but also for measles, scarlet fever and the various forms of pneumonia, which like tuberculosis are primarily airborne.
>
> Particularly in the case of pneumonia has the fall in mortality rate followed a downward course which is almost indistinguishable from that of tuberculosis and [here is the point I want to stress] which began long before the introduction of serum therapy and the use of sulfonamides and penicillin. Clearly, something has happened to the mode of living in our civilisation which has rendered man more resistant to some of his ancient plagues.

Women and children, too.

Medical intervention has dramatically reduced the rates of death from what were once deadly epidemic infectious diseases of childhood, but this was by means of immunisation, not antibiotics. Professor McKeown shows that immunisation has proved effective against diphtheria and (possibly, this is controversial) whooping cough, which are potentially deadly bacterial childhood diseases; and also reduced the rates of death from poliomyelitis and smallpox.

Antibiotics have saved countless lives, and will continue to do so. But antimicrobial drugs, including antibiotics, are not the reason why bacterial infections ceased to be vast epidemics in the UK, America and other industrialised countries in the twentieth century. The tide turned against the infectious public health scourges of the nineteenth and early twentieth centuries before the introduction of antibiotics.

To use a military metaphor that doctors are fond of, the war against bacterial infections was not won by medical means. And these diseases – while no longer rampant in Europe and America, but which break out and become epidemic following industrialisation elsewhere throughout the world – remain unconquered.

'THE CAPTAIN OF ALL THESE MEN OF DEATH'

Take tuberculosis. This foul bacterial infection is like a hidden leprosy; it rots and corrodes the body from within. In the nineteenth century, tuberculosis killed more people in Europe than any other single disease, and two centuries earlier had been called 'the captain of all these men of death' by John Bunyan. The pallor and exhaustion of 'consumptives' gave the disease a perverted glamour, magnified by its effects on creative geniuses. Keats, Shelley, Robert Louis Stevenson and, later, Katherine Mansfield and D. H. Lawrence all travelled abroad to warm countries, trying in vain to escape from tuberculosis; and Sterne, Schiller, Paganini, Chopin, Emily Brontë, Kafka and other great writers and musicians died from the 'white plague'.

The image of blood on handkerchief, red on white, became a theme of European literature, and the languishing consumptive became a characteristic nineteenth-century personality. In the early twentieth century, fewer people were dying from tuberculosis in Europe and North America, but it remained a greatly feared disease, much as cancer is today.

One of the reasons for this fear is that, while the microbiological cause of the disease, *Mycobacterium tuberculosis*, was identified by Professor Robert Koch in 1882, it was not until 1944 that a really effective treatment, in the form of the antibiotic streptomycin, was marketed. Thereafter, the incidence of the disease declined further in Europe and North America.

As a result, it is commonly supposed that tuberculosis has been conquered by antibiotics. But this is not so. First, its decline in Europe and North America had little to do with medical intervention. Second, it has not been conquered.

In *The White Plague*, Professor Dubos traces the history of tuberculosis as a global epidemic, and shows that it is a disease whose fundamental cause is squalor.

> Physiological misery and crowding permitted the explosive spread of the disease among the labouring classes, and from this huge focus, the infection spread through society by means of countless unavoidable contacts . . . Tuberculosis was, in effect, the social disease of the nineteenth century, perhaps the first penalty capitalistic society had to pay for the ruthless exploitation of labour.

In Europe and North America, tuberculosis spread with industrialisation. In Africa and Asia, it spread with colonisation by the industrial powers. As an epidemic disease, it rises and falls according to environmental conditions. Overcrowding and filth breed the disease: virulent epidemics occur in shanty towns and concentration camps, for example. During World War II, much of central Europe reverted to the worst nineteenth-century conditions, and by its end, according to René Dubos:

> tuberculosis had once again become the great plague of continental Europe. But the threat of a lasting epidemic vanished as soon as living conditions improved and people began to live again in relative security. Many of those who had been near to tubercular death in the concentration camps succeeded in overcoming their disease when decent shelter, food and peace of mind were provided.

The most effective weapon in any war against epidemic infectious diseases is public health legislation. In Europe and North America, water-borne diseases such as cholera were successfully countered by the construction of closed sewers, air-borne diseases such as tuberculosis by slum clearance. With or without drugs, infections will dwindle in a clean, spacious environment and will flourish in a dirty, crowded one. Micro-organisms such as bacteria do indeed carry infectious diseases, but whether or not disease develops in the individual, or becomes epidemic, mostly depends on the quality of personal and public health.

Well-nourished and healthy people are resistant to infection; they may be infested with infectious bacteria without ever showing symptoms of disease. This fact was dramatically demonstrated around the turn of this century by the German Professor Max von Pettenkofer and the Russian Professor Elie Metchnikoff, both of whom were sure that germs alone do not cause disease. They put themselves to the test by publicly swallowing vast quantities of cholera bacilli cultured from corpses, and did not suffer significant illness. Conversely, babies and little children in Africa and Asia now, who suffer semi-starvation and a filthy environment through no fault of their own or their parents, die in millions from diarrhoeal infections that are usually trivial in their effects on well-fed, clean babies in Europe and North America.[34]

In this age of AIDS, tuberculosis is not mentioned much in industrialised countries. But on a global scale, tuberculosis remains 'the captain of all these men of death'. About one-third of the world's population harbour *Mycobacterium tuberculosis* and therefore could develop the disease. Every year throughout the world, about eight million people start to show the clinical signs of tuberculosis, and just under three million people a year die from the disease.[35] A report for the World Bank published in 1990[36] concludes that 'the magnitude of the tuberculosis problem is simply staggering'. In absolute numbers, the global death rate from tuberculosis is still rising. In 1994 the World Health Organisation predicted over ten million cases a year, and three and a half million deaths, in the year 2000.[37]

In Europe and North America, the incidence of tuberculosis dwindled until the mid-1980s. But in many cities in the developed world, the disease is now increasing, especially among the homeless and people weakened by the human immunodeficiency virus (HIV). By 1989 about 25,000 people in New York were suffering from tuberculosis, and in parts of the city the disease is out of control. A report published in the magazine *Science* in August 1992[38] said: 'If we do not learn from the current epidemic of TB . . . the tragedy unfolding in New York City could be repeated in any city in America that has homeless people, AIDS, prisons, hospitals and nursing homes.' There are plenty of such cities outside the USA.

In the UK an average of 5,357 cases and 418 deaths a year from TB were notified in 1989–91, mostly among immigrants from the Indian sub-continent.[39] But a report in March 1991 began: 'Tuberculosis, the "disease of the poor" which doctors thought they had conquered, has become common among London's homeless population.'[39] Irrespective of antibiotics and other medical treatment, when social conditions deteriorate, as they have in the USA and the UK since the 1980s, cities once again become breeding grounds for tuberculosis, and incidence of the disease increases.[40]

What's worse, *M. tuberculosis* is now evolving throughout the world in mutant forms that are resistant to drugs. Almost half the new TB patients arriving at New York hospitals late in 1991 were suffering drug-resistant forms of the disease[41] and one strain of the disease was then identified as being resistant to a total of eleven drugs. In 1993 physicians in New York were trying half a dozen or more drugs in attempts to treat TB resistant to both isonazid and rifampicin, two antibiotics on which doctors have mostly relied to treat the disease.[42] A further problem is that tuberculosis is highly infectious: in New York doctors as well as their patients are now dying from drug-resistant TB.

'NEW INFECTIONS DEFY DRUGS WAR'

As with tuberculosis, so also with other bacterial infections. In May 1990, the Royal College of Physicians in London, together with the Royal College of Pathologists, issued a joint statement on infectious diseases, accompanying an expert report.[43] The statement begins:

> Twenty years ago, the problem of infection was thought to be almost resolved by vaccines and antibiotics . . . Today, the medical profession and the public are again aware of, and indeed alarmed by, the dangers of infections. While many infections are well controlled by vaccines, others are causing increasing problems. For example, infections such as salmonellosis caused by food are increasing dramatically, there are recently recognised serious infections such as AIDS, and new infections are appearing in patients whose resistance to infection has been decreased by treatment or disease.

A consequent story in *The Daily Telegraph* was aptly headlined: 'NEW INFECTIONS DEFY DRUGS WAR ON DISEASES.'[44]

The statement continued, 'Major problems in infectious disease remain, quite often in new and challenging forms', and added, 'The widespread use of antibiotics have created their own problems.' In

October 1994 the UK Parliamentary Office of Science and Technology published its report 'Diseases Fighting Back'.[45] This stated:

> Some types of bacteria have acquired resistance to so many drugs that doctors are in danger of running out of effective treatments, and diseases that were regarded as curable ten years ago are emerging as potential killers once again.

The report instanced pneumonia and meningitis as two diseases now increasing in the UK in forms that are resistant to drugs, together with potentially deadly hospital infections caused by drug-resistant staphylococci, streptococci, enterococci and klebsiella species, which are 'potentially lethal to the very young, the very old, and the very ill . . . Minimising the further spread of drug resistance relies very much on the future prescribing behaviour of UK doctors.' The fact is that drugs are not and never have been a complete answer to disease. Antibiotics are often effective individual treatment, but no epidemic bacterial infection has ever been wiped out by drugs. All antibiotics have toxic ill-effects, and their general overuse and abuse is a vast waste of money and causes vast unnecessary suffering.

SUMMARY OF PART 1

Our belief in drugs gives doctors a peculiar power, and profoundly influences our ideas about disease and health – what it means to be ill and to be well. Antibiotics are indeed vital treatment for dangerous, invasive bacterial infections. But reality is very different from the myth of drugs as elixirs. Antibiotics have many ill-effects, some of which may mimic the diseases they are meant to cure. Overestimation of the risks of antibiotics and overestimation of their benefits leads to careless overuse in hospitals and in general practice. And the historic reputation of antibiotics, as the conquerors of the great nineteenth-century epidemic infections, is unfounded.

Part Two

On the Treadmill:
The Drug Era

It is never easy for any organisation whose members share a set of beliefs and attitudes to recognise that they are becoming irrelevant to the needs of the community. In the case of the medical profession, it is made all the more difficult because it is sustained in many of those beliefs by one of the most powerful commercial empires in the world: the pharmaceutical industry. The 'wonder drugs' era from the 1930s to the 1950s forged an alliance between the profession and the industry. It has since led to the industry achieving an unprecedented and dangerous measure of control over the profession.

Brian Inglis
The Diseases of Civilisation; 1981

Our industry produces the enchanted substances that give health care professionals their real power to cure. And actually, prior to the Second World War there really weren't too many things that would help. Doctors could tell you to keep in bed, keep warm, drink a lot of fluids, and they can make you feel better. But because of the investments in research and development that our companies have made, we really are making many diseases obsolete.

Gerald Mossinghoff
President, US Pharmaceutical Manufacturers Association; 1989

4 The ABC of Bugs and Drugs

MODERN MEDICINE

Half a century ago, in the 1940s, and then into the 1950s, when antibiotics were first developed and used in a big way, and more and more natural compounds and synthetic formulations were being discovered and devised, the general mood was euphoric. Medicine had become a science with results as emphatic as those of physics in the atomic age, or so it seemed. Antibiotics appeared to be all benefit and no risk – or little to worry about, anyway. Leading scientists in Europe and North America believed that antibiotics would eventually conquer the great epidemic diseases that have plagued humankind down the centuries. Researchers who developed effective antibiotics were rewarded with Nobel prizes. Some became very rich and famous.

And no wonder. Before the antibiotic age, hospital wards were filled with patients suffering from severe, invasive bacterial infections such as septicaemia, meningitis, rheumatic fever, endocarditis, pneumonia, tuberculosis and syphilis. Many of these patients were young, and they died while physicians watched helplessly. Antibiotics changed all this. They empowered doctors. Bacterial infections were successfully treated in hospitals and in the community. Physicians were generally not aware that the great epidemics were waning in any case, and even if they were aware, what understandably concerned them were the patients in front of them who before antibiotics would suffer and maybe die, and with antibiotics would probably recover.

In the UK, the astonishing phenomenon of antibiotics encouraged the vision of the founders of the state-run National Health Service in the late 1940s, that with provision of free medical services to everybody, disease would wither away – which is rather like supposing that the way to eliminate madness is to build an insane asylum on every street corner. General practitioners and hospital doctors believed that old methods of individual patient care could be replaced with a brave new medical world of drug therapy, with the bedside manner replaced by uniform doses of tablets and injections, giving a uniform cure.

Production of sulphonamides and penicillin, the first antibacterial drugs, was given a colossal boost by the coincidence of World War II: both Allied and Axis governments knew that infection had destroyed armies in the past and that anti-infective drugs are vital medicine in modern war. And the pioneers of the antibiotic industry in Europe and America, their enterprise acclaimed by governments, by the scientific community, by the media and the public, knew they had hit gold. In the twentieth century, what oil is to transport, drugs became to medicine, and with antibiotics, the pharmaceutical industry and the medical profession, hand-in-hand, created modern medicine as we experience it now.

TEN PER CENT HUMAN

To know your way around antibiotics, and understand their effect on human health, you have to know something about two complex areas of medicine – microbiology and pharmacology – which is to say, bugs and drugs. It's no wonder that many people are foxed when they read about bacteria and antibiotics; for a start, there are so many names. It's worth remembering that many general practitioners and other non-specialist doctors are foxed, too.

When Charles Darwin proposed that humans are descended from apes, he took a very short view of evolution: biologists now commonly believe that all living things on earth have evolved from one-cell organisms. Fossils of such organisms, looking very like bacteria and dating back 3.1 billion years, have been found in shale in South Africa. So taking the long view of evolution, human beings are descended from bugs. This proposition would have made Darwin even more unpopular than he became among the churchmen of his day.

So what are bacteria and what do they look like? In the 1950s, a British television quiz show entitled *Animal, Vegetable, Mineral*? was based on the idea that those three words referred to everything on earth. They do not. While certainly not minerals, micro-organisms such as bacteria and viruses are neither animals nor plants.

Bacteria are one-cell living organisms. One key difference between animals and plants on the one hand and bacteria on the other is in the DNA, the nucleic acid that encodes the genetic information of all living organisms. The cells of animals and plants contain a number of chromosomes, loops of double-stranded DNA in complex structures. Human cells usually contain 46 chromosomes, for example; those of bees, 16; those of corn, 20. Cells containing a multiple number of chromosomes arranged in a nucleus are called *eukaryotic*. By contrast, bacteria, which contain just one chromosome without a nucleus, are called *prokaryotic*.[1]

So looking at the world from the bacterial point of view, which in a sense is what microbiologists do, the world is not animal, vegetable, mineral, but prokaryote, eukaryote, mineral: humans are just one eukaryotic structures among others.[2]

Although the structures of bacteria are less developed than that of animals and plants, they are complex. Individual chromosomes encode vast amounts of information, and microbiologists are continually astonished to find just how adaptable bacteria are, notably when attacked by antibiotics.[3]

Bacterial cells usually come in one of four basic shapes, within which the chromosome is encased: round, in which case the bacteria are called 'cocci', as in streptococci (some of which are the microbiological cause of 'strep throat'); rod-shaped and called 'bacilli' (as in lactobacilli, found in the human vagina and in yoghurt); comma-shaped and called vibrios (as in *Vibrio cholerae*, the agent of cholera); or shaped like a joined coil, rather like a chromosome itself, and called spirochaetes. One other type of bacteria, mycoplasmas, has no cell walls. The cover of this book shows a photograph taken under a powerful microscope of *Escherichia coli* (*E. coli*) that lives in profusion in the human gut; this, as you can see, is a bacillus.[4]

Each of us carries more bacteria on and in our bodies than there are, or ever have been, people in the world. Almost all the bacterial species in contact with us have evolved with us, and are ordinarily harmless, or else are actually beneficial to our health.[5]

Your skin carries an average of one million bacteria on every square inch. You can't see them, but they are there, before and after washing. They are most abundant where the skin is warm and moist, but they are everywhere. Take *Staphylococcus epidermidis*, for example, which lives all over us, and usually does us no harm. 'Staphylococci . . . seem to have adapted to conditions in our skin that are uncongenial to most other bacteria,' says Professor Lewis Thomas in his book *The Wonderful Mistake*.[6] 'When you count them up, and us, it is remarkable how little trouble we have with the relationship.'

It may be a horrid thought, that invisible bugs are swarming all over us. But as happens in nature when different species evolve in balance with each other, *S. epidermidis* is normally good for us. Simply by flourishing on our skin, it keeps off foreign micro-organisms that could cause illness; there is no room for them. Further, it benefits us by releasing fatty acids that enhance the natural antibacterial quality of the skin. From our point of view, *S. epidermidis* is itself antibiotic.

The fact that bacteria can protect our health may seem strange, but consider an analogy: ladybirds. Like many other visible bugs, ladybirds do not sting or buzz, get stuck in jam, lay eggs in meat or keep us awake by blundering into lightbulbs at night. Like *S. epidermidis*, they don't bother us. Nevertheless, you might think that, while harmless, it makes no difference to us humans whether or not ladybirds exist. Not so: they are an integral part of nature's balance. Aphids eat garden flowers, which we like to cultivate, and ladybirds eat aphids. Without ladybirds, aphids are liable to multiply out of control, and eat all the flowers. One moral of the story is: be nice to ladybirds.

Likewise, with the normally harmless bacteria that live on or in us. Take another example, a streptococcal species, *S. viridans*, that lives in the mouth. This keeps other bacterial species in check simply by being there – for example, *Streptococcus pyogenes*, the microbiological cause of 'strep throat' and impetigo, and *Staphylococcus aureus*, a baleful bug of which more later, the agent of many unpleasant or dangerous infections including boils and abscesses, and hospital infections of surgical wounds and of blood. In the analogy, *S. viridans* is the ladybird, and *S. pyogenes* and *S. aureus* are the aphids. Bugs that normally predominate on the skin or in the openings of the body, such as *S. epidermidis* and *S. viridans*, are often known as 'friendly flora': by being there, they stop other bacterial species multiplying out of control and doing us harm. And the moral of this story is: be nice to friendly flora.

There are many millions of bacteria *on* us; there are many millions of millions of bacteria *inside* us, in our gut. The average human being is made up of something like 1,000,000,000,000,000 cells, of which around nine in every ten are the one-cell organisms we call bacteria. Counted in numbers of cells, we are therefore around one-tenth human. Bacteria are part of us, they have learned to live with us, and now we know they are there, it is best to learn to live with them.

There are a vast number of bacterial species, grouped into a great number of families (genera). The scientific name for humans is *Homo* (genus) *sapiens* (species). Likewise, and as with animals and plants, the scientific names for bacteria are conventionally printed in italics with an initial capital, family name first (as in *Lactobacillus*) and species name second (as in *acidophilus*). The bewildering array of names of bacterial species sometimes are tributes to the scientists who identified them, sometimes are indications of the diseases of which they are the microbiological cause and sometimes are both. Thus, Albert Neisser identified *Neisseria gonorrhoeae* as the agent of gonorrhoea, and Kiyoshi Shiga identified *Shigella dysenteriae* as an agent of dysentery.

Bacteria are of course not the only type of micro-organism that lives all around and on and inside us. Fungi, specifically yeasts and moulds, live in relatively small numbers on healthy skin and inside healthy guts, normally held in check by the far more numerous friendly bacterial flora. Fungi are structurally different from bacteria; they are primitive eukaryotes, whose cells contain more than one chromosome. Antibiotics designed to check or kill bacteria are usually ineffective against yeasts and moulds, which are therefore liable to multiply out of control after antibiotic treatment, in which case they are treated by other types of antibiotic designed specifically as antifungal drugs.[7]

Viruses are everywhere, too. These are sub-cellular organisms, smaller and simpler than bacteria. Whereas bacteria contain a chromosome in the form of a loop of double-stranded DNA, usually within a cell wall, viruses are made up of simple loops of nucleic acid (DNA or RNA) with a protein coating. They multiply only when they are inside the cells of other living things – bacteria, plants, animals or humans. Outside cells, they are inert, in a state of suspended animation. They are sometimes said to be 'on the threshold of life', having no ability to reproduce on their own.

Some viruses multiply within cells, destroy their hosts and then scatter. Viruses that have this effect on bacterial cells are called 'bacteriophages' – literally, 'eaters of bacteria'.[8] Other viruses evidently are contained stably within their host cells, doing them no harm.

The purpose of viruses on the planet is debated among biologists. An exciting theory is that viruses are the instruments of evolution, reshaping and scattering DNA and RNA fragments within and between their hosts, rather as seeds from dandelion clocks waft over the landscape; more of this later. Some viruses, some of the time, do cause infections, by releasing toxic substances as they multiply within cells. Viral diseases of humans include the common cold, influenza, herpes and AIDS, as well as a number of common childhood infections such as chickenpox, measles and mumps. Some viral diseases can be prevented by vaccination.

Generally, viral diseases run their course and are mostly little affected by medical treatment. Milder viral infections are 'self-limiting': they flare up, are resisted by the body's immune system and eventually fade away. It's sometimes said that, with treatment, a cold lasts a week; without treatment, seven days.

Infections may produce the same symptoms but be caused by any one of a number of bacterial species, or else be viral in origin. Such infections include those of the respiratory tract, from the mouth and oral cavity (such as tonsillitis) to the bronchus (bronchitis) and lungs (pneumonia); and also of the gut, including simple diarrhoea. Meningitis and endocarditis may also be bacterial or viral in origin.

Conversely, one species of bacteria may be responsible for infections of different sites with different names. For example, pneumococci, as their name suggests, are a bacterial cause of pneumonia; and they also can cause middle ear infections (otitis media) and meningitis. These are all reasons why it is vital, in cases of serious infection, that the physician takes samples for urgent laboratory analysis, and positive identification of the micro-organism responsible, so that treatment is appropriate.

HOW ANTIBIOTICS WORK

What exactly are antibiotics, and how do they work? As mentioned in the introduction, the word 'antibiotic' literally means 'against life': the science of biology is the science of living things. Antibiotics are drugs designed to treat diseases caused by microbes.

The first antibiotics were found in nature and extracted from substances that had evolved their own antibacterial defences. Penicillin was originally derived from penicillium mould. Streptomycin and other early antibiotics were extracted from soil micro-organisms. The first cephalosporin, an antibiotic chemically similar to penicillin, was found in fungi growing in a sewage outfall. Later, antibiotics were synthesised in laboratories.

Some antibiotics work by killing bacteria, in which case they are known as *bactericidal*; others stop the multiplication of bacteria, in which case they are known as *bacteriostatic*. A bacteriostatic drug can be bactericidal if used in high enough doses. Another distinction, is between 'narrow-spectrum' antibiotics, which kill or check a relatively small number of bacterial species, and 'broad-spectrum' antibiotics, which work simultaneously against a relatively large number of species. The wider the spectrum, the more species of friendly flora an antibiotic is liable to devastate. Physicians prescribe broad-spectrum antibiotics usually for one of two reasons: first, because they happen to be the most immediate effective treatment for a specific identified infection, second, because they are more likely to work on the 'blunderbuss principle' or as a 'shot in the dark' in the case of an illness such as bronchitis, that may be bacterial, or viral, or not an infection at all ('itis' means inflammation, not infection). For the case of acute, dangerous infections such as meningitis this policy is rational. But the prescribing of broad-spectrum antibiotics is usually inadvisable: they are comparatively more toxic and the risk of breeding drug-resistant bacteria is much higher. Even more than narrow-spectrum antibiotics, they certainly should not be used for relatively trivial infections liable to clear up without drug treatment.

CRACKING THE ANTIBIOTIC CODE

Here is as good a place as any to crack the antibiotic code, by introducing the main classes of antibiotic; more details later in this chapter.[9]

Sulphonamides were first introduced in the mid-1930s. They are bacteriostatic: they starve bacteria of folic acid, a B vitamin vital for bacteria as well as humans. Sulphonamides are now not much used on humans in developed countries except in the mixture co-trimoxazole: they are broad-spectrum, can be very toxic and are often ineffective because many species of bacteria have evolved to become resistant to them.[10]

Penicillin was first used in World War II. It remains the most widely used antibiotic, with over 25 types now on the market in the UK and over 50 branded products. These drugs are bactericidal: they kill bacteria by bursting their cell walls (and therefore do not work against mycoplasmas). Penicillins vary in their spectrum of effectiveness. They are relatively non-toxic, but as already stated, allergic reactions are common, and their massive use has provoked the evolution of many drug-resistant bacterial species, some of which can cause dangerous infections.

Cephalosporins, first marketed in the 1960s, are chemically similar to penicillins and, with them, are classified as betalactams. They are broad-spectrum with similar advantages and disadvantages to penicillins. Older cheap cephalosporins often now are ineffective because of bacterial resistance, and newer versions are expensive.

Before cephalosporins were marketed, three other types of antibiotics were developed in the United States: streptomycin, one of the **aminoglycoside** class; **chloramphenicol**; and the **tetracyclines**. They all proved powerful in their effects on various bacterial species and, protected by patent, were a gold-mine for the drug companies that owned their formula. They may be bactericidal or bacteriostatic, but all work by interfering with the protein synthesis, and thus the genes of bacteria. These relatively toxic drugs are generally now not much prescribed for human use in developed countries, and then usually only for specific serious or potentially deadly bacterial infections.

Other antibiotics include erythromycin, a **macrolide** often still used when patients have become allergic to penicillin; the **glycopeptides**, notably vancomycin, a relatively toxic and expensive drug usually held in reserve by hospitals for use when a serious bacterial infection is resistant to all other antibiotics; the **imidazoles**, notably metronidazole, used against parasitic as well as bacterial infections; the **lincosamides**, including clindamycin, an alternative when betalactams cannot be used; and the **polymyxins**, now not much used.

The one important family of antibiotics to be developed since the antibiotic 'golden age' of the 1940s and 1950s are the **quinolones**, of which the best known is nalidixic acid. They were at first thought to mark an antibiotic renaissance because they seemed to be remarkably safe and effective, and not to breed resistance. In time, though, various ill-effects have been identified, and bacterial resistance is spreading.[10]

Other antibacterials are reserved for specific infections, notably tuberculosis and leprosy. Antimicrobial drugs are also formulated against fungi; the best-known antifungal drug is nystatin. Antibiotics are prescribed to be taken as tablets, capsules or liquids; those used in hospitals are often injected. Other antibiotics are used on the skin; these include some drugs now judged to be too dangerous to take by mouth or injection.

In developed countries, regulatory authorities screen new drugs for safety in use, but evidence of ill-effects caused by older drugs not monitored so carefully at the time of their introduction. With some exceptions, journalists have an unimpressive record as drug watchdogs, partly because few medical correspondents know much about microbiology or pharmacology, and in any case, get much of their information from industry. General practitioners are normally better informed than journalists, but what specialist knowledge they gained as medical students quickly becomes outdated, and they often don't have time to keep up with textbooks and medical journals, commonly relying instead on updates from industry literature and sales representatives. It is, of course, in the interests of both governments and industry to check that drugs are acceptably safe. Physicians are given a lot of guidance on the ill-effects of antibiotics, and both general practitioners and hospital doctors are trained to prescribe the safest possible drug. Nevertheless, antibiotics are problematic.

A BABEL OF NAMES

And there are so many drugs! In the early days of antibiotics, citizens interested in making informed choices could, if they chose, quickly get a fair idea of which drugs were used for which infections, and why. But now, although there are admirable patients' handbooks available in bookshops[11], even the most interested reader is liable to suffer severe information overload. Also, the use of medical jargon and scientific names is part of medical mystique: if not deliberately designed to baffle the lay reader, it certainly has that effect. And when we are excluded from discussion about the drugs on which we may depend, we are alienated from decisions about our health.

So it is worth knowing how drugs, including antibiotics, are named. There are agreed rules. Every drug has three different types of name: chemical, generic and trade. *Chemical names* are used by pharmacologists to indicate the chemical structure or structures of a drug. For example, the chemical names for ampicillin are ampicillinum, anhydrous ampicillin and aminobenzylpenicillin. You will be glad to know that you don't have to remember any chemical names. In this book, only the generic names are used.

Taking the same example, ampicillin is the *generic name* of a broad-spectrum aminopenicillin (one of a number of types of penicillin), commonly prescribed by general practitioners for ear, nose, throat, respiratory and urinary tract infections. In Britain, *trade names* for ampicillin on its own or formulated in combination with other drugs are: Amfipen, Penbritin, Vidopen, Ampiclox, Flu-Amp and Magnapen. As you can see, by convention trade names begin with capital letters. They are the names owned by the drug companies and are printed in large letters on packets and in advertisements to doctors, and tend to be the names best known to patients. Generic names are used in textbooks, but are not promoted by manufacturers, who want doctors to remember the trade names.

Once the patent on a drug expires, that drug may be manufactured and marketed by any pharmaceutical company as a generic drug, without an additional trade name. Thus the generic version of ampicillin, which is also on the market, has passed out of the ownership of any particular drug company and, as usual with generic drugs, is cheaper than the branded versions. In the UK, successive secretaries of state for health have, from time to time, tried to encourage generic prescribing to save taxpayers' money. Manufacturers have always fought against any encouragement of generic drugs, arguing that they need the profits from branded drugs to research new drugs. They have been supported by the medical profession, who believe that doctors need 'clinical freedom' to prescribe the drugs they think are best for their patients, even when this means a relatively expensive branded drug that is effectively identical to the cheap generic version.

The babel of drug names may also have the effect of inhibiting public scrutiny of drug companies. In 1959, a US Senate Committee chaired by Estes Kefauver was set up to investigate the antibiotic trade.[12] Members of the committee were baffled by what seemed to them perverse confusion in the naming of drugs. In their report, the committee said:

> The multiplicity of names for products in the drug industry exceeds the bounds of human imagination . . . A single drug product is represented in the market by such a complex body of nomenclature

> as to intimidate even initiates in the field. And if one can visualize the situation for a single drug multiplied by the thousands of drugs currently marketed, one can get some impression of the chaos existing.

Although trade names are better known than generic ones, this book usually uses generic names. While the formulation, dose and presentation of a drug may vary from brand to brand, judgements on its nature – including what infections it works against, its toxicity, and its possible longer-term ill-effects – usually apply both to the generic drug and to its branded versions. Thus, co-trimoxazole is available in generic form or, for a higher price, as the branded products Septrin and Bactrim. The various branded versions of ampicillin, also available in generic form, have already been listed. Branded versions of metronidazole available as tablets include Flagyl, Metrolyl, Nidazol and Zadstat. The basic point is that the generic and branded versions of antibiotics are much the same in their fundamental nature and effects.

The total number of antibiotics available in the UK on prescription for internal use by mouth or injection is, at the time of writing, just over 100 counted as generics, and somewhat under 200 branded drugs (including the generic versions). Many of these are rarely used or are reserved for serious hospital infections. Betalactams – notably the older and the newer penicillins – are the antibiotics most commonly prescribed by general practitioners for common infections, and some of these, such as penicillin G or benzylpenicillin – in use since the 1940s – are narrow spectrum and, if effective, are relatively safe apart from the risk of allergic reactions.

5 The Trouble with Antibiotics

SUPERINFECTIONS

Naturally enough, the more powerful the dose of any drug, the more problems it can cause. The more courses you take, and the more broad spectrum the formulation, the more likely you are to suffer ill-effects from antibiotics; but just one course can sometimes make you ill. Simple cause and effect is easy to understand. If you take a course of antibiotics and immediately suffer, say, diarrhoea or shock, you or your doctor are likely to guess that the drug is involved.

The trouble with antibiotics, though, is not so much their acute ill-effects as the long-term damage they can do to individual patients and to the community, by a relatively complex process of cause and ill-effect generally better understood by microbiologists than physicians. Antibiotics often are effective short-term treatments for infection but, in the longer term, can be the underlying cause of the same or other infections. That is to say, in curing disease antibiotics may cause more disease. This is partly because of a phenomenon known as *superinfection*.

When you take antibiotics, the drug kills vast numbers of bacteria in your gut and elsewhere, on and in your body, but countless millions remain. The bacteria that survive include species unaffected by the drug, or else (initially rare) drug-resistant variants of a vulnerable species. Non-bacterial micro-organisms such as fungi also survive, unless the drug is specifically formulated against them. After a number of courses of antibiotics, these surviving micro-organisms are liable to multiply and to fill the space created by the drug.

The bacterial species that are normally dominant on and in our bodies are the friendly flora that have evolved in harmony with us. These species are usually resilient. A course of antibiotics may devastate them, but is unlikely to wipe them out totally; and afterwards they are liable to become re-established in the right relationship with each other, especially in normally healthy adults.

But not always. Antibiotics can start a sequence of events in which the naturally protective populations of bacteria are overwhelmed by superinfection with different species of bacteria and other micro-organisms. Professor Marc Lappé of the University of Illinois, explains[13]:

> When antibiotics kill or inhibit harmful bacteria, they also eliminate vast numbers of relatively benign or even beneficial bacteria. When these more benevolent counterparts die off, they leave behind a wasteland of vacant organ and tissue. These sites previously occupied with normal bacteria, are now free to be colonized by new ones. Some of these new ones have caused serious and previously unrecognized diseases.

The people most likely to suffer this malign process include the very young, the old, the weak and the generally ill, as well as those whose immunity to illness has been weakened for other reasons. After courses of antibiotics, our friendly flora in effect have to fight to re-establish themselves as the dominant species. The more drugs we take, and the generally more vulnerable we are, the greater the chance that they will lose this fight against superinfection by other species of micro-organisms liable to cause disease.

The bacteria and other micro-organisms that are liable to be superinfectious can be subdivided into three types. The first normally live harmlessly in profusion on or in the body, notably in the gut, and are capable of harm only when their natural balance with the normally dominant friendly flora is destroyed. The *E. coli* bacillus is an example: it is a menace usually only when it multiplies out of control throughout the gut, or else when it is able to invade other parts of the body, such as the urinary tract, whose opening is normally shielded by friendly bacterial flora.

The second type of potentially superinfectious micro-organism may also live in or on the healthy body, but in small numbers, normally kept down by the dominant friendly flora. These have no known useful function in the healthy body, and, like the normally more common species such as *E. coli*, can be a menace when they multiply. Examples are the *Clostridium difficile* bacillus that can cause a severe and even deadly 'pseudomembranous' colitis, and the *Candida albicans* fungus that can cause thrush after antibiotic therapy. (More of these later in the book.)

The third type of micro-organism does not live in the normal healthy body, and is kept out by the body's natural defences of which friendly flora are an integral part. When these flora are devastated by antibiotics, we become more vulnerable to these foreign bacterial species. Among very many examples are the shigella family of bacilli that are the microbiological cause of dysentery, the *Vibrio cholerae* bacillus that causes cholera, and the *Treponema pallidum* spirochaete that causes syphilis.

Superinfections can usually be checked by further courses of antibiotics formulated for this purpose. Doctors in Europe, North America and other privileged parts of the world, with access to well-stocked pharmacies, can usually check superinfections, although they may not be able to cure them. People in Africa and Asia and other less privileged parts of the world are more likely to succumb, simply because of a lack of appropriate drugs.

Ironically, superinfections have the effect of enhancing the reputation of antibiotics as wonder drugs. If you become ill with thrush, say, or severe diarrhoea, and do not realise that your illness may well be a superinfection caused by a previous course of antibiotics, you will turn to antimicrobial drugs again and, once you recover, will be all the more likely to turn to these drugs once again in future.

THE CHEMICAL TREADMILL

Soon after antibiotics were first used, microbiologists became aware of superinfection. So did industry. Many antibiotics are specifically formulated to treat superinfections caused by other antibiotics. On the one hand, antibiotics are effective against bacterial infection; on the other, more and more antibiotics are used every year. Why? This paradox is partly explained by superinfection: the more antibiotics are used, the more they *have* to be used. This is the drug treadmill.

If you are surprised by the phenomenon of bacterial superinfection, consider its parallel on the land. When farmers use insecticides and other biocides, they disrupt the balance of nature. Sometimes this does no harm (unless, that is, you are concerned not just about pests but also about all the other species of animals, birds and insects that are killed). At other times, though, just as in the case of the ladybirds and the aphids mentioned earlier, biocides may have the effect of turning previously harmless insects into major pests. In the worst cases, new pests created by the use of biocides may cause vast damage. The distinguished entomologist the late Professor Robert van den Bosch explains[14]:

> When applied to a crop, a biocide kills not only pests but also other species in the insect community, including the natural enemies that restrain noxious species . . . Insecticide spraying frequently creates a virtual biotic vacuum in which the surviving or reinvading pests, free of significant natural-enemy attack, explode. Such post-spraying pest explosions are often double-barrelled, in that they involve not only the resurgence of target pests but also the eruption of previously minor species, which had been fully suppressed by natural enemies. The frequent outcome is a raging multiple-pest outbreak, more damaging than that for which the original pest-control measure was undertaken.

A pesticide that kills ladybirds is liable to provoke a plague of aphids. An antibiotic that kills *S. viridans* and other friendly flora found on or in the body is liable to provoke an outbreak of superinfection. Indeed, 'provoke' is really the wrong word. Potentially superinfectious bacterial species are relatively harmless in the healthy body. When antibiotics are a link in the chain leading on to disease, it is really the drug, just as much as the bug, that is the cause of superinfection.

Dr van den Bosch concludes:

> This is the genesis of the insecticide treadmill . . . [which] is magnified and prolonged by genetic selection for insecticide resistance in the repeatedly treated pests . . . Insects become resistant to pesticides, and the more intensive and widespread the poisonous blanket, the more rapid the selection for resistance in the pests. With insecticide resistance plugged into the formula, the treadmill whirrs at full tilt, and the consequences can be awesome.

The phenomenon of resistance is the second parallel between biocides and antibiotics. The fact that, after chemical attack, agricultural pests evolve mutant strains invulnerable to the insecticides formulated to destroy them has been known since 1914.[15] Pesticide-resistant creatures spread; during the 1950s, as the use of agrichemicals multiplied, scientists and farmers found that more and more pests were resisting more and more of the biocides hurled at them. In 1979 in Britain, the Royal Commission on Environmental Pollution[16] reported: 'Resistance to insecticides and fungicides is a matter of serious concern.'

Worse still was the discovery that insects carrying micro-organisms that cause human disease were also evolving mutant strains resistant to biocides. DDT (dichloro-diphenyl-trichloroethane) was identified as an insecticide in 1939 by the Swiss scientist Dr Paul Müller, who won a Nobel price for his discovery, which had proved effective against the malaria mosquito. In 1955, the World Health Organisation announced a $1.3 billion programme for the global elimination of malaria to be achieved by spraying the mosquito's habitat, including houses, with DDT and dieldrin, another insecticide.

Thus the 1950s were the 'golden age' of biocides as well as of antibiotics. Scientists believed that all human diseases borne by insects or animals – including yellow fever, typhus and plague as well as malaria – could be eliminated forever by chemical means. But mosquito resistance to DDT was observed as early as 1950, and to dieldrin, in 1954. Other very toxic insecticides such as malathion and lindane were substituted. These worked, but only for a while, and colossal epidemics of malaria carried by insecticide-resistant mosquitoes broke out all over Asia in the 1970s. Professor Robert Metcalf of the Department of Entomology at the University of Illinois reported[15]:

> some countries have recorded 30–40 fold increases in the case of malaria from 1968 to 1976 . . . By 1986 resistance had been reported in 58 *Anopheles* [mosquito species] recorded as vectors of human malaria and multiple resistance was widespread in more than 30, with 8 species showing resistance to all the five classes of insecticides available for residual house spraying.

The World Health Organisation programme to eliminate malaria was abandoned in 1976. The disease is now uncommon in Europe and North America but has surged once again as a vast epidemic elsewhere in the world. Worse, not only are the mosquitoes that carry the malaria parasite often resistant to insecticides, but now *Plasmodium falciparum*, the species of protozoa that causes the most vicious form of malaria, is also often resistant to chloroquine, otherwise the first-choice anti-malarial drug.[17]

Those suffering from chloroquine-resistant malaria can, if they happen to live in Europe, North America or elsewhere in the prosperous parts of the world, usually be successfully treated after returning home. But insecticide-resistant malaria mosquitoes carrying drug-resistant malaria bugs amount to a public health catastrophe in Africa and Asia, and the cost of biocides and antibiotics – all of which are liable eventually to become useless as pests and bugs develop resistance – is crippling the economies of some already impoverished tropical countries.

In 1989, Professor Metcalf wrote[15]:

> The past 40 years have seen insect resistance to insecticides develop from a scientific curiosity to an immense practical problem that threatens man's ability to control not only the insect pests of agriculture but also the insect vectors that transmit major human and animal diseases.

In the same year, his address to the annual meeting of the American Association for the Advancement of Science resulted in the following headline in the (London) *Independent*: 'MONSTER BUGS THRIVE AS CHEMICAL ARSENAL FAILS:' 'Some strains of insects and microbes have appeared that are resistant to nearly everything in our chemical arsenal,' stated Professor Metcalf, and he warned that 'the world may be returning to the agricultural and medical dark age that existed before the discovery of modern insecticides and antibiotics.'[18]

Superpests, invulnerable to at least some forms of chemical treatment, have emerged and may become epidemic as a result of the use of biocides. Similarly superbugs – which is to say bacteria and other micro-organisms that resist treatment with one, some or even all available drugs – are a new health hazard created by the use of antibiotics; which is why in effect, antibiotics are pesticides used on people.

SUPERBUGS

What antibiotics do, in a phrase used by microbiologists, is to exert 'selective pressure' on bacteria. This distorts and accelerates their evolution, so that previously vulnerable species become drug-resistant. To some extent, this is simply the result of Darwinian chance mutation. When any bacterial species is attacked by antibiotics, only the fittest survive. However, in a population of many millions of bacteria, there will be some chance mutants, maybe one in a million, that just happen to be invulnerable to the drug that kills all the others. These previously insignificant mutants survive, multiply and colonise the space left by the destruction of all the other bacteria in the species that were previously vulnerable to the drug. So in future the drug doesn't work.

The creation of superbugs is not just a matter of chance mutation, however. Although microscopic, bacteria are very complex and adaptable living organisms. Their genetic organisation includes structures that probably evolved in order to resist naturally occurring chemicals contained in rival living things, just as plants, insects, birds, animals and, indeed, we humans have evolved means to resist predators.[19]

These structures – rings of genetic material contained within the bacterial cell wall in addition to the chromosome – are called *plasmids*. I mention them now briefly (more of these later) so that you can see why antibiotics, like biocides, can have such an explosive effect. The codes for bacterial resistance to antibiotics are contained in plasmids. Under selective pressure from drugs, these codes – also known as 'R' (for 'resistance') factors – can be transferred not only within bacteria of the same species, but also from one species to others. And there is more! Plasmids may contain codes for resistance not just to one but to a number of antibiotics. Under pressure from a course of one antibiotic, bacteria may therefore transfer multiple drug resistance within and between species.

What this means is that, as a result of taking antibiotics, you could end up with a gut full of bugs against which any number of future courses of antibiotics will be useless. And drug-resistant bacteria may themselves be the microbiological cause of unpleasant or even deadly infectious disease. If you take antibiotics, such disease may spread from you to me. If I take antibiotics, such disease may spread from me to you. You cannot avoid superbugs by avoiding antibiotics. Superbugs are everywhere.

CAULDRONS OF CONTAGION

So far, superbugs can usually be successfully treated by one or more of the antibiotics in any well-stocked pharmacy. Nevertheless, there are four reasons why they are frightening. First, the next antibiotic you take may be for an infection caused by the last antibiotic you took, which has made you vulnerable to superinfection, so that you get more infections that make you more ill, so that you take more antibiotics . . . and so on and so on, round and round the drug treadmill.

Second, the antibiotic you take, say, for a mild infection, can breed superbugs that may transfer their drug-resistance to more dangerous bacterial species, making you vulnerable to invasive and even deadly infections. In the West, these usually can be treated, but sometimes only with drugs that are expensive, powerful, relatively more toxic and unpredictable in their effects.

Third, it is possible that, one day, antibiotics will breed a superbug that is the microbiological cause of a deadly epidemic infection that resists treatment with all antibiotics. Outside the West, this is now effectively happening countless times, simply because the drugs that can be used against serious infections are not available, or because the victim cannot be reached by a doctor. In the West, this doomsday superbug, everything-resistant enterococci, are now causing disease outbreaks in Western hospitals, and are killing people, but are not yet epidemic[19,20].

Fourth, you may never take antibiotics and yet be vulnerable to disease caused by a superbug, from any chance encounter with somebody themselves infected. The intestines of people who take antibiotics are factories producing drug-resistant bacteria. The next course of antibiotics you take may be for an infection caused by the last course of antibiotics taken by somebody else, which has made them more vulnerable to infection; so then you become more vulnerable and thus suffer another infection, so then you and they take more courses of antibiotics . . . and so on and so on, multiplied countless times across communities, countries and continents.

Overcrowded living conditions, infectious surroundings and constant dosing with antibiotics create ideal breeding-grounds for superbugs. Five examples of such cauldrons of contagion are: factory-farmed animals; hospital patients, including mothers and their babies; school children, especially at nursery school; people with many sexual partners; and countless millions of people living in slums throughout the world. In the August 1992 issue of *Science* magazine, an article on this subject[20] concluded:

> Those who believed a plague could not happen in this century have already seen the beginning of one in the AIDS crisis, but the drug-resistant strains [of bacteria], which can be transmitted by casual contact in movie theaters, hospitals, and shopping centers, are likely to be even more terrifying.

Superbugs are everywhere in the world. 'Each time an antimicrobial agent is used, there is potential for a significant effect on world microbial ecology' – this is Professor Calvin Kunin in an address to his colleagues of the Infectious Disease Society of America in 1984. He continued:

> Most of the world's population is located in the so-called under-developed parts of the world. The greatest proportion of this population live under conditions of poverty, inadequate medical care, and poor sanitation and nutrition . . . These conditions, abetted by often irrational self-administration of antibiotics, have become a fertile ground for resistant micro-organisms . . . Travel is so extensive today that these organisms have gained entry and spread rapidly in Western countries.

In this address and in a report to the World Health Organisation in 1990[21], Professor Kunin gives examples of some of the many strains of drug-resistant diseases that have spread like brushfire internationally or globally. These include: meningitis, 'which spread rapidly throughout the world'; pneumonia in and from South Africa and Spain; and the global epidemic of drug-resistant gonorrhoea that 'appears to have originated in southeast Asia and Africa'.

In a cover feature, 'The end of antibiotics', published in March 1994[22], *Newsweek* magazine stated: 'Every disease-causing bacterium now has versions that resist at least one of medicine's 100-plus antibiotics . . . Already patients are suffering and dying from illnesses that science predicted 40 years ago would be wiped off the face of the earth. The scientists were wrong. Before science catches up with the microbes, many more people will die.'

6 Gold in Them Thar Pills

SULPHONAMIDES: WEAPONS OF WAR

The antibacterial era began in the 1930s, not in the UK with penicillin, but in Germany with sulphonamides. In 1935, the German firm I. G. Farben began manufacturing and marketing Prontosil, the first sulphonamide drug. It had been discovered by Dr Gerhard Domagk, Farben's research director, who was awarded the Nobel prize for medicine.[23]

Sulphonamides were the wonder drug of the 1930s, medically and commercially.[24] By 1941 over 2000 tons had been manufactured and used to treat puerperal fever, pneumonia, meningitis and infections of the gut and urinary tract. Sulpha drugs (as they are known) were vital to the war effort in the late 1930s and throughout World War II. They were used by the American military authorities to treat gonorrhoea among their troops, and by the Japanese to treat their soldiers' dysentery. Ironically, given its German origin, Winston Churchill recovered from pneumonia in North Africa towards the end of the war after treatment with a sulpha drug.

Prontosil was protected by patents, and its success helped to make Farben a vast chemical conglomerate. After World War II, the firm was broken up into three: BASF, now also well known in the plastics industry; and two chemical manufacturers, Hoechst and Bayer, which are today two of the three biggest drug companies in Europe, each with sales in 1993 totalling over £4 billion.[25]

Sulphonamides turned out not to be magic bullets. Some of their ill-effects have already been mentioned. Allergic reactions and diarrhoea are quite common. Less frequently they can also sometimes cause sore gums or tongue, loss of appetite, nausea and vomiting, gut pain, headache, need to sleep, inability to sleep, dizziness and vertigo, numbness and tingling, hallucinations, depression, nervousness, apathy, confusion, nightmares, painful joints and muscles. Rare ill-effects include kidney failure, severe hepatitis, liver damage, severe anaemia, Stevens-Johnson syndrome (which can cause permanent eye damage) and Lyell's syndrome, in which the skin peels off in sheets.[26]

Even in the 1930s, doctors found that sulphonamides increasingly did not work in cases of gonorrhoea: gonococci bacteria were becoming drug-resistant. In those days, drug resistance was a mystery. By the 1950s, around half of all meningococci, bacteria that cause meningitis, were resistant to sulphonamides, as were the *E. coli* that cause urinary tract infections. An analysis carried out in London between 1974 and 1978 found that three quarters of all strains of *Shigella dysenteriae*, the bacterial cause of dysentery, were sulphonamide resistant.[27]

Professor Thomas O'Brien of the Department of Medicine at Brigham and Women's Hospital, Boston, Massachusetts, is a leading authority on antibiotic resistance. I went to Boston to see him, and asked him how bacteria become resistant to sulphonamides. Initially, he explained, the drug works by blocking a bacterial enzyme involved in the synthesis of folic acid. However, in time, the bacteria simply get another enzyme to do the job. 'It's like in a factory – if the lights go out, somebody turns on the emergency generator.'

Because of their toxicity and because they often don't work, sulphonamides (with one exception) are now not much prescribed in Europe and North America, except for meningitis and urinary tract infections. The exception is co-trimoxazole, the combination of a sulpha drug with trimethoprim. As already mentioned, although it has the ill-effects of other sulphonamides, co-trimoxazole is a popular drug, prescribed for many common conditions including bronchitis and other respiratory tract infections, children's middle ear infections, and gonorrhoea, as well as cystitis and more serious infections such as typhoid fever.[26]

SAFE SEX WITH PENICILLIN

Alexander Fleming first noticed the antibacterial power of penicillin in 1928, but he did not take his research far enough to make his discovery useful. This work was done by a team of scientists in Oxford led by Professor Howard Florey and Dr Ernst Chain, who became motivated by the imperative need for drugs for Allied troops in the war against Hitler's Germany.

In early 1940 Florey and Chain used up all the penicillin then manufactured in an attempt to save the life of an Oxford policeman who had developed septicaemia after cutting himself shaving. Despite recycling the drug from the patient's urine, the supply ran out, and he died. Yet within a few years penicillin replaced sulphonamides as the general-purpose antimicrobial drug of choice, for two reasons. First, penicillins (in the original and also later forms) are relatively safe drugs, with fewer and milder ill-effects than sulphonamides. Second, while Florey and Chain did not attempt to take out patents on penicillin, seeing it as a wonderful natural healer, American and then British pharmaceutical firms made it very profitable by patenting the manufacturing processes of as many varieties as they could devise.

Early on, penicillins became the drugs of choice for puerperal fever, bacterial pneumonia and meningitis, and bacterial sexually transmitted diseases. Professor O'Brien explained to me how penicillins work. 'Bacteria are tiny little organisms in a hostile world, that need to be protected,' he told me. 'They have a cell wall around them that protects them against trauma and shock. This is their home. They would swell and rupture without their protective cell wall. Penicillins sabotage the synthesis of the cell wall; so they pop – like popcorn.' All antibiotics in the very large betalactam family, including all penicillins and cephalosporins, work like this.

In the 1960s, women were liberated sexually by the contraceptive pill. Penicillin gave men sexual licence as from the 1940s. Production of penicillin was given a priority in the USA after its entry into World War II, second only to production of the atom bomb. In 1943 a total of 29 pounds of penicillin was manufactured. Ten years later the figure had risen by a factor of around 30,000, to just under 400 tons.

Healthy servicemen were given hefty doses of penicillin as protection against gonorrhoea and syphilis during the later years of World War II, and then later in Korea, Vietnam and wherever else in the world they have been based. Prostitutes were also dosed. Antibiotics thus became used rather like vaccination, prophylactically as a guard against an infection that a healthy person has not got, but might get. American GIs loved penicillin. Safe sex! British troops were pleased, too. In 1943, Churchill was faced with a problem. He was asked whether penicillin, then scarce, should be used to treat venereal diseases or battle wounds. His careful reply was: 'This valuable drug must on no account be wasted. It must be put to the best military use.'

So preference was given to troops with VD who could most quickly be made fit to fight.

Penicillins are still often effective against a range of bacteria that are the microbiological cause of a variety of common childhood infections of the ear, nose, throat and lower respiratory tract, including streptococcal, staphylococcal and pneumococcal species. Paediatricians, the physicians who specialise in childhood medicine, took to penicillins in a big way from the start. In 1950, the British journal *The Practitioner* published a book in which various distinguished doctors contributed their 'Favourite Prescriptions'. The chapter on children was by Dr Philip Evans, then consultant at the Hospital for Sick Children at Great Ormond Street in London. He wrote: 'The most popular prescriptions in paediatrics are of antibiotics, because children so often suffer from acute infections . . . Penicillin is the standby, perhaps because one cannot give an overdose.' After specifying a recommended dose, he added: 'But in babies this amount is usually and harmlessly exceeded.'

In these early years, treatment with antibiotics was an event in the family. In 1950, I was ten years old and, in a letter to my father, wrote: 'I am just recovering from an attack of tonsillitis, and am hoping to be back at school by Monday. The doctor prescribed penicillin lozenges and M&B [a sulpha drug made by May and Baker, hence the 'M&B'] and as you realise, I wasn't exactly looking forward to them. Still, it turned out that the penicillin at least, did the trick.' (Or so I and the doctor thought at the time; later my tonsils, now known to be part of the body's immune defences against disease, were removed. Tonsillitis is usually not a bacterial but a viral infection. Oh, well . . .)

The first penicillins were 'natural', derived from moulds. These include benzyl penicillin (also known as penicillin G) and phenoxymethyl penicillin (penicillin V), both of which are still used, including for common infections of children. But as early as the 1940s, doctors were faced with a growing problem: penicillins increasingly simply did not work. Bacteria had evolved a weapon, known as betalactamase or penicillase, which attacks the drug itself, cutting its betalactam ring. Professor O'Brien explained: 'It's like a Patriot missile. The incoming Scud antibiotic molecules are intercepted.'

By the 1950s, various bacterial species were resistant to penicillin. The most fearful was *Staphylococcus aureus*, which can cause acute and sometimes dangerous sepsis on or in the body, in the blood (septicaemia) and in vital organs.[28] Penicillin-resistant *S. aureus* made open-body surgery once again a hazardous procedure. 'I had a medical student classmate who died of staphylococcal sepsis in the 1950s because it was multi-resistant,' Professor O'Brien told me.

Since the 1950s, drug companies have formulated successive generations of penicillins in an attempt to keep one step ahead of resistant bacteria. 'This vast and very profitable market has been driven by resistance,' says Dr O'Brien. In the late 1950s, the British firm Beecham, not until then a drug company, devised synthetic penicillin specifically designed to combat betalactamase, of which methicillin, cloxacillin and flucloxacillin are still on the market. In due course, though, *Staphylococcus aureus* evolved a new resistance mechanism, and developed into what is known as 'MRSA' (methicillin-resistant *S. aureus*). This superbug is now a major menace, for penicillins of any type now rarely work against it. '*Staph. aureus* that are sensitive to penicillin are collectors' items,' stated a 1990 review.[29]

Other bacteria whose danger to humans is increased by frequent resistance to penicillins include those that cause pneumonia and meningitis, as well as invasive hospital infections. One group of drugs, the carboxypenicillins, have been devised specifically against *Pseudomonas aeruginosa*, now a troublesome hospital pathogen.

The story of the development of penicillins, and of the other betalactam drugs, notably the cephalosporins, is a story of science and industry wrestling with ever-evolving nature. The most popular antibiotics devised for use in general practice are the aminopenicillin family, including amoxycillin and ampicillin. Like other penicillins, these occasionally cause sickness, diarrhoea and allergic reactions[24] but usually work against a variety of bacterial infections. In 1989, the world's top-selling antibiotic was reckoned to be SmithKline Beecham's Amoxil, an amoxycillin, with an annual market value then of US$368,500,000.[30] In the UK, successive generations of cephalosporins, which are increasingly expensive, are mostly reserved for use in hospitals before surgery, and for invasive infections. In the USA, cephalosporins are vigorously promoted by industry for use in general practice.

From the point of view of the general practitioner and the patient in the community, penicillin of one type or another is usually effective treatment. It is true that if you take regular courses of penicillin, in childhood or as an adult, you are sooner or later likely to suffer allergic reactions as your body loses its ability to absorb the poison of the drug, so that the drug becomes unusable. It is also true that 'safer' antibiotics such as penicillin are all the more likely to be prescribed, and this increases the risk of breeding superinfections and superbugs in your gut, which may cause serious untreatable infections. In general practice, penicillins are also often prescribed for illnesses that are not infectious, for infections that are not bacterial, and for bacterial infections better treated with milder remedies, or best left to clear up by themselves.

The use of any antibiotic puts selective pressure on any bacteria to evolve drug resistance. Routine dosing with penicillin of vast numbers of men whose sexual behaviour put them at high risk of sexually transmitted diseases has turned out to have had disastrous consequences, originally unforeseen. In the mid-1970s, drug-resistant *Neisseria gonorrhoeae* spread all over the world. One source was the Philippines, where during the Vietnam war US servicemen and local prostitutes had been routinely given heavy doses of penicillin as protection against gonorrhoea. As a result, the gonococci evolved and acquired a betalactamase that was – and is – resistant to any dose of penicillin. Karma! By the mid-1980s, between one third and one half of all gonococci in many countries had become resistant to penicillin.

In any case gonorrhoea remains a worldwide epidemic and the disease is flaring up within inner-city areas in the United States. A report in *Scientific American* published in 1991[31] states:

> The re-emergence of bacterial sexually transmitted diseases (STDs) in young, black and Hispanic inner-city poor populations, coupled with the rising incidence of AIDS and other viral STDs, has created a demand for public health care and preventive interventions that exceeds the capacity of many systems to provide diagnostic and treatment services.

In plainer language, this means that the environments of inner cities now are such as to create new cauldrons of uncontrollable bacterial contagion. Reports in the 1990s have identified gonococci in Britain, as elsewhere in the world, that are resistant not only to penicillin but also to cephalosporins, tetracyclines, the aminoglycoside spectinomycin, and even to quinolones.[32,33] Widespread multi drug-resistant gonorrhoea, now threatened, would be a public health catastrophe.

Penicillins remain far and away the most commonly used antibiotics. In 1987, a study carried out for the US National Institutes of Health estimated that world production of all penicillin for human and animal use in 1980 was 17,000 tons, almost two-thirds of the 25,000 tons of all types of antibiotic manufactured in that year.[34]

STREPTOMYCIN: PAYDIRT

Back in the USA in the 1940s, streptomycin was the first all-American antibiotic. It was identified at the University of New Jersey at Rutgers by Professor Selman Waksman, a soil biologist, who deduced that micro-organisms with antimicrobial properties would be found in earth. After a meticulous search with a team funded by the local drug firm, Merck of Rahway, Waksman and his collaborators isolated streptomycin in 1944.

Streptomycin, an aminoglycoside antibiotic, was an immediate sensation because, as well as working against a number of bacteria, it can kill *Mycobacterium tuberculosis*. The fortunes of Merck were founded on streptomycin. In 1948, penicillin and streptomycin alone accounted for more than half of the drug industry's total income from the sale of patented drugs, and in that year of the $191 million export sales for all drugs from the USA, almost half came from antibiotics, mostly streptomycin and penicillin.[35] Now merged as Merck Sharp and Dohme, this American-based multinational was in 1994 the biggest drug firm in the world, with annual sales in 1993 of $8,822,000,000.[25,30]

Tuberculosis was identified as a bacterial infection by the German bacteriologist Robert Koch in 1882. This knowledge created over half a century of paranoia: the invisible germ that causes tuberculosis seemed invincible, even though the rates of suffering and death from the disease steadily decreased during the twentieth century. The first scientist to discover a drug that really worked against tuberculosis could expect the tumultuous acclaim that would now be enjoyed by a scientist who found a successful treatment for AIDS. So it proved: Waksman was awarded a Nobel prize in 1952 for streptomycin, following Fleming, Florey and Chain, who had shared one in 1945 for penicillin. Waksman became rich on the royalties from streptomycin, and a massive Waksman Institute was built at Rutgers.

First impressions are often lasting impressions. The first animal and human trials of streptomycin cleared it as a safe drug, and it was acclaimed as the answer to tuberculosis. Nevertheless, streptomycin and other aminoglycosides turned out to be unusually toxic.

As already mentioned, streptomycin can damage the ear, on rare occasions causing progressive and sometimes permanent deafness and the loss of the sense of balance. Other more common ill-effects include nausea, fever, numbness, kidney damage, and allergic reactions. Moreover, bacteria soon developed shields against aminoglycosides; resistant strains of *Mycobacterium tuberculosis* were first reported as early as 1946.

Because of its toxicity and also because it is now often ineffective, streptomycin is no longer much prescribed in developed countries. Once used to treat a multitude of diseases[36] it is now recommended only as one of a combination of drugs or else as a fall-back option for tuberculosis and a few other serious bacterial infections such as brucellosis and bubonic plague.[10]

In the Third World, however, streptomycin is a popular drug, sold over the counter and in markets as a remedy for colds and coughs, and prescribed for trivial bacterial infections. As reported by Dianna Melrose of Oxfam[37], the Indian doctor Mira Shiva has stated that the use of streptomycin, in combination with penicillin and chloramphenicol,

> for ordinary infections is creating increasing problems for developing countries like ours. Primary resistance of tuberculosis to streptomycin which is one of the first-line drugs is a calamity. We can't afford expensive second-line drugs. Further infection of individuals with resistant tuberculosis mycobacteria helps in making the situation worse.

THE CHLORAMPHENICOL GUSHER

After streptomycin, two further types of antibiotic were first developed in the United States in the late 1940s. First was chloramphenicol in 1947, discovered by scientists at Yale University. The research was funded by Parke-Davis, who still market the drug under the brand name Chloromycetin. Next were the first tetracyclines, developed and still marketed by Lederle and Pfizer with the brand names Aureomycin and Terramycin. All these drugs work against bacteria in similar ways to streptomycin, and can be effective against a great range of bacterial species, including some unaffected by penicillins.

In the late 1940s, American drug firms managed to persuade the US Patents Office that antibiotics, even those that are products of nature, could be patented as authentic inventions. This is why there are now such a vast array of antibiotics on the market: every firm wants to own a slice of the action. With the patent rights on chloramphenicol secured, Parke-Davis had capped a drug gusher. The firm went from nowhere in particular to No. 1 in the US market in 1951, with sales of $52 million in that year from Chloromycetin. Sales steadily increased throughout the decade. Physicians loved chloramphenicol – it worked. It can be effective against a great range of bacteria, including those that are the microbiological cause of whooping cough, diphtheria, gastroenteritis, dysentery, meningitis, gonorrhoea, cholera, anthrax, and infections in the body and blood.

But what the original clinical trials had not picked up is that chloramphenicol has a snag. As well as some of the usual ill-effects of antibiotics, it can sometimes kill people. In 1952, alerted by reports from observant physicians, the US Food and Drug Administration, together with the National Research Council, confirmed that chloramphenicol can have a deadly effect on bone marrow. It is now known that anything between one in 10,000 and one in 40,000 people given the drug, develop a severe irreversible 'aplastic' anaemia, caused by suppression of blood-cell formation in bone marrow.[24] A standard textbook states: 'It can appear during treatment, but it often appears long after treatment has ended. It is not related to the dose of the drug. The prognosis is very poor, with a high percentage of fatalities.'[10]

Chloramphenicol is especially dangerous for babies.[24] In the 1950s, hospital doctors were worried by 'grey baby syndrome': occasionally, premature babies were turning grey, going into shock and dying. At first nobody knew why. Then researchers had an idea. In those days – a time of great enthusiasm for antibiotics – premature babies were commonly given 'prophylactic cover' just in case they fell victim to a hospital infection. Initially, it was assumed that the infants were well protected, the thinking being rather like that of enthusiastic growers who spray seedlings with insecticides to keep off pests. But could it be that the antibiotics were killing the grey babies?

The answer was yes. In 1959, the *New England Journal of Medicine*[38] reported a survey in which a total of 126 premature babies were allotted to four treatment groups. Half were given penicillin and streptomycin or else no drug treatment: less than a fifth died. Half were given chloramphenicol alone or with other antibiotics: more than three-fifths died. The findings of the survey were agreed to be conclusive, and babies were taken off chloramphenicol.

The *British Medical Journal* published an editorial in 1952[38] stating, of chloramphenicol, that 'The only absolute and imperative indication for its use is typhoid fever.' In 1961 another editorial[38] written with reference to the 'grey baby' syndrome cited work questioning whether it is possible to define a safe dose of chloramphenicol, and concluded that deaths from aplastic anaemia caused by the drug had probably been under-recorded.

The patent on chloramphenicol has now run out; any drug firm can market it. The data sheets circulated by the pharmaceutical industry to general practitioners in Britain now include an explicit warning[39]:

> Chloramphenicol is a potent therapeutic agent and should not be used for trivial infections. It should be administered according to the instructions of a medical practitioner. It is recommended that chloramphenicol should be reserved for use in typhoid fever, *Haemophilus influenzae* meningitis, serious chest infections and situations where . . . no other antibiotic would suffice.

So in Europe and North America, chloramphenicol is now not much used. Physicians do still prescribe it from time to time, though, for an ironic reason that applies to all antibiotics. If an antibiotic is cheap and relatively safe, like penicillin, it will be used a lot. The result is that drug-resistant superbugs become epidemic and so the drug is liable to become progressively useless. On the other hand, if an antibiotic is expensive, or relatively hazardous like chloramphenicol, and its dangers are well known to physicians with access to safer alternatives, it will be used only occasionally. The result is that bacteria are less likely to develop resistance to this drug, and so it is most likely to work against infection. Antibiotic chemotherapy obeys a version of Sod's Law: as time goes by, safe drugs don't work, and the drugs that do work may well be dangerous. Sometimes the drug that is most likely to damage you is most likely to damage bugs.

By contrast with Western countries, chloramphenicol is still a common drug in the Third World, where typhoid is endemic, and it is marketed by many manufacturers, foreign and local. Dianna Melrose reported that in 1981 she was offered the drug in Yemen for uncomplicated diarrhoea. A World Health Organisation worker in Ethiopia noted in 1977 that a hundred people attending one health station got through 5000 capsules and vials of tetracycline, streptomycin and penicillin, and 2000 capsules of chloramphenicol, in three months. A VSO worker in Nepal, also quoted by Dianna Melrose, reported in 1979 that it was commonplace to see people buying capsules of tetracycline and chloramphenicol for children with fever or diarrhoea. In the 1990s chloramphenicol remained a common drug in Africa and Asia.

The consequences have been disastrous. The shigella and *Salmonella typhi* bacilli that are the microbiological causes of dysentery and typhoid have developed superbug versions resistant to chloramphenicol and other antibiotics all over the world. Dysentery, a major worldwide epidemic killer in the nineteenth century, faded and had become uncommon by the 1920s, but starting in the 1960s, explosive outbreaks caused by drug-resistant superbugs have killed tens of thousands of people in Central America, Asia and Africa. In 1988, the World Health Organisation reported in its *Guidelines for the control of epidemics due to Shigella dysenteriae*[40]: 'As resistance to sulfonamides, streptomycin, tetracyclines and chloramphenicol is common, these drugs should never be used until strains have been demonstrated to be susceptible to them.' In developing countries, dysentery is now often close to untreatable with any available antibiotics.

TETRACYCLINES: THE MAGIC BOMB

Throughout the 1940s, research scientists in America and Europe searched for the superdrug: an antibiotic active against the greatest number of bacterial species. Imagine! A drug that kills all known germs, dead! The quest for the ultimate germicide was initially rewarded with chlortetracycline, isolated in the USA like streptomycin and chloramphenicol from soil samples. The successful team who struck the drug equivalent of oil this time was led by Professor Benjamin Duggar, working for Lederle. Chlortetracycline, first marketed in 1948, and then later tetracyclines, proved to be the broadest spectrum antibiotics yet identified and accepted by regulators as safe in use.

From the start, physicians loved tetracycline, using it not so much as a magic bullet as a magic bomb. Marketed as the most powerful and effective antibiotics, which indeed they can be as treatment of many bacterial infections, tetracyclines are now second in world sales only to penicillins. They remain commonly prescribed for ear, nose and throat, gut, urinary tract and sexually transmitted bacterial infections, and also for acne. The 5000 tons of tetracyclines manufactured worldwide in 1990, for use as human medicine and also for use on animals and on plants, is expected to double to 10,000 tons by the year 2000.[34] In the UK over 20 branded tetracyclines as well as generic versions are on the market.

In his remarkable book *The Prize*,[41] Daniel Yergin argues that more than any other resource, oil has, for better or worse, shaped the modern world and our place in it. A similar claim can be made for antibiotics. Certainly, the vision of the American industrialists responsible for the commercial exploitation of antibiotics in the 'golden years' beginning in the late 1940s, was as focused as that of the oilmen of the previous century.

Antibiotics are treasure that is consumed. Like other treasure such as gold and art, the value of drugs is maximised by control of supply. Like other consumer goods such as cars and computers, the value of drugs is sustained by obsolescence. In the case of drugs, ownership and control involves patenting and branding, and obsolescence enables the development of successive new patented branded products. The pioneers of the modern pharmaceutical industry believed with reason that this could be the realisation of their dreams, the secret of their success.

In 1948 Cyanamid/Lederle owned chlortetracycline, branded as Aureomycin (which is still on the market). In 1949 Pfizer developed a new tetracycline, oxytetracycline, owned and branded as Terramycin (also still on the market).

From the start, Pfizer marketed Terramycin with phenomenal energy.

In 1935 the firm's total sales had been $5 million. By 1953 it was the market leader in the UK. In 1957 its total sales were $200 million, with profits of $23,900,000, almost all from broad-spectrum antibiotics.[42] In 1990 Pfizer was the twelfth biggest pharmaceutical company in the world, with annual sales of over $3.5 billion.[30] The fortunes of Cyanamid/Lederle similarly depended on tetracycline: in the early 1950s their profits were entirely from broad-spectrum antibiotics, whose sales between 1954 and 1961 totalled over $300 million.[42]

The tetracycline story became more complex and dramatic in the 1950s. The race was on to develop new versions of tetracycline that could be protected by patent.

In 1952 scientists working for Pfizer isolated tetracycline itself by removing the chlorine atom from chlortetracycline, and applied for this new formulation to be patented. In 1953 Cyanamid and two other companies, Heyden and Bristol, also claimed patent rights on tetracycline. Industry had reason to fear that the US Patent Office would insist that tetracycline was unpatentable, on the grounds that it was not sufficiently different from chlortetracycline, in which case the profits of the initial market leaders would be liable to collapse. In the event, the Patent Office upheld industry's ownership of tetracycline.

As long as tetracycline in its various forms was protected by patent its branded versions were immensely profitable. However, in 1961 the UK business was disturbed by a new company, DDSA Pharmaceuticals, who marketed what was in effect a generic version of the drug with the apt name Econamycin, at a tenth of the price charged to the National Health Service by companies owning other branded versions.

Enoch Powell, then UK Minister of Health, gave DDSA a contract to supply hospitals. Pfizer challenged the UK government; the case eventually went to the House of Lords, then the ultimate court of appeal in the UK, where in an extraordinary decision the government's right to override a drug patent in the national interest was upheld.

In the early 1970s the patents on tetracyclines expired; they are now cheap drugs, in branded as well as generic versions.

Unfortunately though, like other early antibiotics, tetracyclines have turned out to be troublesome drugs. Apart from their ill-effects on teeth and bones, which make them inappropriate for pregnant women and children, they can affect kidney function, as well as causing nausea, diarrhoea and allergic reactions in common with many types of antibiotic. Other ill-effects include sore tongue, difficulty in swallowing, sore anus, and green/yellow faeces.[24] The immediate toxicity of tetracyclines is less problematic than their longer-term ill-effects. Because they are so very broad spectrum and penetrative, they can devastate gut flora, and superinfections with invasive bacteria or fungi such as *Candida albicans*, are common consequences of tetracycline treatment.

While tetracyclines check or kill bacteria in much the same way as aminoglycocides like streptomycin or chloramphenicol, the mechanism by which bacteria develop resistance to tetracyclines is different. 'It's like a bilge pump,' Professor O'Brien explained to me. 'The bacteria develop this marvellous ability: the bacterium expels the drug right out of the cell again.' What this means is that, when bacteria become resistant to tetracyclines, the drug is not absorbed and degraded, but is ejected into the outside environment.

Because of their ill-effects, tetracyclines are now not so often used in many European countries and in North America. However, they are massively used by farmers, to prevent and treat bacterial infection in intensively reared animals, and also as growth promoters. They are also used in horticulture. In addition, and in common with all potent antibiotics that are out of patent and therefore cheap, tetracyclines are used in massive amounts throughout the developing world. Thus, every year, an unknown fraction of some thousands of tons of tetracycline is being pumped out of humans and animals into the environment, in biologically active form. What effect this is having on us and the planet is also unknown.

THE GOLDEN AGE FADES

After tetracycline, other antibiotics, mentioned briefly earlier in this book, were identified and marketed. Erythromycin, in the macrolide group, remains a valuable drug. The relative toxicity and high cost of vancomycin has given it a clinical advantage: it still works against the *Staphylococcus aureus* superbug. Hospital doctors in Europe and North America usually now hold some antibiotics in reserve, specifically for use against dangerous superbugs, which is lucky for hospital patients in rich countries.

The lincosamides, including clindamycin and lincomycin, gained a bad reputation after the discovery that they can (rarely) cause potentially deadly pseudomembranous colitis which in rare cases kills people, but other antibiotics can also cause this vicious infection.[25]

And in the late 1950s the first antifungal, nystatin, was marketed.[9]

QUINOLONES: GENE GENIES

With one exception, since the 1960s no new group of antibiotics has been marketed. As the patents on older products have expired, much of the commercial thrill of the golden age, when antibiotics dominated drug sales, has gone. Now, the top-selling drugs are for non-infectious diseases. But antibiotics still have a big share of the world drug market: 11 percent of all drug sales in 1980, projected to rise to 15 percent in the year 2000 as the vast new markets in the developing world are thoroughly penetrated.[34]

Quinolones are the one new family of antibiotics. These synthetic drugs include nalidixic acid, ciprofloxacin and norfloxacin. In the 1980s and 1990s they have been and are vigorously promoted for use against a great variety of bacterial infections. Quinolones work by wrecking the integrity of the bacterial chromosome. Scientists are generally confident that, while quinolones attack the DNA of bacteria, they have no effect on human DNA. If they did, the consequences would be extremely serious, because damage to DNA, the building blocks of life, in one generation will cause deformities in the next. So far, though, the argument that quinolones may be mutagenic is only theoretical.

The main agreed use of quinolones is for urinary tract infections. But industry has argued for them to be used for other common 'indications' (which is to say diseases). Interviewed in Bristol for this book, microbiologist Professor David Reeves, chairman of the working party on antibiotic use of the British Society for Antimicrobial Chemotherapy, said that industry 'has pushed quinolones very hard'. He explained that, 'with any new drug, the companies want to realise the return on their investment in the shortest possible time. So they will go for the widest range of indications.' In his opinion, 'Many quinolones are marginal antibiotics for treating respiratory infections. Yet the drug companies were keen to get respiratory infections as an indication, because if they were confined to urinary tract infections, you would be looking at a far smaller market.'

Accepted uses for quinolones now include, as well as urinary and respiratory tract infections, those of the skin, soft tissue, bones, joints, gut, eyes, ears, nose and throat, and gonorrhoea. A recent indication being argued for is travellers' diarrhoea.

Industry and many scientists were at first very enthusiastic about the safety of using quinolones, but as so often happens with drugs, in time reports of ill-effects on patients have accumulated. While quinolones seem not to be particularly toxic, they do have a number of occasional ill-effects, including nausea, diarrhoea, stomach pain, skin reactions, headache, disorientation, visual disturbances, hallucinations, fits and, rarely, psychosis.[10,43]

Methods now used to regulate and monitor the safety of drugs cannot be perfect. In 1991 a new quinolone, temafloxacin, was licensed for use in the UK, and around 20,000 prescriptions were issued for its branded version, Teflox, between October 1991 and June 1992.[44] In September 1991, the journal *Hospital Doctor*[45] had reported that: 'A tough new generation of quinolone antimicrobials is about to emerge in the UK . . . Much hope is being pinned on the first of the arrivals, temafloxacin, already licensed elsewhere in Europe.' Indications for use included urinary and respiratory tract infections (including pneumonia) and drug-resistant hospital bugs.

Then, on 6 June 1992, Dr Christina Carnegie, medical director of Abbott Laboratories, wrote to all physicians in the UK stating that Teflox had been withdrawn worldwide 'as a result of reported serious adverse reactions'.[46] These included blood disorders, liver and kidney problems, anaphylactic shock, and death. 'Although the reports of these serious adverse events are rare,' wrote Dr Carnegie, 'you should discontinue treatment in any patient currently receiving temafloxacin and replace it with an alternative therapy.' So happily, this unusually toxic quinolone is now off the market.

The main worries about quinolones are not, however, concerned with their toxicity. Could they conceivably be mutagenic in humans? It seems utterly unlikely; but as Professor Richard Lacey puts it[47], 'the question of mutagenicity is not resolved.' Conservative microbiologists such as Dr Lacey feel some unease about any drug that works by interfering with bacterial DNA, particularly when, as with quinolones, the drug is synthetic, with no analogy in nature. Although it is accepted by virtually all microbiologists that damage to bacterial DNA has no bearing on the integrity of human or any other eukaryotic cell structures, nature is still capable of nasty surprises.

Second, quinolones are similar to tetracyclines in two respects. First, the drug is not fully absorbed; some is excreted unchanged into the environment. Second, bacteria evolve resistance to quinolones by means of the 'bilge-pump' mechanism that expels or 'spits out' the drug. So what happens to the quinolones? Dr Tore Midtvedt is worried about this question. Writing in *Lancet* in 1989[48] he said:

> More than ten million patients [have already] received ciprofloxacin, just one quinolone. Some of these drugs are used in veterinary medicine and in fish farming. The worldwide production of quinolones is not available but it seems reasonable to suppose that it runs into several thousands of kilograms.
>
> It is astonishing that so little is known about their fate . . . If not broken down, quinolones must end up somewhere, but I know of no studies of their ultimate fate. I am surprised that drug registration authorities have allowed introduction of such potent drugs . . . without asking this question. The potential hazardous biological effects of quinolones should not be underestimated.

Talking to Dr Midtvedt in his laboratory at the Karolinska Institute in Stockholm, I asked him to elaborate. 'We now have drugs that are not broken down by any microbial enzymes – I'm talking about the quinolones,' he told me. The coastal fish farms in his native Norway are the most extensive in the world, and by the time of my visit in 1992, he had established that between 10,000 and 20,000 kilograms (11–22 tons) of quinolones had already been used to prevent or treat the infectious diseases inevitable when fish or any other creatures (humans included) are grossly overcrowded. 'In all environments in which it has been investigated, the quinolones will stay active in the water, just below the surface, for months and for years,' he told me. 'They will stay partly inside the wreck of the microbes they have inactivated and partly outside.' With what effect on marine life? And on human health? He couldn't say.

Dr Midtvedt was equally concerned about the use of quinolones to prevent and treat travellers' diarrhoea. Although quinolones work against diarrhoea, prophylactically and therapeutically, as already stated, taking any kind of antibiotic for simple diarrhoea is usually a bad idea: the condition, while often intensely unpleasant, is best left to resolve itself, or if severe, treated by rehydration. And the after-effects of antibiotics, quinolones especially, could be troublesome.

'Now, about a hundred million people travel north to south every year,' said Dr Midtvedt. In many countries, quinolones are available without prescription. 'All those people going north to south will produce quite a lot of faeces down there, and they are not bringing their faeces back with them. And in the faeces you will have a substantial amount of quinolones. And the development of resistance will start in the south. And it has started. There are now many reports of resistance to some quinolone anti-diarrhoeal agents in those countries. Because the mechanism of resistance to quinolones is efflux – spitting out the active drug, like tetracycline – the drug will go from one microbial species to others.' The result is that quinolones are becoming ineffective against serious bacterial diseases. How many people in the African and Asian countries visited by those tourists who were anxious to settle their stomachs will suffer from infections made drug-resistant by quinolones imported into their environment? There is no way of knowing.

Like other antibiotics before them, quinolones may cause superinfections, in which normally friendly or harmless bacteria become dangerous by spreading into parts of the body where they normally have no place. A short report to this effect, from the Public Health Laboratory Service in Portsmouth, appeared in the *Lancet* in April 1992.[49] Lactobacilli, normally friendly flora that live in profusion in and around the vagina, and which protect women against invasion by potentially dangerous bacteria, were turning up in the blood of severely ill hospital patients. Because quinolones are regarded as unusually safe drugs, they are now often used extensively on hospital patients. They have a very broad spectrum, and wipe out many friendly and harmless bacterial species – but not lactobacilli, which happen to be invulnerable to quinolones. So, in the opinion of Dr Rosalind Maskell, consultant at St Mary's Hospital, Portsmouth, and an authority on urinary tract infections: 'The nearly uniform resistance to the quinolones suggests that the lactobacilli in the commensal [friendly or harmless] flora of patients treated with these agents, to which most other commensal species are sensitive, may multiply and assume a pathogenic role.' In other words, quinolones can turn women's most intimately friendly flora into enemies.

Dr Midtvedt regularly contributes the chapters on antibiotics to the annual *Side Effects of Drugs* edited by Professor Graham Dukes, lately of the World Health Organisation European region office in Copenhagen (who kindly wrote the Preface to this book).[50] I asked him this question: 'As now used, do antibiotics do more harm than good?' He thought for a while, and then said: 'If you are taking the whole consumption – humans, animals, fish farming and so on – they are doing more harm than good.' I asked him when he himself used antibiotics. 'I have used them seldom: I have good health,' he said. 'Once in my lifetime I had a urinary tract infection. I took antibiotics for three days. I took the cheapest and the most narrow-spectrum one. It worked.' And for the future? 'The way we are using antibiotics, we are increasing our problems. We must reduce total consumption, and we must reduce the drugs that most promote resistance. And we have to find other treatments for infectious diseases.'

DOSING EVERYBODY ON THE PLANET

From industry's point of view, antibiotics are not now the most promising class of drug. But the market for antibacterial drugs continues to expand worldwide. The annual market value for antibiotics for human and also for animal use worldwide, was estimated by an expert group convened in 1984 by the US National Institutes of Health at US$8,250 million in 1980 and US$18,000 million in 1990, with a projected figure of US$40,500 million in the year 2000.[51]

Annual production of antibiotics for human use worldwide has been estimated at around 25,000 tons in 1980 and 35,000 tons in 1990, with a projected figure of 50,000 tons in the year 2000.[52]

The amount of drug in different courses of antibiotics varies. But given a rough average of seven grams for an average seven-day course, 35,000 tons a year works out at five billion courses of antibiotics every year: enough for one course every year for everybody on earth in the year 1990. Indeed, it was stated in 1982 of penicillin alone that: 'Today there is sufficient fermentation and production capacity worldwide to provide every individual on this planet with sufficient penicillin for one therapeutic treatment each year.'[53]

People living in developed countries may have the impression that doctors are more cautious in their use of antibiotics nowadays. In general though, the trend is upwards. In England, the total number of prescriptions issued by general practitioners for antibiotics in 1980 was just over 43 million, which averages out at just under a course per person per year. Eleven years later the figure had increased remarkably, to just under 70 million, or close to one and a half courses per person per year.[54]

At this rate, and given a 75 year lifespan, everybody in the UK will on average be taking antibiotics for around 750 days or over two years, during their lives. And this excludes antibiotics prescribed in hospital and by dentists, and any purchased over the counter in other countries.

These remarkable statistics of production and consumption would be testimony of unqualified benefit to humanity, if antibiotics were harmless, or at least almost always appropriately prescribed. But they are not.

7 The Infection Business

WHO SAYS DRUGS ARE SAFE?

Everybody wants drugs to be as safe as possible. Nobody wants drugs to injure or kill people. The trouble is, sometimes they do. Industry is proud of its reputation as a health-giver and a life-saver; and its executives have families, are themselves liable to fall ill and be prescribed drugs, and want their products to be safe and to work. However, sometimes drugs turn out to be dangerous or deadly only after they have been put on the market.

With drugs, the only way to protect the public interest is by means of an independent regulatory agency, responsible for licensing drugs and judging their safety in use. In the USA, the Food and Drug Administration does this job. The FDA, a branch of the US Department of Health and Human Services, is the nation's oldest federal consumer protection agency. Set up soon after the US Pure Food and Drug Acts were passed in 1906, the FDA is now a vast organisation, with an annual budget of well over $500 million and a staff of 8000. In 1991, the new FDA commissioner, Dr David Kessler, announced his intention to hire an additional 100 investigators to enforce the US food and drug laws.[55] Standards set by the FDA formally apply only in the USA, but they do influence the judgement of governments round the world.

The British system of drug regulation is different. The Department of Health has a joint responsibility both to the consumers and to the producers of drugs. The Department is the official 'sponsor' of industry, and reconciles this responsibility as best it can with that of looking after the interests of patients. It is officially advised by the Committee on Safety of Medicines (CSM), a body of 21 people, a majority of whom have some connections with the drug industry.[56] Are industry consultancies against the public interest? Questioned by the Yorkshire TV programme *First Tuesday* in November 1990, a

Department of Health spokesman said that consultancies help to keep CSM members 'abreast of the new developments'. As quoted in the *Guardian* in June 1990, a member of the CSM explained that almost all pharmacologists are bound to be associated with industry: 'If you take the holier-than-thou approach, there would be no one to sit on the Committee. Our job as pharmacologists is to research drugs. Who makes drugs? The drug companies.'[56]

The CSM is enjoined to follow the European Community directive that states of any drug that 'Therapeutic advantage should outweigh clinical risk' – which means that drugs should do more good than harm to the individual patient. How is this assessment made? A CSM member explained, to the *Guardian*:

> In the population there will be groups who will benefit, groups who will have some side-effects, and some who will suffer. We try to eliminate the group who will suffer from receiving the drug, but there's no scientific formula of risk to benefit.

The same is true for the doctor in the community. A general practitioner should not give you a drug for a trivial problem unless that drug is believed to be relatively safe. On the other hand, if you have a condition that a doctor believes is serious, you may be given a drug that is also dangerous, but which is judged to be less dangerous than the condition itself (like the example of typhoid and chloramphenicol given earlier). It's a matter of human judgement, and sometimes doctors will make the wrong choice. Those who are well informed, by their patients as well as by the literature, will make more reliable judgements.

The Committee on Safety of Medicines is a fairly new creation. Until the 1960s, the drug industry in the UK was more or less trusted to regulate itself. Then came the thalidomide catastrophe, as a result of which the 1968 Medicines Act gave government formal responsibility for the licensing and regulation of drugs.

All the research and development on a drug, and its testing on animals, human volunteers and hospital patients, is funded and organised by industry. The total cost of developing and marketing a new drug can, in the 1990s, be anything up to £150 million.[57] Matching or even monitoring the toxicity testing carried out by industry is thought not to be a sensible use of public money. The industry safety data – which, in 1988, averaged 170 books of research for each drug submitted for licensing – are assessed by the scientists who work part-time for the CSM, and the decision whether or not to license a drug is taken on their advice.

To protect their interests, pharmaceutical companies take out patents on new formulae as soon as they think they may be on to a winner, even before the process of toxicity testing begins. Drug patents generally expire after twenty years; but what with research and development, testing and the time taken for drugs to be approved, a new product may be on the market for only a dozen years or so before the patent runs out and other companies may compete and drive its price down. So scientists working for industry are naturally under intense pressure to complete toxicity testing as fast as is practicably possible.

The Community's Pharmaceutical Industry, a report prepared for the European Commission in 1985[58], stated that 'British policy makers are very aware that the UK industry is highly competitive and that it has improved its international standing during the past decade.' The report pointed out that, while the Department of Health has an interest in the safety of drugs, the Department of Trade and Industry sees British drugs as a high-technology growth sector and a major source of foreign earnings, and the Department of Employment sees them as a source of jobs.

Drugs are the UK's outstanding industrial success story. In January 1995 the UK-based Glaxo announced its takeover bid for Wellcome, set to make Glaxo by far the biggest pharmaceutical firm in the world, with annual sales of well over $10 billion a year.[59] Drugs are very big British business. In 1989 the drug approval process in the UK was speeded up. The Department of Health Medicines Division was hived off, to become the Medicines Control Agency (MCA), a free-standing public body. This change was good for business: the time taken for initial approval of drugs was dramatically speeded up, from five-to-six years to as little as 75 days. The MCA is wholly funded by licence fees paid by industry, and its policy is to attract more business as the main centre for drugs approval within the European Union, whose drug laws are now subject to harmonisation.

This new initiative may not be in the public interest. According to *The Economist* in April 1991[60]:

> The MCA now vets new drugs faster than almost any other drug agency in the world . . . Because it works so fast, and yet still provides a powerful endorsement for a drug, pharmaceutical companies are

> submitting their products to it for approval before approaching other European or American agencies. In contrast, America's Food and Drug Administration often does not approve a drug until after it has first been accepted in another large market.

The Economist continues:

> But the MCA's success could backfire. The British may not like becoming guinea-pigs for new drugs. And according to *Scrip*, a London-based trade magazine, other European regulators are uneasy about the MCA's unabashed commercialism. The agency, they growl, is behaving more like an advertising agency touting for clients than a government guardian of good health.

The Economist report was also concerned about the closeness to industry of the drug regulators in Britain: 'The danger of too much cosiness is the greater because in Britain, unlike other countries, the information that passes between the drug industry and its regulators is confidential.' In the US, hearings on drug safety are held in public; whereas in the UK, section 118 of the Medicines Act makes breaches of confidentiality a criminal offence, subject to a maximum term of two years in prison.

SHOWING THE YELLOW CARD

Once a drug is in use in the UK, the CSM relies on doctors to give warnings of ill-effects, through what is known as the 'yellow card' system. Printed on yellow paper and headed 'IN CONFIDENCE ... REPORT ON SUSPECTED ADVERSE DRUG REACTION', these slips are distributed to doctors, who are asked to fill them in and send them to the CSM, who may by this means be informed of any drugs evidently causing a lot of ill-effects. A recent count showed that less than 20,000 slips are sent in every year: an average of less than one per general practitioner. Four in five general practitioners in the UK never send in yellow cards.

Professor Bill Inman, director of the Drug Safety Research Unit at the University of Southampton, is sceptical about the yellow card system.[61] Most doctors don't use it, for a variety of reasons. As he sees it:

> They fear litigation and ridicule if a subsequent investigation suggests that the adverse reaction was caused because they prescribed an inappropriate drug. Other GPs complacently believe that the authorities already know about any problem they may have spotted, or they doubt their own ability to distinguish between a true reaction to a drug and an unconnected event.

The £180 million a year that industry spent on promoting its products in the UK by the end of the 1980s amounted to around £7500 for each of the 24,000 physicians in the country. As required by the Medicines Act, some industry money is spent on the distribution of data on their drugs to doctors by the trade's representative body, the Association of the British Pharmaceutical Industry. The *ABPI Data Sheets* are detailed, and have been used as a resource for this book. However, information supplied by industry tends to be rather less explicit about the dangers of drugs than that to be found in independent publications.

Another *Economist* report, in January 1990[62], stated that, in 1988, the drug industry spent 80 times more keeping British doctors informed than did the Department of Health. The report went on to say that 'The 1980s have shown the rewards of good marketing and sales muscle.' Averaged out, the turnover of industry divides roughly equally between research and development (23 percent), manufacture (25 percent), marketing (24 percent) and profits (an awesome 28 percent). Investment in marketing pays off. According to *The Economist*:

> A recent survey conducted by Dr Justin Greenwood of Teeside Polytechnic among British physicians found that six out of ten decide to prescribe a product solely on the basis of what a drug salesman has told them.

PUSHING THE PRODUCT

Physicians and microbiologists sometimes say that industry pushes the medical profession too hard, with the result that drugs – antibiotics included – are overused and abused by any standards. Professor Stuart Levy of the Departments of Medicine and Microbiology at Tufts University, interviewed for this book in Boston, said: 'Once antibiotics have come to market, the company has invested millions of dollars in research. They want and need to get their profits and they want to get them as quickly as possible. So they will push the drugs: and the drugs will be overused.'

Interviewed for this book in Chicago, Professor Marc Lappé said: 'A physician's clinical judgement cannot be questioned. And drug companies tune in. If I want to market an exotic, expensive antibiotic – say, a latest generation cephalosporin – do I want it kept in a hospital safe as a drug of final resort? No. I want it used up. I want to sell as much of it as I can. The drug salesman will come around to the physician with little buttons and pins and pens and briefcases and stethoscopes with the drug company's name and brand on them. Crystal paperweights, notepads, doctors' kits, all with the name of the new antibiotic on it.' He smiled ruefully. 'And then you expect physicians not to prescribe it?'

Professor Richard Lacey believes that government as well as industry is responsible for promoting drugs in ways that are good for business but bad for public health. Also interviewed for this book in Leeds, he said, 'Today's technology makes it easy to manipulate molecules, creating an almost endless array of chemicals that are really much the same, but different enough to be patented. The development and introduction of new drugs is largely determined by market forces, such as the expiry of patents, identification of new "growth areas" such as surgical prophylaxis and, above all, the ability to "defend" the new product with patents.'

Regulatory authorities are mainly concerned with safety, and not whether the drug is less toxic or more effective than drugs already on the market, or whether there is any real need for the new drug. So the market becomes flooded with what are known as 'me-too' drugs, virtual copies of each other. With drugs, the profit is in the patented product; industry is much less interested in products whose patents have expired. Companies push hard to introduce new drugs, in order to make more profit.

The system works like this. Suppose a company – let's call it Omnicure – owns the patent on the (fictitious) antibiotic Whizzomycin, the patent for which is about to expire. When patents expire, other companies can market the drug, and so the price will go down. Omni want to maintain a patented drug, so its scientists manipulate the molecules of Whizzomycin just enough to create a 'new' antibiotic – let's call it Bugbiffen. And if, according to the testing carried out by Omni, Bugbiffen is evidently sufficiently safe, the Committee on Safety of Medicines is bound to approve it.

So now there are two antibiotics on the market where there was one: Whizzomycin, which Omni is losing interest in, and Bugbiffen, the potentially very profitable drug, promoted with fanfare. The result? Some doctors stick with Whizzomycin. Others are impressed by the promotional *ta-rah* for Bugbiffen, and so they give it a whirl. Thus, both drugs are used, and more likely than not, the total sales of both drugs are greater than they had been for Whizzomycin alone. This encourages Omni – and the rest of industry – to manipulate more molecules. Professor Lacey comments: 'While this approach is successful in maintaining profits, including exports, it has resulted in antibiotic chemotherapy becoming unacceptably complex.'

CALLING THE SHOTS

The patenting and pricing of drugs is a hot political issue throughout the world. In the mid-1980s, the British Conservative government once again tried to cut the costs of drugs to the National Health Service, and thus the taxpayer, partly by encouraging physicians to prescribe cheaper generic drugs, partly by trying to limit the list of drugs approved for prescription. This initiative was successfully opposed by the pharmaceutical industry and by the medical profession, both of whom claimed that the interests of the patient are best protected when physicians are free to prescribe any drug. In truth, though, the interests are not so much of the patient as of the patent.

Industry controls or influences every decision taken about antibiotics, from the moment research is started on a new formula, to the moment you take the drug, and beyond. The decision to research a new antibiotic is taken by industry. The animal and human trials on which the judgements of regulatory bodies are based are funded by industry and carried out by scientists employed or hired by industry. Once a drug is licensed, it is heavily promoted by industry and advertised in journals that are either published by or heavily dependent on advertisements from industry. Conferences to launch new drugs are funded by industry, and most of the information about antibiotics, on which physicians base their clinical judgements, comes from industry salespeople, marketing and advertising.

So does the pharmaceutical industry control the medical profession?

If the question means, do drug industry executives give instructions to doctors, the answer is, of course, no; formally, the stance of industry is fairly deferential. Its influence is rather more subtle. Asking if industry controls the medical profession is a little like asking if the United States controls the United Nations. On the one hand, the great majority of doctors in the field, not only in Europe and North America, but throughout the world, are trying to do an effective job. On the other, industry does have strategic goals for marketing its products, and is remarkably successful in achieving these goals.

If all goes well, antibiotics work with no ill-effects. But if you are unlucky, here's how you can get caught on the antibiotic treadmill. You have an infection and go to the doctor, who prescribes an antibiotic. Probably it works; at least, the symptoms subside. You are pleased, the doctor is pleased. But the antibiotic causes the breeding of superinfectious bacteria; so you go back to the doctor with another infection, and are prescribed another antibiotic. It, too, evidently works. You are pleased, the doctor is pleased. Meanwhile, micro-organisms on and in you develop resistance to the antibiotics you have been given; they grow, spread and cause more infection. Back you go to the doctor, who prescribes another antibiotic, perhaps an anti-fungal agent. This time perhaps the disease is more obstinate, so you are given broader-spectrum drugs.

By now, some or much of your normal healthy gut flora have been destroyed; and when disease-carrying bacteria (or viruses) drift in from the outside world, you suffer another infection. Back again to the doctor. This time, nothing works. The doctor is stuck. At this point, you may get the impression that you have become a nuisance. But then maybe a new antibiotic comes on the market, licensed to kill your infections. The doctor is impressed by the advertisements for this new weapon in the never-ending war against infection. It works. You are pleased, the doctor is pleased – until your next infection. This process may continue until you become allergic to many antibiotics and your gut flora become generally drug-resistant.

It is reasonable to suppose that industry is aware of this phenomenon. The agrichemical industry says it manufactures biocides for the benefit of the farmer. This is true; and at the same time, the agrichemical industry is in the pest business. Likewise, the pharmaceutical industry says it manufactures antibiotics for the benefit of the patient. This is also true; and at the same time, the pharmaceutical industry is in the disease business.

If antibiotics really were magic bullets, bacterial disease would now be extinct. As it is, the disease business is booming: in the United States, people now pay more for medicine than they spend on either food or housing.[61] Industry and science constantly proclaim that there are always new diseases to conquer, and so there are. But where are these diseases coming from? And what really causes them?

Of course antibiotics are not developed, marketed and prescribed with any intention of causing illness. But good intentions can have bad effects. Take Brazilian cattle ranchers. They have a bad name, but their intention is to rear cattle. That is why they cut down the rain forests; it is not their purpose to disturb the world's climate. Besides, how can any one rancher have such an effect? Likewise, the intention of the pharmaceutical industry and the medical profession is to develop, market and prescribe antibiotics to treat infections. The physician's attention is on the recovery of the patient, just as the rancher's attention is on the growth of the cattle. They mean no harm. They may not perceive the eventual effect of their actions. Besides, would you stop a doctor giving an antibiotic to a child with a potentially deadly infection?

SUMMARY OF PART 2

Antibiotics founded the fortunes of the modern pharmaceutical industry and the reputation of the modern medical profession. Before the antibiotic age, drug companies were small business. During the 'golden age' after World War II, new antibiotics, protected by patent, were industry's equivalent of oil: endless demand, vast profits. The enthusiastic commercial development of antibiotics transformed industry into what now are transnational giants, with individual companies turning over more money a year than some small countries. For industry, antibiotics are dream drugs: the more they are used, the more bacteria develop resistance. So industry patents and markets ever-more expensive products, which in turn become obsolescent . . . and the drug treadmill turns ever faster.

Part Three

Bug Wars:
How Bacteria Protect Health

SIR RALPH BLOOMFIELD BONINGTON: If you're not well, you have a disease. It may be a slight one: but it's a disease. And what is a disease? The lodgement in the system of a pathogenic germ, and the multiplication of that germ. What is the remedy? A very simple one. Find the germ and kill it.
SIR PATRICK CULLEN: Suppose there's no germ?
SIR RALPH BLOOMFIELD BONINGTON: Impossible, Sir Patrick, there must be a germ; else how could the patient be ill?

Bernard Shaw
The Doctor's Dilemma; 1906

The germ theory of disease developed during the gory phase of Darwinism, when the interplay between living things was regarded as a struggle for survival . . . This attitude moulded from the beginning the pattern of all the attempts at the control of microbial disease. It led to a kind of aggressive war against the microbes, aimed at their elimination from the sick individual and from the community. No place here for the biological concepts now prevailing in other fields of natural history . . . The view that some sort of biological equilibrium can be achieved between the microbes and their potential victims has not been popular among physicians and medical scientists.

Professor René Dubos
Mirage of Health; 1960

8 The Germ Theory of Disease

ZAPPING THE BUGS

We hate bugs. Advertisements on television remind us that the little blighters still lurk in sinks and toilets, but, in one memorable phrase, 'Domestos kills all known germs. Dead!' And we have come to believe that doctors have the same power over disease-causing bacteria as we have over household germs. *Zap!*

In his essay on 'Germs', Professor Lewis Thomas, a wise observer of medical science, writes[1]:

> We are instructed to spray disinfectants everywhere, into the air of our bedrooms and kitchens and with special energy into bathrooms, since it is our very own germs that seem the worst kind. We explode clouds of aerosol, mixed for good luck with deodorants, into our noses, mouths, underarms, privileged crannies – even into the intimate insides of our telephones . . . We live in a world where the microbes are always trying to get at us, to tear us cell from cell, and we only stay alive through diligence and fear. Watching television, you'd think we lived at bay, in total jeopardy, surrounded on all sides by human-seeking germs, shielded against infection and death only by a chemical technology that enables us to keep killing them off.

This is so, isn't it? We accept the idea that we are encircled by disease that is 'out there', and without a second thought, we equip our lavatories with Harpic, our bathrooms with Zamo, our kitchens with Vim, our medicine cabinet with Dettol and other disinfectants whose mission to annihilate bugs is advertised on television with images of elemental power.

Having exterminated the bugs in the sinks and drains of our homes with cheap, pungent chemicals, we then devastate bugs in our own nooks and crannies with expensive, perfumed chemicals. When these small-arms attacks on bacteria fail, and we suffer infectious disease, we go to the doctor for the magic bomb – antibiotics.

It is, of course, sensible to guard against disease, if no harm comes from the precaution. What is striking, though, is just how aggressive we are with bacteria and, in contrast, just how uninterested we seem to be in the reasons why bacteria may become infectious. Indeed, we evidently assume that all bacteria are out to get us. Besides, prevention requires some forethought; treatment does not.

In Britain, one remarkable recent example of the way in which the war on bugs is waged has been the decision by government to allow industry to blast food – which may be contaminated by *Salmonella enteritidis* or *Listeria monocytogenes* – with gamma irradiation. These two bacterial species are the microbiological cause of the food-borne infections that hit the national headlines in 1989. Gamma irradiation does not, as some fear, make food radioactive, but it does destroy some of the nourishment in food, and is liable to be used by reckless 'cowboys' in the food industry to reduce the 'bug-count' of contaminated food. It also does not address the fundamental issue, which is that salmonella and listeria infection is bred by the factory-farming of animals, and by unsafe methods of pre-preparing processed food.[2] But just as doctors use the magic antibiotic bomb on us, industry can now use the magic atom bomb on our food.

The military metaphor of the 'magic bullet' remains a touchstone for Western medicine. From their first days in medical school, doctors are encouraged to think of themselves as warriors in a war against disease, and the tight discipline and rigid hierarchy that hospital doctors endure is modelled on army lines. Like generals in the field, the medical élite such as consultant surgeons do not expect their life-and-death decisions to be questioned. Many women are repelled by this military culture, and few top physicians or surgeons are women.

It isn't only doctors who are trained to think of modern medicine as a form of war. We are all indoctrinated in this way. Here, for example, is the text of an advertisement for the Imperial Cancer Research Fund, the leading British charity, which was published in national newspapers in 1988. Its headline read: 'NOW WE'VE DEVELOPED A CANCER-SEEKING MISSILE, WE DON'T NEED TO ATTACK THE WHOLE BODY.' It continued:

> The line between destroying cancer and destroying the patient can be a thin one. But now, monoclonal antibodies will home in on cancer cells and stick to them. So they can be used both as an early-warning system and a powerful weapon . . . Attach drugs or higher doses of radiation and the missiles have their 'warheads' . . . This is one arms race where there is hope.

Such a concept, as fantastic as Star Wars, depends on our belief in drugs as magic bullets, and our faith in the ability of doctors to bombard us for our own good. Ironically, the military men whose language is used by the medical profession now themselves use medical language as a reassuring metaphor, referring to the bombing of villages in Vietnam and cities in Libya and Iraq as 'surgical strikes'.[3]

'We are the most aggressive physicians in the world' – this is what Professor Marc Lappé of the University of Illinois thinks about American doctors. Interviewed in Chicago for this book, he continued: 'Across the street from here, Benjamin Rush, a nineteenth-century physician, said: "We rely too much on thinking that we can use nature to cure disease. We have got to be more aggressive. We have got to cure disease by battling." It's a battleground. If we are battling microbes, then we use chemical warfare, we say, "Let's knock it out." It's the same mentality as war. Remember what we did in Vietnam? "Bomb the village in order to save it."' But the more antibiotics – these chemical weapons – are used, the more drug-resistant superbugs will be bred, especially in the closed environment of a hospital. 'The medical community so often fails to think about the impact that every decision made on behalf of the individual patient has on the whole population of patients, and on the community.'

LITTLE HITLERS

The military vocabulary and attitude we share with the medical profession and the drug industry, when we think and talk about the 'war on disease', is based on the germ theory: that diseases are caused by entities, invisible living things that must be killed in order to restore our health. And these unseen enemies are germs. Bacteria, viruses and other micro-organisms are taken to mean disease; indeed, it's as if they actually *are* disease.

The germ theory of disease is embedded in our thinking. Look at the following definitions from the *Shorter Oxford Dictionary*:

> **Bacterium.** Microscopic . . . organism found in all decomposing animal and vegetable liquids. Hence *bacteritic*, marked by the (morbid) presence of bacteria.
> **Germ.** In early use, vaguely, the 'seed' of a disease. In modern usage, a micro-organism or microbe, especially one which causes disease.
> **Microbe.** An extremely minute living being, whether plant or animal, chiefly applied to the bacteria causing diseases and fermentation.

Popular medical handbooks give much the same impression. For example, here is what the *Family Medical Adviser*, published by Reader's Digest in 1983, says about infectious diseases:[4]

> An infection occurs when harmful organisms known as pathogens invade the body. These organisms include viruses, bacteria, protozoa, rickettsiae, fungi and worms . . . Harmful organisms lie in contaminated food and drink or the soil, and may enter the body through the mouth or an open wound.

And treatment? 'The success of medical treatment for infectious diseases depends on the organism responsible. Antibiotics, such as penicillin, eliminate bacteria.' Later on in this handbook, the body's own defences are described, in military language.

> *How the body fights infection.* A vast army of cells is on constant alert to counter any attack by agents of disease. Most of the germs that invade the body are bacteria and viruses intent on releasing toxins that will cause disease.

So it seems not only are doctors engaged in an unending fight against germs; our bodies are, too. Germs are identified as the universal enemy. And, by analogy, universal enemies are identified as germs. A popular cartoon of Hitler, devised by the British government and published in wartime newspapers and magazines, showed him as a horrid virulent bug, whose planned invasion of Britain would be foiled by the British germicide.

According to the germ theory, disease is 'out there' and invades us.

We are more or less chance victims of the external agent, the 'bugs' or 'germs' – that is, bacteria, viruses and other carriers of disease that come 'out of the blue'. We may make ourselves more vulnerable to disease by the way we behave – by travelling in the tropics (malaria, dysentery), crowding together in trains (the common cold) or by having many sexual partners (gonorrhoea, syphilis) – but on the whole, disease is an accident, something we 'catch'.

This attitude has roots in history. From the seventeenth to the nineteenth century, micro-organisms had been observed through microscopes but their significance was generally unrecognised. The leaders of the great public health movement that began in Europe in the 1830s fought visible dirt, and were convinced of the importance of decent working and living conditions and nourishing food. Their work created a cleaner and safer environment. In the half-century between the 1830s and the 1880s, the public health movement was led by engineers who built the great waterworks and underground sewage systems that made cities such as London and Paris comparatively safe places. The epidemic death rates from infectious diseases dropped, without anybody knowing much about the causes of these diseases, let alone their effective treatment.

The 'microbe hunters' of the late nineteenth century, of whom Louis Pasteur is now the best known, told a new story. They identified micro-organisms as the cause of infectious disease. In their day, infections were the great killers – of royalty, nobility, leaders of society and armies in the field, as well as the common people. For practical purposes, in those days 'disease' meant 'infection'.

The discovery of germs and their significance in disease was the beginning of the end of the public health movement of the early and mid-nineteenth century. For it was evidently not enough to eliminate open drains, refuse in the streets, filth, stenches and overcrowding: the newly discovered germs, microscopic agents of disease, could penetrate any *cordon sanitaire*. Water, air, earth and hands might seem to be clean, but actually be swarming with bacteria, a sort of invisible filth.

The germ theory of disease suggests that a clean environment is useless if disease-bearing bacteria survive, and – even more subversive – that if the bacteria are killed, a clean environment is agreeable but medically unnecessary. And so, starting around the 1880s, power in public health passed from the engineer to the scientist; from the protection of public health to the treatment of individual disease.

PASTEUR'S THEATRE OF PROOF

The microbe hunters sought the cure as well as the cause of disease. Pasteur became the founding father of modern drug-based medicine as a result of spectacular trials in which he demonstrated the power of vaccines to check infection.[5]

In France, the story of Pasteur's sheep is as celebrated as Fleming's chance discovery of penicillin is in Britain. In the spring of 1881, Pasteur, a self-publicist of ceaseless energy, had gathered together a great throng of French politicians, scientists, farmers and journalists in a field at Pouilly-le-Fort for a series of demonstrations designed to show the power of his anthrax vaccine. After a series of rehearsals in the laboratory, he was sure of success; his *coup* was effectively to turn a farm into a laboratory, and to conduct a scientific experiment in public, in front of leaders of French society.

In the field at Pouilly-le-Fort were 48 sheep. On the first day, Pasteur's assistants injected half the sheep with vaccine in which the disease organism was weakened so as not to cause the disease, but to produce an immune response protective against the disease. Twelve days later, this process was repeated. Subsequently, all the sheep were injected with a concentrated dose of *Bacillus anthracis*, the bacterium that carries anthrax. Finally, three days later, Pasteur and his assistants walked on to the field to enthralled applause from the distinguished audience. The carcases of 22 unvaccinated sheep lay on the grass, and the remaining two were in the final stages of anthrax, with blood oozing from their muzzles. By contrast, every one of the 24 vaccinated sheep were evidently in perfect health.[6]

This astonishing 'theatre of proof'[7] gave medical science a supreme status. Pasteur believed that he held the fate of nations in his syringes. Just as great battles change history, after Pouilly-le-Fort and other *coups* staged by Pasteur, medicine changed for ever. The germ theory of disease triumphed. And in the public mind, the germ *was* the disease. Find the germ, kill the germ, and cure the disease: that was what people came to believe over a hundred years ago, and still believe today. Pasteur himself at one point believed that his experiments would be extended until, in his words: 'All infectious diseases might be made to disappear from the face of the world.' And for all anybody knew at the time, perhaps all diseases were infections.

In the euphoria that greeted the work of Pasteur and his followers, it seemed possible that, one day, the secrets of all diseases would be revealed. Medicine became exalted to a science, with the power over the human mind of a religion. The revelation of the germ theory remained a mystery invisible to the uninitiated, perceived only by a specially qualified and equipped élite who spoke in a language only they understood. Scientists became explorers of the microscopic world of the microbes or, as they became known, the bacteria, viruses and other micro-organisms. The germ theory of disease has enabled doctors to gain the oracular authority both of scientists and of priests.

EHRLICH'S MAGIC BULLET

The half-century between the 1880s and the 1930s was an anxious time, because knowledge of the microbiological causes of infections generally came before knowledge of how effectively to treat the diseases. In those days, doctors might have a good idea of what was wrong with you and would give a confident diagnosis using long scientific names, but usually without being able to be of much practical help beyond offering a bedside manner and (in the days before the National Health Service in the UK) proffering a bill.

Nevertheless it was hoped and believed that, one day, science would have the answer. In 1895, Dr Émile Trélat wrote in the leading French journal, *Revue Scientique*:[8]

> If we could know the microbe at the source of each disease, its favourite haunts, its habits, its way of progressing, we might with good medical supervision catch it in time, stop it in its tracks, and prevent it continuing in its homicidal mission.

In the war against disease, the late-nineteenth-century scientist was seen as some sort of spy for the forces of light, following every move of the germ, the secret agent of the forces of darkness that, like some unseen assassin, flits through every barrier. In this paranoid period after the identification of bacteria as agents of disease, but before the discovery of sulphonamides, people felt pretty apprehensive not only about disease but also about doctors.

This mood is reflected in *The Doctor's Dilemma*, Bernard Shaw's satire on the medical profession, first performed in 1906. In the preface to the play, Shaw writes:

> The popular theory of disease is the common medical theory: namely, that every disease had its microbe duly created in the garden of Eden, and has been steadily propagating itself and producing widening circles of malignant disease ever since . . . Doctors . . . conceive microbes as immortal until slain by a germicide administered by a duly qualified medical man.

The motto of the profession, he proposed, was: 'Find the microbe and kill it. And even that they do not know how to do.'

During this period, people felt that bacteria were a threat 'out there' that could not be seen or heard or touched, but which could invade at any time, rather like the Soviet Union in the minds of Americans (and the United States in the minds of the Soviet people) during the Cold War.

Such paranoia was gradually reduced with the discoveries by other microbiologists such as Alexandre Yersin, Robert Koch, and, above all, Paul Ehrlich, not only of the microbiological causes of other deadly infections such as plague, diphtheria, syphilis and tuberculosis, but also of their possible effective treatment, with the drugs that came to be known as 'magic bullets'.

The term 'magic bullet' was coined by Paul Ehrlich, the founder of modern chemotherapy, who worked in Berlin a generation after Pasteur. He used the term to describe drugs which, as he put it, 'strike only the objects against which they are targeted'.

In 1905, the microbiological cause of syphilis was identified as *Treponema pallidum*, a bacterium now usually attacked with penicillin. In the pre-penicillin days, Ehrlich and his assistants tested hundreds of arsenic compounds, and found that No. 606, arsphenamine, which he later called Salvarsan, killed *T. pallidum*. In 1910, just five years after the discovery of its bacterial target, Salvarsan was put on the market, followed by an improved version, Neosalvarsan. The salvarsans were no magic bullets; they are intensely toxic. But they saved lives.

The glamour and power of the germ theory of disease, which developed between the 1880s and the 1930s, were then magnified by the discovery and mass application of sulphonamides and penicillin as treatments for many infections previously beyond the skills of doctors. And an overblown version of the germ theory became a persistent myth: not just that germs cause disease, but that *all* germs cause disease, and maybe even that *all* diseases are caused by germs. Therefore, the way to health was by means of waging war on germs.

Doctors have not done as much as they might to dispel this myth. They gain authority by evidently not only knowing the cause of disease but also its cure. And while doctors may agree that good food and clean surroundings are the essential means to prevent disease and promote health, modern medicine is not greatly interested in public health. What excited doctors in the first half of the twentieth century were specific causes of disease and specific cures – bugs and drugs, targets and bullets. You go to the doctor, who finds out what's wrong with you and gives you your medicine and you are well again. Above all, antibiotics still seem to be the magic missiles that seek out and destroy the invisible enemies that afflict us.

And generally speaking, that's how things are now. We have medicalised our health. This is the context of the spectacular growth of the pharmaceutical industry and of high-technology medicine in the second half of the twentieth century.

'THERAPEUTIC THUNDERBOLTS'

The germ theorists championed by Pasteur were aligned on one side of a great nineteenth-century debate on the nature of health and disease. They marshalled their evidence with vigour and style, and overwhelmed their opposition – so much so that the voices raised against the germ theory at the time faded into obscurity.

The other side of the debate is associated with another Frenchman, Pasteur's contemporary, the great physiologist Professor Claude Bernard. He saw disease not as 'out there', but 'in here', caused not so much by invasion from outside as by disturbances and weaknesses within the body which we ourselves may be able to put right. Bernard believed that good health depends on a proper balance within the internal environment of the body, which he called the '*milieu intérieur*' – that is, he thought ecologically.

According to this theory, we can strengthen ourselves not only against non-infectious diseases, but also against infections, by means of a healthy lifestyle. Thus, disease is not so much a medical but a social issue, best prevented rather than treated. This way of looking at disease can be called the 'earth theory', which (or so the story goes) Pasteur accepted on his deathbed with the words: 'The germ is nothing; the earth is everything.'

The French word attributed to Pasteur, translated here as 'earth', was '*terrain*', which can also be taken to mean 'environment'. If your external environment is healthy, and if your body is well nourished, like well-cultivated soil, you are best able to resist disease. By contrast, an abused body is most vulnerable to disease, just like exploited soil. Health is not merely the absence of disease; it is positive well-being.

Such ideas are as old as the healing arts. They form the philosophical basis of traditional Indian and Chinese medicine. They inform the great tradition of Western thinking about public health, from Hippocrates to the World Health Organisation Declaration on 'Health for All', made in Alma Ata in 1978.[9] By contrast, the germ theory, an intellectual underpinning of modern Western medicine, is novel.

A practical difference between the earth and the germ theories of disease, is one of responsibility. If you accept that disease is best prevented, you are liable to take care of your own health and that of the other people in your life. However, if you think that disease is best treated, you are liable to become a spectator of your health, and give away its care to a doctor. Thus, you change from being a person to being a patient.

It is understandable why the germ theory was so compelling in the nineteenth century, at a time when the great killer diseases were epidemic infections. And, of course, there is something to be said for the theory; some germs are sometimes a cause of some diseases. But bacteria, viruses and other micro-organisms are only one part of the story of any infectious disease. Nobody now would consciously propose the germ theory as a universal explanation of disease. It has not stood the test of time. For a start, most of the diseases we now suffer and die from are not infectious. Besides, if all that matters is the germ, the human race would have been wiped out long ago, extinguished by some primeval pandemic infection. With all that we know now about the nature and causes of disease, a great debate held now would be won by Claude Bernard, not Louis Pasteur.

Yet we mostly remain beguiled by the germ theory of disease, and act as if the cancers and diseases of the heart and circulatory system that kill most of us in the West are infections. Most of us do little or nothing to protect ourselves against such diseases, and when we suffer symptoms, we go to the doctor or the surgeon in the hope that a drug or an operation will cure us. Symptoms of non-infectious diseases can be quietened with drugs, and heart disease and cancers can sometimes be cut or burned out of the body. But such treatments are not magic bullets either: they leave scars and increase the chance of other illness; and the underlying disease is likely to recur.

Around the 1880s, the germ theory was the means whereby medical scientists, concerned with the treatment of disease, won their power struggle with social reformers, concerned with the prevention of disease. Beginning in the 1930s, the drugs that work against germs gave the medical profession unique authority. Doctors were 'armed with the therapeutic thunderbolts of Jove,' wrote Sir Derrick Dunlop, first chairman of the British Committee on Safety of Medicines, in 1972. He had seen 'greater advances in medical treatment than have appeared in all previous aeons of time, and there is no saying what the majesty and splendour of its progress will be in the remaining years of this century.'[10]

Our faith in antibiotics is bound up with our aversion to germs. We are all brought up to believe that it is best to be germ free, sterile. We don't want bacteria near us, and use an arsenal of chemical weapons designed to keep them at bay. We believe in the Domestos theory of human health. We need to kill all bacteria. Dead.

9 Living with Bacteria

GUT FLORA: A VITAL ORGAN

Most of our resident bacteria are in our guts. The human colon contains something like 400 to 500 species, altogether weighing around 1.5 kg (3 lb); the bulk of faeces is made up of bacteria. The populations of bacterial species that live in the human gut have evolved in balance with us and with each other; almost all are beneficial, contributing to the vital processes of the body in much the same way that worms turn over and enrich soil.[11]

Until recently, few biological scientists were interested in the contents of the gut. High-flyers did not reckon much on a career spent looking down a microscope at shit. The gut remains the body's Africa, its dark continent. In 1990, Professor Michael Gurr, then editor of the *British Journal of Nutrition*, wrote in an editorial[12]: 'We know very little about the 400–500 or so microbial species in the gut. We are particularly ignorant of how nutrition affects the balance between the species and the significance of minor or even major changes in diet.'

Scientists have much to learn about the effect of drugs, as well as food, on gut flora. In October 1985, Sir Christopher Booth, then head of the Medical Research Council's Clinical Research Centre in Harrow, Middlesex, gave the opening address at a conference on gut flora held in Rome.[13] He said that interest in gut flora has gone through three stages. First, when the colon was found to be full of bacteria in the late nineteenth century, the knowledgeable public were horrified, physicians identified a new disease which they called 'intestinal toxaemia', and the royal surgeon Sir Arbuthnot Lane obliged his fashionable patients by cutting the colons out of their bodies.[14] Then, after the 1920s:

> Interest in the bacterial flora of the gut declined dramatically . . .

> There began to be rather a complacent view that all diseases due to bacteria had already been discovered, and in the days before antibiotics, people did not realise the problems of the bacterial flora of the gut, which developed as a result of antibiotic treatment. And it was not really until the end of the Second World War that interest in the intestinal flora was rekindled.

That is to say, in the first golden years of antibiotics, in the 1940s and into the 1950s, physicians used antibiotics with less idea of what these drugs were doing to the bacteria in the human gut than the average gardener has of the effect that pesticide sprays have on ladybirds.

Microbiologists are now keenly interested in gut flora. What do they do? What are they for? A Microbial Research Group was set up at the Clinical Research Centre in Harrow; Dr Peter Borriello was its head in 1990. He is interested in the vital functions of gut flora which, as he says, can be seen as 'an organ of the body in its own right'.

Like Professor Gurr, Dr Borriello is modest about his knowledge of how gut flora work in the body. As he and colleagues from the British Public Health Laboratory Service say[15], the bacterial population inside our bodies amount to 'an ecosystem of the highest complexity, and our knowledge of it is still only rudimentary'.

It may seem amazing that leading scientists should confess ignorance of the functions of gut flora; but their intricacy is mind-boggling. The hundreds of species of bacteria in the gut can be grouped into at least seventeen types, all of which interact with each other, have countless sub-species and variations, and can and do mutate. 'The enormous complexity of the intestinal flora makes it extremely difficult to study,'[16] says microbiologist Professor Sherwood Gorbach of the New England Medical Center in Boston.

> The bacterial population of the human gastrointestinal tract constitutes an enormously complex ecosystem . . . It is estimated that more than 400 bacterial species can be isolated from the feces of a single individual. Detailed microbiologic analysis of such a heterogenous mixture is a monumental task. Indeed, a complete bacteriologic characterization of a fecal specimen could take up to one year to complete.

Imagine: one year, studying one turd!

Scientists now are sure, though, that our gut flora – the bacteria that live in teeming profusion within our intestines – are an integral part of our digestive system. They assimilate the contents of the gut, notably fats and fibrous material, and thus help to turn food into nourishment. (In much the same way, bacteria living in the earth's soil and water process plant, animal and human wastes, turning silage and sewage into fodder and compost.) Gut flora generate B vitamins and also vitamin K. They are interdependent with the gut wall and its lining of mucous membrane: they stimulate the renewal of cells within the gut wall, scavenge debris from its surface, and also stimulate peristalsis, the muscular pulsations of the gut which move food through the body.

In a review published in 1989[17], the Norwegian microbiologist Professor Tore Midtvedt wrote: 'Statis is death – motility means life. In creating normal movements of intestinal content, the flora is fulfilling its main function: just to keep us alive.' Interviewed for this book in London, Dr Hendrik van Saene of the Department of Medical Microbiology at the University of Liverpool told me: 'You need your gut flora for peristalsis, for mucosal cell renewal and for the generation of vitamins. It is a living organ system.'

So within the twentieth century, there has been a complete revolution in thinking about the bacteria in our bodies. At first, scientists assumed that these germs must be toxic. Then, interest faded: scientists couldn't work out what gut flora are for, and dismissed them as insignificant. During this period, antibiotics were developed. And now the bacteria in our gut are known to be a vital part of our digestive system. It takes time to get used to the idea that we need our gut flora for good health, and that they amount to a vital organ of the body. But so it is.

BARRIERS AGAINST INFECTION

The second reason why gut flora are vital to our health is that they protect us against infection and therefore are also part of our immune system. They work in just the same way as the friendly flora that live on the surface of the body, in driving off or keeping down the micro-organisms that cause disease.

Professor David Hentges of the Department of Microbiology at Texas Tech University is editor of a textbook on gut flora and their role in human health and disease.[11] In a chapter he himself contributed, he writes: 'The stability of the intestinal flora is an extremely important factor in the natural resistance of humans and animals against infections produced by bacterial pathogens in the intestinal tract.' In other words, our friendly resident bacteria keep out other trespassing micro-organisms that bring disease with them.

Young children and old people are relatively vulnerable to infection, because the gut flora's microbiological barrier is not fully formed at the beginning of life, and is fragile at its end, as it can be in illness. But ordinarily, in adult life it is remarkably strong. 'Only the most extreme stress situations, such as antibiotic administration, have a major effect on the stability of the flora,' says Dr Hentges. 'Antibiotics frequently produce profound changes in the composition of the human intestinal microflora, permitting overgrowth of resistant endogenous bacteria or colonization by exogenous organisms acquired from the environment.'

What this means in simpler language is that antibiotics are liable to devastate the bacteria that are normally dominant in a healthy gut, leaving room for potentially dangerous ones that also live in the gut but are normally held in check. These pathogenic bacteria multiply, make us ill, acquire resistance to antibiotics and so become more dangerous. Also, the destruction of the normally dominant healthy flora leave room for dangerous bacteria to enter the body from the outside environment; these also can multiply, make us ill, acquire resistance and so become more dangerous – the drug treadmill.

Dr Hentges concludes that, once antibiotics have broken down the body's natural barriers to infection, 'even a small number of pathogenic organisms can produce serious infection in the host. Clearly, the integrity of the intestinal flora is important to the well-being of the host, and antibiotics, which upset it, should be used with extreme caution.'

What all this means is that antibiotics are a health hazard not just when they are overused and abused, but also when they are prescribed by physicians who follow accepted guidelines for their use. Regulatory bodies such as the British Committee on Safety of Medicines believe that, properly prescribed, the benefits of antibiotics almost always, or at least usually, outweigh the risks. But the ill-effects of antibiotics on gut flora are not always included in this risk–benefit equation. They should be.

What is revealed here is a division within medical science, as fundamental as the nineteenth-century debate between Louis Pasteur and Claude Bernard. Now, a century later, leading physicians are aligned on one side, and leading microbiologists on the other. The responsibility of physicians is to the infected patients in front of them, who can be effectively treated with antibiotics. Microbiologists have a broader concern with the effect of these potent drugs on other people, on the environment and, indeed, on the very same patients in the longer term. Microbiologists think ecologically. They are right, of course, but what they are saying is not being well communicated to the world at large: in the late twentieth century, scientists have got into the habit of speaking only in jargon. Thus there is no great debate about antibiotics – not yet, anyway.

An irony of our time is that knowledgeable people who take a thoughtful interest in global ecology will swallow or let themselves be injected with antibiotics without any thought, ignorant of the damage these drugs can do to their own personal ecology – to the micro-organisms that live within us all, on our skin, in our mouths and throats, in and around our genital organs and, most of all, inside our gut. A further irony is that the doctors who give us the drugs usually have little training in microbial ecology.

IMMUNE DEFENCES

The bacteria that live within the inner passages of our bodies, do not just float about. As I've mentioned, the muscular walls of the entire respiratory and gastrointestinal tracts, from the mouth to the anus, are lined with mucous membrane, a soft tissue that is one line in the body's defences not only against infection, but against other diseases, too. This membrane produces mucus, a thick fluid that acts rather like oil, lubricating and protecting our inner passages. This protection is not just mechanical; mucus, like saliva, contains substances that are natural antibiotics, protecting against infection by foreign micro-organisms.

The bacterial species that are dominant inside a healthy body themselves form a protective coating, interpenetrated with mucus and its underlying membrane. As the distinguished Dutch microbiologist Dr Dirk van der Waaij puts it, these bacteria 'appear to adhere particularly to the mucosal lining of the ileum [the lower third of the small intestine] and the colon [the large intestine], forming "living wallpaper".'[18]

In 1971, Dr van der Waaij coined the term 'colonisation resistance' to refer to the system of defences within the body designed to keep out micro-organisms liable to cause disease.[19]

Colonisation resistance includes four barriers. The first is the body's own resident bacteria. The second is the mucosal lining of our inner passages. The third is the inner walls of these passages, which constantly renew themselves, eliminating toxins along with dead cells and other debris. The 'living wallpaper' incorporating the bacteria that have evolved with us is an integral part of all these three barriers. Then, if these fail, the body's fourth barrier against infection is its inner defences, involving immunoglobulin and phagocyte cells that circulate in the bloodstream and become concentrated at the point of infection.

It is conventionally believed that only this last barrier is part of the body's immunity to disease. Certainly, if the term 'immune response' is taken to refer only to that part of the response to infection that involves immunoglobulin, then this is true by definition. But the first three of the four barriers that together make up our resistance to disease-carrying micro-organisms are clearly also part of the body's immunity to infection. It therefore follows, in a broader and more logical sense, that our resident bacteria are part of our immune system.

Here is an explanation why the two most common ill-effects of antibiotics are diarrhoea and allergic reactions; these are both the result of the body's resident bacteria being attacked by drugs. With diarrhoea, colonisation resistance is working; peristalsis speeds up, as does the process by which the cells in the gut wall, together with the mucosal lining, renew themselves. The gut seems to be working flat out to eliminate the toxic drug, to prevent infection by dangerous micro-organisms, and to bring the bacterial populations within the gut back into a healthy balance. Usually, this works: simple diarrhoea, while uncomfortable and sometimes acutely painful, is a healthy reaction of the body's outer immune defences.

With allergic reactions, colonisation resistance is breaking down; the 'living wallpaper' of bacteria and mucous membrane is stripped away, and the body's exposed inner defences go into a state of shock. Usually, once the drug is withdrawn, the healthy gut flora restore themselves, but the victim is liable to become allergic to any future doses of the same or related antibiotics.[20]

The integrity of the gut is vital not only as protection against infection, and for the health of the gut itself, but also as protection against non-infectious diseases. However, the importance of the intestines as a vital organ system of the body has been relatively neglected by modern medical science, whereas research into diseases of the cardiovascular system, notably coronary heart disease, has been the glamour area, attracting leading scientists and massive funding in the last half-century.

If the gut is injured, we are liable to suffer general bad health. We tend to think of our intestines just as carriers of waste matter, rather like sewage pipes. But there is more to them than that. The gut turns food into nourishment. If it is not working properly, after a time the whole body becomes starved. Also, the intestines are not impenetrable. Agents of disease that pass through the gut wall can reach the interior of the abdomen and, from there, the bloodstream, and thereby infect any organ of the body.

Just as cut skin normally heals quickly, the healthy gut normally repairs itself after injury. But as with all other parts of the body, regular injury and insult may cause breakdown of the repair mechanisms and result in serious disease. A diseased gut makes us vulnerable to other diseases, infectious and non-infectious. The best way to ensure that your gut remains healthy, and that its defences against disease remain strong, is to treat it, and its resident bacteria, with respect.

10 Our Inner Ecology

BACTERIA: THE ORIGINAL SPECIES

The human-centred view of bacteria and viruses as nothing more than irritants or bad accidents is understandable, since we can't see them and usually are aware of them only as causes of disease. But a more helpful view is an ecological one, looking not just at what micro-organisms do to us, but at how they have evolved with each other, and with the soil, water, plants, animals and humans. We should then get a better idea of what they can do for us.

From our point of view though, as hosts to bacteria, a key distinction is between those bacterial species that are aerobic and those that are anaerobic. Aerobic bacteria need the oxygen in air to survive and flourish. It follows that the bacteria that live on us – for example, *Staphylococcus epidermidis* – are aerobic. Many anaerobic bacteria need an absence of oxygen to survive and flourish; and the bacteria that live inside us, including the many bacteroides and bifidobacteria 'friendly flora' species that dominate in the healthy human gut, are anaerobic.[21]

So put simply, aerobic bacteria live outside us, and anaerobic bacteria live inside us. Many of the bacteria that are agents of disease are aerobic species carried in food or on animals, insects or dust. The reason that many are invasive and can survive inside us is that they are adaptable. They are known to scientists as 'facultative aerobes' – they prefer an environment with oxygen, but are still able to flourish without it. One reason why open-body surgery is hazardous is that it exposes whatever is being operated on to facultative aerobic bacteria that can adapt and flourish once the wound is sewn up, but which have no place inside a healthy body.

Bacteroides, bifidobacteria and other bacterial species dominant in the healthy gut are known as 'obligate anaerobes': these are the type that require an absence of oxygen. Other bacteria that live in the healthy gut in smaller numbers, of which *Escherichia coli* is an example, are 'facultative anaerobes' – their usual habitat is mostly empty of oxygen, but they can adapt to an environment containing it. Many facultative anaerobes that live in the gut are normally harmless, but can be a cause of disease when they move outside the body and then inside again to a site foreign to them. This is why *E. coli* are normally harmless inside the gut, held in check by the obligate anaerobes, but potentially harmful when they are able to move out of the gut into, for example, the female genital and urinary tract.

Similarly, obligate anaerobes are harmless and indeed beneficial contained within the gut, but are potentially harmful if the gut becomes injured or ulcerated, enabling them to move around inside the body. Generally speaking, bacteria are a cause of disease when they are, for some reason, in the wrong place.

As well as oxygen (or the lack of it), bacteria need nourishment and the right range of temperature and acidity to survive and multiply. In test-tubes, fast-multiplying bacteria can double, by the process of cell division, once every half-hour: so a single bacterium can become 1000 in five hours, and 1,000,000 in ten hours. If nothing stopped this process of multiplication, the world would have become a compacted mass of bacteria aeons ago. However, bacteria multiply only as long as their nourishment lasts, the conditions are right and they are unchallenged. When one or more of their essential nutrients runs out, bacteria stop multiplying and, after a while, start to die. The general laws of nature that determine the balance between bacteria and other living things in the world are the same laws that govern human populations.

For many hundreds of millions of years, bacteria lived in their own world. Early bacteria, known as autotrophs, lived in water or earth and, as plants now do, fed off carbon dioxide and either light or inorganic compounds. Later heterotrophic bacteria evolved; these live off organic compounds which means that before the evolution of plants and animals, they lived off other bacteria. Later, but still hundreds of millions of years ago, fungi (including yeasts and moulds) and other primitive eukaryotic (multiple-chromosome) organisms evolved.

The planet would not have developed as a support system for plants, and thus for animals and humans, without micro-organisms. The soil of the world was formed by bacteria and fungi, and the process of decomposition, not only of earth, but also of all living matter from which all new life springs, is carried out by bacteria. Without bacteria, life would stop. Without bacteria as the original living things, life as we understand it, including ourselves, would never have started. Human beings are not only descended from but also dependent on bugs. What links earth, plants, animals and humans is bacteria.

ANTIBIOTICS IN NATURE

We are accustomed to think of antibiotics as an invention of modern science, whose sole purpose is to treat bacterial infection of humans and animals. However, substances with antibacterial properties were originally evolved by bacteria themselves for their own protection, before the evolution of plants, animals and then humans.

As soon as bacteria developed the ability to live off other bacteria they must also have developed attack and defence mechanisms, like living things in all ecosystems. And this is how antibiotics evolved, in nature.

In his book *Modern Meat*, Orville Schell describes this process[22]:

> Millions of years ago, certain single-celled organisms dwelling in the soil developed the ability to produce within themselves compounds that could either inhibit the growth of or kill competing micro-organisms. This ability, which was acquired through random genetic mutation, was an extraordinary evolutionary development. The micro-organisms that could produce these compounds, which have come to be known as 'antibiotics', a term derived from the Latin meaning literally 'against life', gained an immense advantage in the struggle for survival.

Hence the discovery of penicillin by Alexander Fleming in the Penicillium mould, and the later discovery of streptomycin and other antibiotics, following Selman Waksman's deduction that these would be found in soil. The same logic led to the discovery of the first cephalosporin in sewage. Depending on your attitude towards nature, you can see the original evolution of nature's own antibiotics in bacteria either as a weapons system in a war where only the fittest survive, or else as a balancing mechanism in the global ecosystem.

The healing power of antibiotic substances found in nature has been known for thousands of years. In China, mouldy soya beans have been used to heal wounds for the last 3000 years. There is a reference to mould cures on ancient Egyptian inscriptions and in the Talmud. Baker's and brewers' yeasts have been used for surface infections since antiquity. In his book on antibiotics, *Miracle Cure*[23], Dr Martin Wainwright comments:

> Most medical historians have tended to dismiss these claims for the curative properties of moulds as merely old wives' tales; however, the fact that such practices took place on all continents and in all ages suggests that they must to some extent have been successful.

One story in Dr Wainwright's book comes from just such an 'old wife' in Cork, Ireland, who seemed to know what she was talking about:

> Many years ago an old aunt (who was some 82 years old), who appeared to be quite learned in cures, read one day in a magazine of Professor Fleming's discovery of penicillin, which was described as resulting from research on mould. My aunt said in her inimitable way: 'I had that cure before he did.' I knew that one of her cures was to collect ten or twelve oranges and place them somewhere where they would get mouldy as soon as possible. She would then carefully remove the greenest mould and make it into some kind of infusion and use it on abscesses, whitlows, boils, or other forms of pustule. She would then administer it orally, all apparently with complete success.

It may be that the origin of the Easter hot-cross bun was as a natural antibiotic. Throughout Britain, buns baked around the time of the new spring season were traditionally hung up and left to go mouldy, and the mould scraped off later in the year and used as a cure. Perhaps the cross was added at some time, with the sanction of the Church, as an emblem of the power of Jesus to heal suffering humanity.

In 1925, an editorial in the *Lancet* suggested that 'Medicinal properties attributed by tradition to certain fungi may possibly represent an untapped source of therapeutic value.' Just three years later, Alexander Fleming noticed the antibacterial effect of the penicillium spores blown into his laboratory. He might have appreciated the practical value of his discovery sooner had he contemplated the healing powers of mouldy buns hung up by custom in British pubs.

Vegetables, fruits, herbs and their products have also evolved to incorporate antibiotic qualities to guard against their own infections, and some of these can also be effective against human diseases. Eventually, it may be that anti-infective substances will be identified in all living things. So far, foods, drinks and herbs known to have useful antibiotic qualities include cabbage and onion, cranberries and other fruit, and wine. Raw carrots can work against *Listeria monocytogenes*. A species of fig used medicinally by the people of New Guinea is now known to contain an antimicrobial substance. Honey is a useful medicine for children: it can kill species of salmonella and shigella that cause diarrhoea. Olive oil can be effective against infections of the gums. Tea can work against camplylobacter, bacteria that now cause even more food poisoning than salmonella. And the antibacterial properties of garlic have been recognised since Pasteur's day.[24]

The healthy human body is protected against infection not only by its own resident bacteria, but also by natural antimicrobial and antiseptic secretions. Lysozyme, an enzyme contained in tears, keeps the surface of the eyes sterile by killing bacteria; it is also contained in nasal secretions and saliva, protecting the nose, mouth and throat. Lactic acid, contained in sweat and secreted by the lactobacilli in the vagina, confers protection throughout the surface of the body and within the female genital organs. Hydrochloric acid in the stomach prevents any aerobic bacteria that may have managed to get down the throat from passing into the intestines. The function of fatty acids on the skin and that of mucus in the digestive tract have already been mentioned.

Babies are protected against infection by their mother's breastmilk, rich in antibodies which protect against foreign bacteria. Breastmilk is the best protection a mother can give her baby against infection, together with plenty of intimate cuddles: the closer the physical bonding between mother and child, the better the child is able to resist dangerous bacteria.

When humans evolved, first healers, then doctors learned to use antibacterial substances against those micro-organisms that infect humans. Scientists then synthesised antibiotics to give humans further supremacy over other living things, and pharmaceutical companies mass-produced these drugs to gain competitive edge over each other and over other industries. We humans probably evolved from bacteria, and owe our existence to them. And we owe antibiotics to bacteria and other micro-organisms. They are a treasure of nature and, like all treasure, valuable only when used very carefully and sparingly.

THE BUGS THAT LIVE WITH US

We are inclined to think of bacteria as parasites; indeed, they are often so called in textbooks. This is a mistake. In the usual sense of the word, a parasite is a burden, something unpleasant, better not there. And this does not describe the typical relationship we have with bacteria. For a start, the autotrophic bacteria, which live like plants, have evolved in balance with other organisms in the global ecosystem, but are no more parasites on us than are fruit or flowers. These bacteria do not affect us.

The bacteria that do affect us, one way or another, including all the types and species so far mentioned, are the heterotrophs, which live off organic compounds. Heterotrophs do indeed live on, or in or with other organisms, but then so do animals, including humans. Our felt need for antibiotics is influenced by our assumption that bacteria are parasitic, but they are usually no more parasitic on us than we are on them. Typically, the bacteria that live on or in us are better described as commensal or else as symbiotic with us.

Both these words mean 'living together', but in rather different senses. Commensals dwell together harmlessly. Symbionts live together to each other's benefit.

So, for example, *Staphylococcus epidermidis*, which lives on our skin and keeps off bacteria that can do us harm, is symbiotic with us; the relationship is mutually beneficial. Similarly, the anaerobic bacilli that make up over 99 percent of the micro-organisms in the human gut are almost all friendly, symbiotic flora, not just occupying space and therefore keeping off unfriendly flora, but also acting as part of the digestive process. And the aerobic *Lactobacillus acidophilus*, well known as a fermenting agent in yoghurt, is abundant in the female genital tract, where its secretions of lactic acid make it symbiotic with its human host.

In their natural environment, these bacteria never do us harm.

However, bacteria that are commensal in a healthy gut, such as *Escherichia coli* and *Clostridium difficile*, become harmful when they multiply out of control, as they may when the symbiotic bacteria also usually present in the gut are destroyed by antibiotics. A symbiont can become a parasite just as a plant can become a weed, simply by growing out of control or growing in the wrong place.

Another analogy is people. Somebody living in your spare room is commensal with you. People get married in order to live together in a symbiotic relationship. A commensal lodger becomes a parasite by outstaying his or her welcome or by not paying the rent. Similarly normally commensal bacteria become harmful and therefore parasitic only when they become dominant in the gut, or else when they are able to move from inside the gut (where they are confined in a healthy person) into the urinary tract, where they should not be.

You might think it would be better to have a gut inhabited only by symbiotic bacteria that never do us any harm in their natural environment. Well, for a start, we don't.

In addition, our friendly flora, the obligate anaerobes, flourish in our gut in the presence of our less friendly flora, the adaptable facultative anaerobes. Bacteria evolve not only to become symbiotic with us; they also become symbiotic with each other. The bacteria in our gut live in a tube closed at one end by the stomach, whose fluid secretions shut off almost all air from above, rather like the U-bend in a water closet, and at the other by the anal sphincter that blocks off the back passage. Nevertheless, some air does get into the gut – we swallow air with our food, for example. So a symbiotic function of the adaptable facultative anaerobes (such as *E. coli* and *C. difficile*) is to absorb the small amounts of oxygen that do enter the gut, thus enabling the obligate anaerobes (notably the bacteroides and the bifidobacteria) to flourish and remain dominant.

This mutual dependence between facultative and obligate anaerobes explains why antibiotics are liable to devastate our friendly flora, if not directly, then indirectly. Antibiotics targeted against the facultative anaerobic species that are the microbiological cause of many infections will also tend to create an unnatural environment in which oxygen is not eliminated and therefore one in which our friendly flora cannot flourish. As with pesticides, the use of antibiotics has unforeseen consequences.

It may also be that the relatively unfriendly facultative anaerobes in our gut are particularly good at protecting us against invasion by disease-carrying aerobic micro-organisms that have no place in a healthy body, but which can enter us, borne on water, food, dust, animals and (in the case of viruses) within bacteria themselves.

If this seems unlikely, consider an analogy from business. A majority of directors of a company may be friendly with each other, make their shareholders prosperous, and take care that their disagreeable colleagues, a minority on the board, ordinarily never get their way. However, it may be that this unfriendly minority are particularly good at repelling hostile takeover bids from other companies. Anybody with experience of working closely with other people is likely to have come across interactions like this, which are infinitely simpler than the microscopic interactions involving hundreds of species of bacteria within our bodies.

Which species of gut flora protect us best against invasion by dangerous micro-organisms? This is an issue of great interest to microbiologists – as indeed it is to everybody. But there is no way to know for sure. Because the obligate anaerobes that are dominant inside the gut die once exposed to the oxygen in air, analysis of bacteria excreted in faeces is a bit rough and ready. Researchers think it likely that the populations of bacteria in samples of faeces are much the same as those living in the lower gut, but they are not sure.

Also, how bacteria work in the body (*in vivo*) and how they work in the laboratory (*in vitro*) are two different stories. In the gut, any one bacterial species lives in a complex relationship with other species and with the gut wall and its mucosal lining, as well as with the contents of the gut, which are always in movement. The laboratory environment cannot hope to mimic that of the body; scientists can only try to make their experiments as apt as possible.

THE BUGS THAT ARE BUILT INTO US

Friendly, symbiotic bacteria do not only live on plants, animals and humans, and inside the guts of all creatures with digestive systems. They are also built into us. In his essay on 'Germs'[1], Professor Lewis Thomas gives examples of the integration of bacteria into other living worlds. For example, the metabolism of leguminous plants such as peas and beans depends on bacteria that are incorporated into root hairs 'with such intimacy that only an electron microscope can detect which membranes are bacterial and which plants.' And insects have bacteria living inside them 'like little glands, doing heaven knows what, but being essential'.

Within all human cells are structures called mitochondria, which are essential as a means of converting food into energy: mitochondria are, in effect, the body's power plant. Professor Thomas sees them as astounding evidence of our evolution in symbiosis with bacteria. He writes:[1]

> A good case can be made for our non-existence as entities. We are not made up, as we had always supposed, of successively enriched packets of our own parts. We are rented, shared, occupied.
>
> At the interior of our cells, driving them, providing the oxidative energy that sends us out for the improvement of each shining day, are the mitochondria, and in a strict sense they are not ours. They turn out to be little separate creatures, the colonial posterity of migrant prokaryotes, probably ancestral primitive bacteria that swam into ancestral precursors of our eukaryotic cells and stayed there. Ever since, they have maintained themselves and their ways, replicating in their own fashion, privately, with their DNA and RNA quite separate from ours. They are as much symbionts as the rhizobial bacteria in the roots of beans. Without them, we could not move a muscle, drum a finger, think a thought.

We are not solid. Looked at through a powerful microscope, we are interpenetrated with bacteria and, it seems, with the living fossils of bacteria, working in ways which microbiologists are only beginning to understand. Such discoveries should surely make us see bacteria and other micro-organisms in a new light, and with new respect. If the scientists who first developed antibiotics just over half a century ago knew as much about our interdependence with bacteria as you know now, they might have been altogether more cautious, less aggressive, in their public statements. But like the scientists who first developed the atom bomb, they did not know the full meaning of what they were doing and, in any case, soon had their discoveries taken out of their hands by industry and governments.

Soon after birth, all of us, all of the time, live with bacteria, some of which may cause disease. That is the way of things. Bacteria are the foundation of the living planet: they are as universal as earth – and, indeed, there would be no soil without bacteria. Towards the end of his life, the billionaire Howard Hughes developed intense paranoia about germs, and tried to seal himself in a chamber of his own design: an act of utter futility. There's no getting away from bacteria.

The bacteria all around and inside us are rather like the people in our lives: there they are, and how they behave, how they react, and what effect they have on us depends to a large extent on us. Just as a key to a good life is learning to live with people, a key to good health is learning to live with bacteria.

11 Bombing Bacteria into Retaliation

WHY WE SUFFER INFECTION

What of those bacteria that invade us and cause disease? Why do they do us harm? For it does not suit parasites to kill their host. 'There is nothing to be gained, in an evolutionary sense, by the capacity to cause illness or death,' says Lewis Thomas.

> A man who catches a meningococcus [a cause of meningitis] is in considerably less danger of his life, even without chemotherapy, than meningococci with the bad luck to catch a man. Most meningococci have the sense to stay out on the surface, in the rhinopharynx [inside the nose and throat]. During epidemics this is where they are to be found in the majority of the host population, and it generally goes well. It is only in the unaccountable minority, the 'cases', that the line is crossed, and then there is the devil to pay on both sides, but most of all for the meningococci.

The same is true during all epidemics: with rare exceptions such as the medieval Black Death, for every person who suffers from infection, many people are infected but do not suffer. Infection is not the same as disease.

Almost always, with infectious disease, what is significant is not just the micro-organisms that carry infection, but their relationship with us. Most of the time, when we are healthy, we shrug off pathogenic bacteria, those that can be a cause of disease. Sometimes, though, the bacteria multiply fast, unchecked, perhaps because the virulence of the bacteria temporarily overcomes the body's immune defences, or perhaps because these defences are already weakened. In such cases, the body may rally its forces, so that we feel only a flicker of malaise. At other times, the bacteria may become embedded in us, causing acute illness for a while, until our bodies recover, the bacteria die off and the symptoms of disease subside.

Sometimes, though, infectious disease persists, and we may become ill for a long time, and even die. Dangerous infections may be caused by very virulent pathogenic bacteria that invade vital organs. When this happens, it is, of course, sensible, once the disease is known to be bacterial, to use antibiotics.

By why does serious and potentially deadly infectious disease happen? 'Most bacteria are totally preoccupied by browsing,' says Lewis Thomas.[1] 'The micro-organisms that seem to have it in for us in the worst way – the ones that really appear to wish us ill – turn out on close examination to be rather more like bystanders, strays, strangers in from the cold.' Or, he might have added, strangers that come in through a door that is better kept closed.

Young children and old people are prone to infection, and at any time of life, our bodies can be weakened by other illnesses, by injury and by surgery. When we are vulnerable, we are in most need of the inner strength of an intact immune system, complete with its resident friendly flora.

Lewis Thomas, who is a fund of fascinating and significant information about microbes and us, points out that some diseases are caused not so much by bacteria as by an over-reaction of the body's inner immune defences, so that it, in effect, attacks itself: 'Our arsenals for fighting off bacteria are so powerful, and involve so many defence mechanisms, that we are in more danger from them than from the invaders. We live in the midst of explosive devices; we are mined.' But why should bacteria trigger off self-destructive auto-immune reactions that, in extreme cases, kill the victim? And why have auto-immune diseases become more common in the last half-century?

It seems unlikely that the human body, faced with bacterial invasion, has evolved to incorporate a self-destruct mechanism which by sheer chance is causing more suffering and death now than two or three generations ago. It seems much more likely that something has happened in recent history to make the inner immune defences located in the human gut oversensitive when exposed to toxins. We know that antibiotics are capable not only of stripping bacteria (with their underlying 'living wallpaper' of mucous membrane) off the inside of the gut wall, but also of causing infection of the gut with new populations of bacteria to which it is not adapted and which are toxic in profusion. Therefore, the obvious explanation is that antibiotics can be an underlying cause not only of superinfections and allergic reactions, but also of auto-immune non-infectious diseases.[20]

WHY FOOD GETS POISONED

Germs are a necessary but not a sufficient condition for disease. What matters more than the germ is the environment. An outstanding example is the gastroenteritis now endemic in Britain, carried by *Salmonella enteritidis*, and the less common but more dangerous infection carried by *Listeria monocytogenes*, which can cause still-birth. Both are food-borne diseases.[2]

Salmonella and listeria are examples of bacilli which have become a menace to public health because the conditions which normally control their growth have changed. Both have always been present in some foods, in small numbers. What has made them a hazard are the conditions in which animals are now reared and in which food is now prepared and stored. For example, factory-farmed chickens are often infested with salmonella because they are crushed together in cages, and because chicken manure and the remains of other chickens are included in their feed, creating a circle of infection. After slaughter, chicken carcasses slung in long lines on hooks are dunked in a tank of water, creating a warm soup in which bacteria can multiply and infect every chicken passing through the slaughter and packing house.

As another example, the 'cook–chill' method of food preparation is liable to breed both salmonella and listeria unless the food is kept at strictly controlled low temperatures; above these, the bugs multiply out of control. This is why pre-prepared food such as sandwiches and pre-cooked snacks and meals, which sit on shop counters at or near room temperature, are best avoided. The warm moist food lying around for many hours, or days, provides ideal nourishment for bacteria, just like the culture dishes used to breed microbes in laboratories.

Healthy people are extremely unlikely to suffer if they eat food containing a few pathogenic bacteria. Some of the screaming national newspaper headlines seen in the UK in 1989 and 1990, which reported laboratory analyses of bacteria in fresh and dairy produce as if every single bug was a microscopic cruise missile, were examples of nonsensical germ-theory paranoia.

Modern methods of food manufacture encourage salmonella, listeria and other bacteria that can cause food poisoning to multiply very quickly, out of control. Hence, in the UK, the Conservative government's Food Safety Act of 1990, which among other things is meant to ensure that any food liable to become infested with pathogenic bacteria is kept in properly controlled cold cabinets, and sold in shops subject to careful regulation. It would, of course, be better if animals were kept properly and fed decently, and if food made from animals and their products was not manufactured by methods that are ideal for the breeding of bacteria that carry infectious diseases.

People most vulnerable to food poisoning are those with weakened immunity. The UK government's Chief Medical Officer of Health has issued warnings meant to put people with cancer and AIDS, and also pregnant women and old people, on guard against foods liable to be infested with salmonella and listeria. These warnings do not point out that anybody on antibiotics is also more vulnerable to infection because of the microbiological void these drugs create in the gut, which is liable to be filled with bugs invading from outside.

VIRUSES: MOBILE GENES

Viruses have a bad name. The word 'virulence' derives from 'virus', which itself comes from the same root word as 'weasel' and 'ooze'. We assume that the world would be a better place without viruses: anybody who says, 'I've got a virus' feels ill.

However, like bacteria, viruses were not evolved as the agents of human disease. They have another purpose on the planet. Lewis Thomas thinks they may be the means whereby genetic codes are transferred from one life form to another: the instruments of evolution. He writes[1]:

> The viruses . . . now begin to look more like mobile genes. Evolution is still a long and tedious biologic game, with only the winners staying at the table, but the rules are beginning to look more flexible.
>
> We live in a dancing matrix of viruses; they dart, rather like bees, from organism to organism, from plant to insect to mammal to me and back again, and into the sea, tugging along pieces of this genome, strings of genes from that, transplanting grafts of DNA, passing around heredity as though at a great party. They may be a mechanism for keeping new, mutant kinds of DNA in the widest circulation among us. If this is true, the odd virus disease, on which we must focus so much of our attention in medicine, may be looked on as an accident, something dropped.

As with bacteria, we can be infected with pathogenic viruses without suffering disease; and viral disease is often caused, not so much by the virus itself, as by the reaction of the body's immune system to the virus. There is no effective medical treatment for most common viral diseases, which therefore usually run their course.

Modern medicine trains doctors, and therefore everybody, to think in rigid, isolated categories about health and disease and, likewise, to break down the body into sets of separated parts. This mechanical attitude misleads us into overlooking our own ecosystems. Because bacteria and viruses are different types of micro-organism, and because antibiotics are useless against almost all viral diseases, we are led to believe that bacterial and viral diseases have nothing to do with each other, and that the use of antibiotics cannot affect our vulnerability to viral diseases.

This is not so. There are certainly two ways in which antibiotics alter the internal environment of the body that lay us open to viral as well as bacterial diseases.

First, the bacteria that are normally dominant on and in our body are an integral part of the body's defences, evolved not only to keep out foreign bacteria, but also other micro-organisms: fungi, parasites – and viruses. When these friendly flora are wiped out by antibiotics, we are more vulnerable to any type of infection.

Second, the 'living wallpaper' of bacteria and mucous membrane covering the walls of the respiratory and digestive tracts have a double function: shielding the gut from penetration by toxins, and insulating the inner immune defences. When this covering is stripped away by antibiotics, we are doubly at risk, not only of penetration of the gut wall by dangerous micro-organisms, including viruses, but also of damage to the inner immune defences. A number of viral diseases that have emerged and even become epidemic in recent years, notably AIDS, are diseases that attack the immune system.

There is a third conceivable hazard. Viruses live and multiply inside bacterial cells, as well as human cells. Is it possible that, when antibiotics kill bacteria inside *us* which have viruses inside *them*, these viruses may migrate into the nearest human cells, lining your throat, say, or gut, or in your bloodstream? And could it be that species of viruses that have evolved to be commensal within bacterial cells are dangerous parasites within human cells? If so, the use of antibiotics to treat bacterial diseases could unleash any number of viral diseases.

Happily, it is agreed by microbiologists that viruses cannot make a bridge between bacterial, prokaryotic cells and human or other eukaryotic cells. 'There's been no case that I know of,' said Dr Richard Novick of the New York Public Health Research Institute, when I went to interview him for this book. 'Maybe I've lost something in the literature somewhere, but I've never heard of that.'

None the less, one cause of viral diseases may well be disturbance of microbiological ecosystems by systematic use of antibiotics, just as one cause of plagues of insects is disturbance of entomological ecosystems by systematic use of pesticides. A good defence against viral as well as bacterial disease is a healthy body whose immunity is complete with intact resident bacteria.

IF IN DOUBT, WIPE THEM OUT

Physicians sometimes forget that antibiotics cause as well as treat disease, because their focus is on the patient and the infection in front of them. They tend not to see toxic reactions or resistance to drugs as red lights, but merely as 'side-effects' – an indication to try another drug. Although standard medical textbooks now refer to the damage that antibiotics do to gut microbial ecology, physicians seem not altogether to accept, or strange the idea that a drug used to treat a disease in one part of the body can cause a disease in another part of the body, or in other people.

Faced with the certainty of an infected patient, the probability that the infection will be stopped by antibiotics and the unknown effect of the drugs on microbiological ecosystems, it is easy to see why busy physicians and surgeons will go for antibiotics. The thinking is just the same as that of farmers faced with pests.

One difference, though, is that farmers who live on the land are able to notice changes in their environment caused by pesticides and other biocides. By contrast, much of the responsibility for patients' care has now passed from family doctors, who have the opportunity of getting to know them personally, to hospital physicians and surgeons, who typically will only see patients briefly, as 'cases'.

So the cumulative ill-effects of antibiotics may become evident to the medical profession only when superinfections and superbugs cause plagues of infection in hospitals and in the community. Doctors (and patients) are likely to notice immediate, dramatic ill-effects of antibiotics. However, long-term damage is likely to be overlooked or misunderstood, and the vital importance of the integrity of resident friendly flora ignored.

Not so long ago, doctors had no idea that the tonsils and the appendix are both part of the body's immune defences, and surgeons often removed these organs casually, assuming they were redundant, some sort of mistake made by nature. If in doubt, whip them out! Similarly, doctors now, who know little about the functions of the protective bacteria that have evolved with us, often destroy them with antibiotics even in cases of trivial infection. If in doubt, wipe them out! One common justification for this recklessness is the claim that friendly flora will recover and establish new healthy ecosystems. But, as with wildlife devastated by biocides, sometimes they won't recover.

Broad-spectrum and combination antibiotics are especially popular, not only with the drug industry and the medical profession, but also with anybody who goes to a doctor wanting to get rid of an infection easily and quickly. They work! But these drugs are most likely to cause microbiological chaos: they are the fastest way to create superinfections and superbugs. Systematic use of broad-spectrum and combination antibiotics is like the slash-and-burn method of agriculture used by small farmers in the Third World, who cut down and burn brush and trees to fertilise their crops and then, when the earth is exhausted, move on and slash and burn again, leaving devastation behind them. The difference is that we cannot move on from our own bodies, as long as we are alive.

We humans seem to have a built-in need to control our environment. We tend to hate and fear anything out of our control. Untamed animals are called 'wild' and seen as vicious and liable to attack and harm us, whereas almost all animals avoid humans, unless provoked by abuse. Native peoples are called 'savage' and are often seen as malevolent, whereas almost all indigenous peoples, including those still surviving in the Americas, Asia and Africa, avoid contact with industrialised people, unless terribly persecuted. And similarly, what we are now doing with bacteria, by systematic use of antibiotics, is bombing them into retaliation.

Certainly, just as there are some evil people in the world, there are some bacteria that carry deadly diseases, such as *Clostridium botulinum*, the bacterial cause of botulism, and *Yersinia pestis*, that of plague. But generally, the aggressive male language used by scientists

– of invasion, fighting, bullets, bombs, explosions, minefields and war – mislead us. With almost all bacteria, the best protection for good health is to learn how best to live with them: not war, but peace.

We strengthen our bodies by maintaining the same stance that well-balanced people maintain in order to live in harmony with each other: by mutual recognition, understanding and respect. And as with other people and as between nations, violence against bacteria breeds violence. Just as people are sometimes right to fight, and nations are sometimes right to declare war, sometimes we do need antibiotics.

But our best guard against infectious disease is our bodies' own immune strength, well-nourished and resilient.

In the futile war against bacteria, we are the losers. Saturation bombing of bacteria breeds drug-resistant superbugs, which, like an intelligent guerrilla army, become transformed, battle-hardened, dug-in and ineradicable. The more that antibiotics are overused and abused, the greater the threat to personal, communal and global human health. In modern wars, the only winners are the manufacturers of the weapons of war – and even they may be bombed one day.

Chemical farming and chemical medicine are parallel stories. At any point, the farmer is likely to enjoy an immediate benefit from the use of chemical weapons. The pests die; the crop grows. But every year the land becomes more dependent on biocides, and more vulnerable to superpests bred by the biocides. These new pests become a disaster when they multiply out of control, unchecked by their natural predators that have been killed by the chemicals. In the short term, the farmer gains. In the longer term, the whole agricultural system of his country and community, including his neighbours, his family and himself may lose.

We are now accustomed to headlines about the disastrous effects of pesticides on crops, the land, wildlife and the environment. We have seen many television programmes about the meaning to us and the world as a whole, of the destruction of the Brazilian rainforests and the erosion of the Antarctic ozone layer. We know that governments all over the world have accepted that the greenhouse effect may amount to a human-made global catastrophe and could even wreck the lives of future generations. We have now gained understanding of the place of nature in the world outside, of our own place in the world, and of the dangers – to the planet, to others and to ourselves – of disrupting that balance.

Curiously though, we still have little understanding of the balance of nature within us. It is time that we thought green about the last ecological frontier, the bacteria on and inside our bodies. We need our friendly flora.

Modern medicine still follows the obsolete germ theory of disease, developed by Louis Pasteur and the other 'microbe hunters' more than a century ago, according to which the only good bacteria are dead bacteria. The ascendancy of the germ theory, and its grip on our ideas about the meaning of health and disease, is the unfortunate result of a titanic nineteenth-century power struggle in which the wrong side won. Its myth persists.

SUMMARY OF PART 3

Countless millions of millions of bacteria live on our skin and within our bodies. These are almost all 'friendly flora' that have evolved in harmony with us, as an integral part of our digestive and immune systems. They preserve our good health, protect us against disease invasion by the micro-organisms that carry and are, in effect, a vital organ of the body. Unfortunately though, antibiotics were developed at a time when bacteria were typically thought to be unclean agents of disease. The war on germs, which has been waged by doctors with antibiotics for over half a century, is liable to devastate our protective bacteria and to make us more vulnerable to disease.

Part Four

Apocalypse Now:
How Antibiotics Breed Disease

Residing in the mouth and intestines, in the nose, in the skin – indeed, on practically all the surfaces and in practically all the orifices of the body – are myriads of bacteria. In the main they are harmless, but among them are forms which are capable of producing serious inflammations or disease. The most potent immediate protection against these harmful forms is an intact and healthy body surface. Only when the skin is broken or cut, only when the mucous membrane is weakened or damaged, are the conditions favourable for the invasion of our bodies by these foreign enemies.

Professor Walter Cannon
The Wisdom of the Body; 1932

In years to come, the story of antibiotics may rank as Nature's most malicious trick.

Professor Sandy Raeburn
Antibiotics and Immunodeficiency; 1972

12 Women and Children First

CYSTITIS: WOMEN'S SECOND CURSE

Girls and women now are vulnerable to infections of the urinary tract and bladder that are treated with antibiotics, and then sometimes recur and get worse. The second most common use of antibiotics in the UK is for urinary tract and bladder infections, notably cystitis, the medical term for inflammation of the bladder.

The urinary tract, leading from the exterior of the body to the bladder and then on to the kidneys, should be sterile. But nowadays, around two and a half million women in the UK suffer from cystitis in any one year, and about half of all women are sufferers at some time in their lives. Of these, around 100,000 are estimated to be 'problem patients', with symptoms recurring four or more times a year. In the USA it is reckoned that the cost of treating cystitis is around $2 billion a year.[1]

The symptoms of cystitis are a constant need to urinate, a burning and often intensely painful sensation when urinating, and pain in the lower back and groin. The disease is much more common in women than in men, because the female urinary tract is much shorter, and its opening in the vaginal area more vulnerable to infection. The most common infectious agents are bacteria, notably *E. coli* and others such as *S. epidermidis*, moving into the genital and then urinary tract, quite often after sexual intercourse, although females of all ages and all sexual backgrounds suffer from cystitis.

The pain, misery and embarrassment of cystitis is made worse when the disease constantly recurs. Antibiotics are the almost invariable treatment. The *Merck Manual*[2], used as a guide to prescribing by many general practitioners, states: 'For an initial course of therapy of uncomplicated infections, sulphonamides, tetracycline, ampicillin or amoxycillin, trimethoprim, or trimethoprim/ sulphamethoxazole [co-trimoxazole] usually are adequate.' For relapses, higher doses and longer courses, for up to four to six weeks, are suggested. If this doesn't work, a 'prophylactic regimen' is recommended, meaning a dose of drugs every day, or three times a week, or after sexual intercourse as a preventive measure. Because of the wide range of antibiotics used, cystitis therapy has many ill-effects.[3]

Doctors who follow the advice in their reference books and continually prescribe antibiotics to women with cystitis seem not to realise that the bifidobacteria and lactobacilli normally resident in a healthy vagina, including at the entrance to the urinary tract, protect against infection. Antibiotics may wipe out these friendly bacteria. Consequently other species, including normally harmless inhabitants of the gut, notably *E. coli*, and of the skin, notably *S. epidermidis*, can pass into the urinary tract, where they cause superinfectious disease.

Dr Gregor Reid, director of urology research at the University of Toronto, works on the effects of antibiotics on cystitis. With colleagues, he has carried out a study of 70 women, published in 1990.[4] Its conclusion is that antibiotic treatment of cystitis is liable to destroy protective bacteria, which are then replaced by dangerous species. 'Examination of the urogenital flora post therapy showed that an indigenous lactobacillus population had not been restored in the majority of patients. Rather, uropathogenic bacteria were found to dominate.' And these superinfectious bacteria became superbugs, developing resistance to various antibiotics. They also mutated in other ways, developing an adhesive quality; this makes them much harder to treat.

Antibiotics can and do cure cystitis. But they can also make the disease recur, and they can make it worse. In the case of recurrent cystitis, antibiotics are, in a sense, drugs of dependency. The more that women take antibiotics to treat cystitis, the more they may have to take them, to keep the infection at bay. Women with cystitis too often turn to antibiotics – 'that little bottle by your bedside' – almost as women given prescription drugs for anxiety crave tranquillisers. The difference is that antibiotics are still generally believed to be benign drugs.

THE WORST START IN LIFE

Natural resistance to infectious disease is developed from the moment of birth. At birth, a baby's gut is sterile, empty of bacteria.

Then, in the first few days of life, the gut becomes populated with countless millions of bacteria. What matters is whether the species of bacteria that colonise the infant gut protect health or cause disease.

We are all so indoctrinated with the Domestos theory of human health, with the idea that, for babies and young children above all, the only healthy environment is sterile, that the thought of bacteria teeming inside a tiny baby is likely to be a worrying one. But the right type of bacteria are crucial to the baby's ability to resist disease.

As in adults almost all the bacteria in the gut of a healthy normal breastfed infant comprise two types of bacillus: bifidobacteria, including lactobacilli; and bacteroides, the bacteria that also protect the vagina and cervix against infection. They colonise the newborn baby as it passes through the vagina of its mother. Bifidobacteria are themselves nourished by breastmilk, and produce lactic acid that has an antibiotic effect on potentially harmful bacteria by keeping the infant gut relatively acidic.[5]

So mother and baby are bonded together in a wonderful eco-system, with the mother's body and milk protecting her baby's health. And the *vernix caseosa*, the greasy substance that covers the baby's body at birth, is itself a natural protection against infection. The passing of bacteria from mother to child, and the nourishment of these bacteria with breastmilk, which also contains important anti-bodies from the mother, are all vital to the baby's resistance to infection as it grows. What all this means is that the health of the infant is best protected by an old-fashioned messy birth, by the baby's physical bonding with its mother, and by breastmilk.[6] The more that birth is a natural process, with mother and baby given support without interference, the better.

A lot can go wrong with this process. Birth by Caesarean section increases the chance of colonisation of the infant gut with pathogenic bacteria. Infant formula milk used instead of breastmilk does not nourish bifidobacteria; a bottle-fed baby is much more likely than a breastfed baby to become superinfected with coliforms such as *E. coli* and clostridia such as *C. difficile*, which cause diarrhoea.[7]

Antibiotics have a profound effect on the gut flora of infants. Several studies have shown that antibiotics given to protect infants against infection actually cause superinfection not only with *E. coli* and clostridia, but also with species of klebsiella that cause pneumonia and meningitis, and of pseudomonas and proteus bacilli that cause various bacterial diseases.[3]

Such superinfections may be caused by antibiotics used not only as medicine for the infant, but also for other purposes. The mother's vagina and nipples may be treated with antibiotic creams or sprays. If she herself takes antibiotics in pregnancy or when nursing, these will pass into her baby's body in the womb or later in breastmilk. When a nursing mother uses antibiotics, their concentration in her milk will be much the same as in her blood.

Worse news for a newborn baby are the dangerous bacteria that infest hospitals. These may be hardy superbugs, resistant to many antibiotics, that breed in hospitals and on hospital doctors and nurses, who thus become unwitting carriers of disease. A baby born in a hospital whose microbiological environment has gone haywire as a result of incessant use of antibiotics over the years, to a mother who herself may well be using antibiotics, is prey to infections themselves treated with antibiotics. And so the baby takes its first steps on the drug treadmill.

When newborn babies suffer serious infections in hospital, and their lives are saved by dedicated doctors and nurses, grateful parents are not told that the essential underlying cause of the infection may well have been antibiotics that disrupt microbial ecosystems both in the hospital and in the human gut.

Childbirth in hospital is relatively safe now, thanks largely to hygienic practice; few newborn and young babies die from bacterial or other infections. And like older children and adults, babies generally recover a healthy balance of resident gut bacteria after individual courses of antibiotics. But not always. And repeated courses are dangerous, especially at vulnerable times of life: an infant constantly exposed to antibiotics may grow into a child constantly suffering from infections. What makes antibiotics insidious is that infections suffered in childhood or as an adult can never certainly be traced back to infancy. Parents know their children are vulnerable to infections; but why, they don't know.

SUFFERING LITTLE CHILDREN

Children now are vulnerable to infections of the ear, nose and throat that are treated with antibiotics, and which then may recur and get worse.

'But what would you do if you were a parent and your child woke up in the middle of the night in agony from pain caused by infection?' Alternatively: 'But if you were a doctor and a mother brought her child to you crying out in pain, what would you do?' I am often asked questions like these. They invite the answer: 'Well, of course in such circumstances I'd forget all these theories about antibiotics being a problem. Of course a doctor should give antibiotics to a child in great pain.' But is this the right answer?

The common childhood infection most often mentioned in this context, especially by parents I know, is otitis media – inflammation of the middle ear, specifically of the Eustachian tube, the passage between the nose and throat and the eardrum. Middle-ear inflammation is now very common, afflicting around one in five British children under the age of four every year, and is often treated not only with drugs but also, in severe cases, with surgery.[8]

Antibiotics are indeed the treatment chosen by physicians for middle-ear infections. An indication of recent British medical practice is given in the 1981 edition of *Black's Medical Dictionary*:

> Treatment consists of the immediate administration of an antibiotic, and the one of choice is usually penicillin . . . It cannot be emphasised too strongly that if otitis media is treated immediately with ample doses of the appropriate antibiotic, the chances of any permanent damage to the ear or to hearing is reduced to a negligible degree.

General practitioners are reckoned to prescribe antibiotics for 97 per cent of cases diagnosed as otitis media. The drug of choice for young children is now amoxycillin.

Middle-ear inflammation is one of a number of childhood diseases, such as asthma, childhood (type 1, insulin-dependent) diabetes and eczema, now much more common in the UK than they were in the early twentieth century. Drug and other therapy may work for individual cases of these diseases, but have not been able to reduce their overall incidence.

Children commonly suffer from various viral or bacterial infections of the respiratory tract – the passage from the mouth to the lungs. Otitis media is a complication of such infections. Like the digestive tract, the upper respiratory tract is richly populated with bacteria. Because the mouth and nose are open to the atmosphere, immune defences against invasion of the respiratory tract are strong. Saliva and mucus in the mouth and throat contain the natural antibiotic lysozyme. Tiny hairs in the nose and throat sweep out foreign particles. The inner immune system operates everywhere in the body, as needed. But the chief protection that children – like adults – have against infections of the respiratory tract are their own resident bacteria. Like those in the gut, these live on and in the respiratory tract lining, have evolved so that they are not affected by lysozyme, are not identified as invaders by the inner immune system, and resist colonisation by foreign bacteria.

A healthy body fights infection, but every now and then, anybody is liable to suffer inflammation of the respiratory tract, which may cause a runny nose, aches and pains in the head, throat or chest, cough, fever and/or general malaise. Inflammation may be caused by infection with viruses or bacteria. The common cold is a viral disease. Other infections – such as tonsillitis, laryngitis, pharyngitis or bronchitis, named after the sites of inflammation, and the plainly named sore throat, are usually caused either by viruses or by smoke and other toxic irritants, less often by bacteria. Simple infections usually last only a week or two; the best treatment, especially for a child, is rest, and loving care and perhaps a painkiller. Natural recovery from infection involves a natural learning process during which the body's immune system becomes more resilient, better able to resist future infection.

But the microbiological ecosystems that naturally protect children against infection are disrupted by antibiotics. Many young children are frequently given a course of antibiotics, sometimes for illnesses that are not bacterial in origin, sometimes 'just in case' a simple bacterial infection becomes invasive. Few children avoid antibiotics nowadays. The result of continual disruption of the natural balance of bacteria in the body, including the respiratory tract, can be vicious superinfections and the breeding of multi drug-resistant superbugs, not to mention direct ill-effects of the drugs; and the prospect of continual infections not only of the respiratory tract but also the gut and elsewhere in the body, which the immature immune system of a child struggles to overcome.

Babies and young children are also exposed to antibiotics not only from breastmilk (if the mother is taking antibiotics) but also at very low levels from cows' milk and from meat and dairy products (from animals treated with antibiotics). It is generally thought that trace amounts of drugs in food are not a problem to human health.

If middle-ear infections are bacterial, the infectious agent is almost always *Haemophilus influenzae*, *Streptococcus pneumoniae*, or *Streptococcus pyogenes*. These may all be found, in small quantities, in the normal healthy ear, nose, mouth and throat. But when the resident symbiotic bacteria are wiped out by an antibiotic, normally commensal bacteria such as *Strep. pneumoniae* or *pyogenes* may survive, multiply, stick to the mucous membrane and invade the Eustachian tube. Sometimes this superinfection will develop with no ill-effects, or just with a mild stuffed-up feeling, and then fade away as the invading bacteria are dissolved naturally. At other times, the bacteria continue to multiply, creating sticky bacterial debris (pus) inside the middle ear; pressure builds up, the eardrum becomes inflamed, and the child may suffer intense pain. This is the point when a doctor is likely to diagnose otitis media and prescribe more antibiotics.

Both parents and doctors want to relieve a child's pain and prevent complications, and antibiotics do check or kill bacteria. However, antibiotics are not painkillers. The quick, practical way to relieve pain caused by middle-ear infection is to give decongestant nosedrops and, if necessary, an analgesic (painkiller) formulated for children. By these means, and a warm heating pad, plus tender loving care, pain may be relieved in half an hour, and the infection will clear up by itself, usually within two days.

So what about antibiotics? Four reports published in the British medical press[8] have all come to the same conclusion: that antibiotics are usually the wrong treatment for middle-ear infections. A large Dutch trial has suggested that most children not given antibiotics recover just as quickly with painkillers and nosedrops. Another study using the records of general practitioners from nine countries came to a more radical conclusion: children not given antibiotics are, if anything, more likely to recover. And in 1990, the opinion of specialists at Leicester Royal Infirmary was: 'Antibiotics have no place in the initial treatment of acute otitis media because they have no effect on the long-term recurrence of the disease over the succeeding twelve months.'

I asked medical microbiologist Professor Richard Lacey for his opinion. He told me: 'Painkillers should be the mainstay of any drug treatment. Anxious parents should be told that antibiotics are very rarely helpful, and indeed might be damaging both in the short and long term.

As with cystitis, the best way to avoid otitis media is to stay off the antibiotic treadmill, or else to get off it. This is often easier said than done.

What about the common sore throat? Professor Lacey's recommendation is much the same.[9]

> About 80 per cent of sore throats are viral. Most of the remainder are due to *S. pyogenes*. Antibiotics are prescribed as a safeguard, in case the disease is due to bacteria. Of course, antibiotics have no effect on viruses. The main reason given for prescribing antibiotics is actually not because they have any major effect in lessening symptoms, but in order to reduce the risk of the serious complication, rheumatic fever. But rheumatic fever is now virtually extinct in the UK. The case is now overwhelming for not treating the great majority of sore throats, or tonsillitis, with antibiotics.

13 Superinfections of the Gut

BREAKING DOWN OUR DEFENCES

Microbiologists have known for half a century that antibiotics create superinfections and superbugs – that is, for almost as long as biologists have known that pesticides cause superpests. Curiously, though, while the ill-effects of pesticides have been publicised for 30 years[10], almost all discussion about the ill-effects of antibiotics on microbial ecology and thus on human health has been confined to the scientific literature.

Some of the studies showing that antibiotics break down the body's defences against disease have been reviewed by Professor David Hentges in the textbook *Human Intestinal Microflora in Health and Disease.*[11] To check what he said, I obtained copies of some of the key research papers he cites. They make disturbing reading.

Diarrhoeal diseases range from simple diarrhoea and gastroenteritis caused by food poisoning to dysentery and the potentially deadly cholera. In the 1950s, Professor Rolf Freter, head of the department of microbiology at the University of Michigan, showed that experimental animals given antibiotics become vulnerable to drug-resistant strains of *Shigella flexneri*, a carrier of dysentery, and of *Vibrio cholerae*, the carrier of cholera.[12] In 1959, Professor Philip Miller, head of the Department of Medicine at the University of Chicago, reported the results of a classic experiment.[13] Half of a group of mice were given the antibiotic streptomycin by stomach tube; the other half were given saline solution. Then *Salmonella enteritidis* bacteria, the carriers of one of the food poisoning epidemics in Britain, were introduced. The result was that, while mice normally need to absorb between 100,000 and a million salmonella bacteria before showing signs of infection, the number needed after the dose of streptomycin was just ten bacteria. In other words, antibiotics made these animals at least 10,000 times more vulnerable to infection. Penicillin, ampicillin and tetracycline can also make people more vulnerable to salmonella infection.[14]

Laboratory experiments have demonstrated that antibiotics cause superinfections. A number of studies have shown that antibiotics wipe out anaerobic bacteria in the guts of animals, allowing *Candida albicans* to multiply.[15] Other experiments have shown that ampicillin, cephalosporins, clindamycin and other antibiotics make both animals and humans vulnerable to pseudomembranous colitis, caused by superinfectious *Clostridium difficile*.[16] It is also likely that healthy gut flora protect against superinfection with *Clostridium botulinum*, the agent of botulism, a deadly infection.[17]

With colleagues, Dr Hentges has himself demonstrated that a series of antibiotics – including streptomycin, ampicillin and metronidazole – make animals vulnerable to superinfection with *Pseudomonas aeruginosa*, the agent of septicaemia that sometimes kills cancer patients and other seriously ill people in hospital.[18]

Cautious experiments on human volunteers support the animal work. For example, Professor Sherwood Gorbach and colleagues have studied the ill-effects of four broad-spectrum betalactams given by injection to healthy volunteers. Two of the drugs caused superinfection with bacteria; the other two caused fungal superinfection. In the case of one drug, a cephalosporin, 'the normal flora was essentially replaced by yeasts.'[19] Dr Hendrik van Saene and colleagues have given volunteers doses of amoxycillin, followed by the pathogenic *Klebsiella oxytoca*, which, in five out of the nine cases, 'were able to colonise the intestine, with clinical symptoms of severe diarrhoea in one'.[20]

Antibiotics do cause superinfections and superbugs. There's no doubt about that. But how great a threat is this to human health?

The body does have natural healing powers. As already stated, the bacteria that protect healthy people are generally resilient, and usually become dominant again after a course of antibiotics is finished. Courses of properly prescribed antibiotics for serious bacterial infections, taken very occasionally – say, on average once every five or ten years – are unlikely to do any lasting damage to normally healthy adults. The risk increases with broad-spectrum antibiotics, and with heavy, long or repeated doses. The most vulnerable times of life are during infancy and old age. Hospital patients are also vulnerable, particularly if they are very ill or debilitated, and surgical patients most of all.

COLITIS THAT CAN KILL

Acute gut disorders caused by antibiotics may be painful, but are usually transient: after some days of diarrhoea, and maybe also sickness, fever or cramps, the body rids itself of poison. Sometimes, though, superinfections caused by antibiotics are harder to shake off.

The most acutely dangerous superinfection of the gut is pseudomembranous colitis. It can be a horrible and occasionally fatal disease whose symptoms virtually begin during or just after a course of antibiotics. The first sign is severe, often bloody diarrhoea. In severe cases the colon becomes grossly inflamed and, in bad cases, scarred and rotten, and may even break, flooding the abdominal cavity with poison (peritonitis). In the worst, fatal cases, autopsy shows that the mucosal lining of the colon has become covered by a sheath of dead and rotting cells – hence, 'pseudomembranous'.[21]

Incidence of pseudomembranous colitis increased in the 1960s and 1970s, and its cause was agreed in 1977. In killing off the friendly resident flora, antibiotics can cause superinfection of the gut with *Clostridium difficile*, which without antibiotics is occasionally present in the healthy gut in insignificant numbers. Very toxic strains of *C. difficile* do the damage.

At first it was thought that lincomycin and clindamycin, two antibiotics developed in the 1970s particularly to treat infections caused by anaerobic bacteria, were the sole cause. Between 1964 and 1978, 23 deaths were reported to the UK Committee on Safety of Medicines.

It turns out that not only lincomycin and clindamycin but most antibiotics can cause pseudomembranous colitis: notably penicillins (ampicillin and amoxycillin in particular) and cephalosporins and also chloramphenicol, sulphonamides, tetracyclines, metronidazole and quinolones.[22] To guard against the disease, the *Merck Manual* warns doctors: 'If significant diarrhoea occurs during antibiotic administration, the antibiotic should be stopped immediately, unless its use is absolutely essential.'

Most victims of pseudomembranous colitis are old and very ill people in hospital. Dr Peter Borriello, now of University Hospital, Nottingham, who has made a special study of *C. difficile*, sees the colitis it causes as a remarkable example of why preservation of colonisation resistance in the gut is so vitally important. Interviewed for this book, he said: 'What is so interesting about *C. difficile* is that it will only infect following compromise of the normal gut flora, classically with antibiotics, or with anything else having antimicrobial activity. I could give you ten to the power of 12 [i.e. 10 million million] organisms of *C. difficile* and nothing would happen. I could give you one of a number of antibiotics first and then give you ten organisms of *C. difficile* and you would go down with diarrhoea. With *C. difficile*, the colonisation resistance is everything or nothing. We don't know why that is.'

Constant use of antibiotics in hospitals has turned *C. difficile* into a menace, infecting millions of patients a year.[22] One study in the USA has found that over one in five in-patients became colonised with potentially toxic *C. difficile* while in hospital. A UK study has found that one in three elderly hospitalised people were similarly colonised.

The bacterium is carried from ward to ward by hospital staff on their hands, under rings, and on stethoscopes. It lives on hospital floors and in bedding, furniture, mops, bedpans and toilets. The incidence of suffering and death from *C. difficile* colitis increases in the colder months of the year, when elderly and infirm people are treated with broad-spectrum antibiotics for respiratory diseases like bronchitis and pneumonia. The very expensive and relatively toxic antibiotic vancomycin normally works against *C. difficile* colitis, but the disease is thereafter liable to flare up again, and also to recur whenever other antibiotics are used by hospital doctors or general practitioners for other infections.

The UK Department of Health has identified *C. difficile* colitis caused by antibiotics as an urgent and important public health problem. A consequent special expert meeting held in London in March 1993 reported that the disease as measured by toxins identified in laboratory examination has steadily increased from 121 cases reported in 1982 to 1,643 in 1992. There will be an estimated one million people aged 85 or over living in the UK in the year 2000, of whom around 75,000 will at any time be in hospital on broad-spectrum antibiotics for respiratory diseases. The expert meeting concluded: 'There is no doubt that *C. difficile* will be a major problem in the 21st century'.[23] So will broad-spectrum antibiotics.

THE INFLAMED BOWEL MYSTERY

Are there other diseases of the gut that may be caused by antibiotics? Any such disease would have become more common in the last half-century. Three candidates are irritable bowel syndrome, ulcerative colitis and Crohn's disease.

Irritable bowel syndrome – also called simple colitis or spastic colon – is at some time now suffered by up to one third of British people, and by twice as many women as men. Commonly, the disease starts in early life, and never clears up. Half of all the people in the UK who go with gut disorders to general practitioners are suffering from irritable bowel. The symptoms include stomach ache, bloating, flatulence, alternating diarrhoea and constipation, headache and fever. Some physicians believe it is 'all in the mind'.[24]

Much more serious are ulcerative colitis and Crohn's disease, both of which are also known as 'inflammatory bowel disease'. Together, they afflict up to 100,000 people in the UK. They also commonly start in early life, and usually do not clear up; one review in the *British Medical Journal* has said: 'Crohn's disease will remain a life sentence until a specific treatment is found.' Symptoms include severe pain and bloody diarrhoea. Ulcerative colitis is confined to the colon (lower part of the large intestine); Crohn's disease may spread throughout the colon and ileum (lowest part of the small intestine) and sometimes throughout the entire digestive tract. Both diseases inflame the intestines and can wreck them. Drugs and diet are used with some success to calm symptoms. In severe cases, surgery with or without colostomy or ileostomy (involving an artificial anus constructed through the abdominal wall) is used, to cut out the diseased portion of the gut, and often has to be repeated as the illness spreads. The number of British children under the age of sixteen suffering from Crohn's disease tripled between the 1960s and the 1980s. People with ulcerative colitis are vulnerable to bowel cancer.[25]

Irritable bowel syndrome can be severe, and ulcerative colitis and Crohn's disease can be mild. On autopsy, they look different, but general practitioners often find it difficult to tell which disease is which. They also baffle modern medical science. The *Merck Manual* says of irritable bowel syndrome: 'No anatomic cause can be found', and classifies the disease as 'functional', which is medical code for: 'We can't find anything physically wrong.' Of inflammatory bowel disease generally, the *Manual* says: 'The etiology of this group of diseases is unknown,' which means: 'We can see there's something physically wrong, but we don't know what's causing it.' Irritable bowel syndrome, Crohn's disease and ulcerative colitis are all mystery diseases.

It is unlikely that any of these diseases has one sole cause. Many things can irritate, injure or corrupt the gut. Five theories have been proposed in the medical literature in recent years. One, stress. The problem with this theory is that, while emotion and anxiety do affect the gut, stressed people in many parts of the world rarely suffer inflammatory bowel diseases. Two, that the cause is allergy to wheat (gluten intolerance) or to cows' milk (coeliac disease). The problem here is that, while both wheat and cows' milk can cause irritation and inflammation of the gut in people who as babies were weaned prematurely on to solid foods, this doesn't account for ulcerative colitis or Crohn's disease; besides which, many people with irritable bowels do not improve on a diet without wheat or cows' milk. Three, that many gut diseases are caused by chemicals such as those contained in smoke, pesticides and some food additives: and it is true that patients sometimes do improve in a pollution-free environment.

Some specialist physicians believe in either a fourth theory, that any or all of these diseases may be caused by the typical Western diet, notably a diet heavy in sugar; or in a fifth one, that the problem is multiple food allergy to any of a great number of foods containing natural chemicals to which the body reacts as if they are poisons. Both these theories have some therapeutic value; people with gut diseases often do improve on a wholefood diet with allergenic foods removed. But the sugar theory does not explain why twice as many people suffer from Crohn's disease now, given that sugar consumption in the 1950s was much the same as it is now. And it seems very unlikely that many common foods – including whole fresh foods that have nourished people all over the world and throughout history – should suddenly become toxic in Western countries without any underlying cause.

None of these five theories is altogether convincing. The medical profession is baffled: when drugs fail, the treatment on offer includes the same sort of surgical mutilation performed by Sir Arbuthnot Lane a century ago. A general review in the *Lancet* says:[26]

> Colitis can introduce uncertainty into every plan, may restrict activities or ambition, and poses questions for which there is often no medical answer . . . The public knows little of colitis and finds it hard to understand and accept the disability. Doctors do not know the cause of colitis, may give conflicting advice about diet (which seems an obvious form of treatment) and cannot relieve uncertainty about

the future course of the illness. Most patients are aware of a cancer risk but repress this fear . . . A frank talk often reveals that a patient fears cancer and dreads an ileostomy.

INFECTIONS THAT ARE NOT INFECTIOUS

'Colitis' is a vague diagnosis; it is a name for a range of disorders and diseases of the colon that may cause moderate or severe pain in the gut. Can antibiotics sometimes cause irritable bowel which persists after the course of drugs is complete? Judging from the work of Dr John Hunter, a consultant gastroenterologist at Addenbrooke's Hospital in Cambridge, who with colleagues has been studying colitis for some years, it looks as if the answer is yes.[27]

Dr Hunter noticed that many of his patients suffered irritable bowels after either a bout of diarrhoea or a course of antibiotics, or else after surgery – during which they were likely to have been given antibiotics. So he decided to check out whether antibiotics were a possible cause of the disease. In one study, he kept a check on a total of 113 women who had been admitted to hospital for a hysterectomy (removal of the womb). Of these, 74 were operated on by surgeons who, as routine prophylaxis, used the antibiotic metronidazole, an imidazole that works specifically against anaerobic bacteria – the type that dominate in the healthy gut. The other 39 women had surgeons who did not use antibiotics for this purpose. Six weeks after their operations, 12 of the 74 women who had been treated with antibiotics had developed irritable bowels; whereas of the 39 without antibiotics, only one had similar symptoms.

Further work by Dr Hunter has shown that people with irritable bowels usually have more – sometimes vastly more – aerobic bacteria in their gut compared with healthy people. This suggests that one important cause of irritable bowel is bacterial superinfection: when the normally dominant gut bacteria are killed off, there is room for more adaptable species to flourish, and these may give off toxins that damage the gut wall.[27]

What about the more serious inflammatory bowel diseases? Diarrhoea, when caused by adaptable aerobic bacteria invading the body, is infectious – it is passed on from one victim to another. But ulcerative colitis and Crohn's disease, together with irritable bowel syndrome, are not infectious. So it's safe to say that these diseases are not caused by micro-organisms from the outside environment. For this reason, scientists have until recently assumed that inflammatory bowel diseases have nothing to do with bacteria. However, infections may not be infectious. If inflammatory bowel diseases are caused by superinfection with bacterial species normally found in small quantities in the gut, and if these bacteria are causing damage because of changes in the internal environment of the individual, they would not be infectious.

Starting in the 1950s, scientists became interested in the part that altered gut flora may play in bowel diseases. The bacterial species most studied is *Escherichia coli.* As you now know, *E. coli* lives in relatively small numbers in the normal healthy gut. It is adaptable, able to live without or with oxygen. Just as a flower becomes a weed when it grows in the wrong place or multiplies out of control, *E. coli* is a cause of disease when it moves from the gut into open surgical wounds, causing septicaemia, or into the urinary tract, causing cystitis, or when it becomes superinfectious in the gut. *E. coli*, together with streptococci and some other species, were the bacteria found in abnormal profusion in the guts of Dr Hunter's irritable bowel patients.

There are two other circumstances in which *E. coli* and other normally harmless bacteria can damage the gut. First, under selective pressure their genetic structure can change, subtly, in ways that may make them more virulent and more invasive not only in quantity but also in quality. Dr Richard Dickinson of the Hinchingbrooke Hospital in Cambridgeshire has identified what he describes as 'adhesive or invasive' strains of *E. coli* in the guts of people suffering from ulcerative colitis.[28] Also, if the mucous membrane lining the gut and the gut wall itself become damaged, then *E. coli* and other bacteria can penetrate into such lesions and may cause extensive damage.

What can cause such dangerous changes in normally harmless bacteria living in the gut and the mucosal lining of the gut wall? One answer is antibiotics themselves. They can penetrate the mucous membrane and irritate the gut wall. Further, in Dr Dirk van der Waaij's words, they can 'peel the "anaerobic wallpaper" off the gut wall', leaving bare patches which become attachment sites for superinfectious bacteria. Dr van der Waaij proposes that 'colonisation by potentially pathogenic bacteria is perhaps only possible when they have found open patches in the otherwise confluent "anaerobic wallpaper" of the colon.'[29]

A word of caution. Antibiotics cannot of course be the sole underlying cause of irritable and inflammatory bowel diseases. Apart from Crohn's disease, identified by Dr Burrill Crohn in the 1930s, these diseases were well known before the development of antibiotics, and like inflammation or ulceration elsewhere on or in the body, will have many causes. For example, invasive aerobic bacteria from the outside environment can alter the microbial ecology of the gut and damage the gut wall: as one example, Dr Dickinson and colleagues noted in 1989 that ulcerative colitis can be a complication of gastroenteritis caused by *Salmonella enteritidis* or *S. typhimurium*[30] (although what bred the salmonella and made them invasive is another story connected with antibiotics). Chemical pollutants and other drugs such as anaesthetics can also damage the gut wall.

However, the proposal that antibiotics, especially when taken in heavy doses over a long period of time, are one key underlying cause of a number of serious, crippling, and even on occasion eventually fatal non-infectious diseases of the gut is biologically plausible, consistent with known facts, and explains some otherwise puzzling features of these diseases.

Put it this way. It is known that antibiotics are liable to devastate gut flora and can, especially as a result of prolonged doses, damage the mucosal lining of the gut wall. It is also known that an exposed gut wall is liable to become inflamed and all the more so if continually exposed to the source of inflammation. On the other hand, much of what happens inside the gut of living people remains a mystery to medical science. More well-designed research is of course needed. Meanwhile it is surely a matter of elementary prudence in the case of anybody who has taken antibiotics, especially over a long period of time, and who also is suffering gut disorders, to suspect the drugs.

WHEN THE GUT EATS ITSELF

The idea that inflammatory bowel diseases are caused by deranged gut flora has been around for a long time. Papers published in scientific journals by leading researchers, as long ago as 1950 and then in 1972, proposed that these diseases are caused by *E. coli* and other normally harmless gut flora not only penetrating the mucosal lining of the gut wall, but also interfering with its inner immune defences. In the mid-1980s, other scientists, including teams from St

Bartholomew's Hospital in London and from the applied microbiology department of the British Public Health Laboratory Service, came to much the same conclusion.[31]

In 1982, Dr Hendrik van Saene summarised this theory in his book *Pathogenesis of Inflammatory Bowel Diseases*[32]. He proposed that a combination of superinfectious bacteria and an exposed gut wall can indeed cause auto-immune diseases of the gut. The body's own inner immune defences go haywire and cannot distinguish between 'self' and 'non-self', food and poison. The result is that the gut eats itself. And it looks as if one key initial cause of this disaster is antibiotics.

The theory that ulcerative colitis and Crohn's disease are both auto-immune diseases is controversial but powerful. It explains why these diseases are sometimes triggered by emotional stress, which can make a vulnerable gut more sensitive. It explains why common features of these diseases are allergic-type reactions to normally healthy and nutritious foods or, to be more precise, to constituents of these foods that antagonise an exposed inner immune system. And it explains why inflammatory diseases of the gut often react unpredictably to drugs, that may relieve symptoms but then cause more microbiological imbalance.

Auto-immune diseases sometimes clear up, as the body succeeds in healing itself. More often they drag on, as the damage and the healing in the body reach a kind of balance, with periods of relapse and recovery. Sometimes they get steadily worse, causing irreversible damage and even eventual death. These are all features of inflammatory bowel diseases. The evidence that antibiotics are involved is strongest in the case of Crohn's disease; the history of this disease coincides with that of antibiotics. Also, Crohn's disease attacks the gut in a peculiar patchy way; the diseased parts may be those in which superinfectious bacteria have stripped off the protective 'anaerobic wallpaper'.

The mucosal lining of the gut is certainly a vital protection, not only against diseases of the gut itself, but also against invasion of dangerous micro-organisms through the gut wall, and friendly gut flora are an integral part of this protection. Anybody who regularly takes antibiotics that kill the anaerobic bacteria that dominate in a healthy gut certainly runs a risk of gut disease. As ever, prudent advice is to use antibiotics only when you really must, for genuinely dangerous bacterial infections.[33]

If antibiotics are an underlying cause of inflammatory bowel diseases they may also be a cause of allergic-type reactions. Most people with irritable bowel syndrome are liable to suffer ill-effects from normally nourishing food. Symptoms include headache, fatigue, anxiety, depression, nausea, itchy skin and rashes, running nose, aching joints and diarrhoea.[34] Victims improve on 'exclusion' diets in which the foods that cause the symptoms are gradually eliminated from the diet. This condition is commonly called 'food intolerance', sometimes diagnosed as a mental illness.

According to a paper published in the *Lancet* in 1991, Dr John Hunter thinks that a more likely explanation is that 'patients with food intolerance have an abnormal gut flora.'[35] I asked Professor Richard Lacey what he thought. He wrote:

> When a patient swallows an antibiotic – for example, for a sore throat – some of the antibiotic will persist in the intestine and destroy some of our useful bacteria. This can then permit unusual or foreign bacteria to proliferate. This is generally agreed. The following is somewhat more speculative. The theory goes that, if we radically alter the balance of bacteria in the gut, the newly dominant species can react with chemicals in food in the gut, in such a way as to make the body's immune system react to them as poisons. The result is that foods containing these chemical compounds will make us ill.

ARTHRITIS: ANOTHER MEDICAL MYSTERY

A remarkable number of serious diseases are officially classified as mysteries, with no known cause. Two more examples are rheumatoid arthritis, and another form of arthritis called ankylosing spondylitis, both of which have become common in the twentieth century, now afflicting up to two million people in Britain, and both of which often start to cause stiffness, inflammation and pain in early adult life.

Rheumatoid arthritis erodes the joints throughout the body, particularly in the arms, hands, legs and feet. It is over twice more common in women than in men. Ankylosing spondylitis has a similar effect at first on the pelvis and then on the spine (*spondylos* is the Greek word for vertebra). It is three times more common in men.

For decades now, scientists have been inclined to believe that arthritic conditions in their various forms are auto-immune diseases, causes unknown. Now, after more than ten years of research, Dr Alan Ebringer and colleagues at King's College, London, believe they may have the answer. Their story is a remarkable extension of that already told in the case of inflammatory bowel diseases.[36]

In the 1970s, Dr Ebringer found that the bodies of people suffering from ankylosing spondylitis produce an immune response to *Klebsiella pneumoniae* bacteria – a parallel finding to that of Dr van Saene, who found that the bodies of people suffering from inflammatory bowel disease produce an immune response to *Escherichia coli*. Like *E. coli*, *K. pneumoniae* is a bacillus that normally inhabits the healthy gut in small quantities. An immune response to a bacterial species that is normally harmless suggests that it has changed its nature and become invasive. Dr Ebringer, a reader in immunology at King's, concludes that anakylosing spondylitis is caused by deep penetration of *K. pneumoniae* through the gut wall, and thence through the lymphatic tissue connecting the gut to the pelvic wall, and thence on to the backbone.

In the mid-1980s, Dr Ebringer and his colleagues made a parallel discovery in the case of rheumatoid arthritis. They think that the cause of this disease may be invasion of the body by *Proteus mirabilis*, also an inhabitant of the normal healthy gut (and after *E. coli*, the most common cause of urinary tract infection). In the case both of ankylosing spondylitis and of rheumatoid arthritis, the erosion of bone and the pain in joints are, in Dr Ebringer's view, caused by constant inflammatory responses to the invading bacteria.

In December 1990, a paper in the *British Medical Journal* by a team from the Department of Infectious Diseases at the University Hospital in Linkoping, Sweden[37], proposed that another form of the disease, reactive arthritis, is caused by repeated inflammatory responses not to the body's own flora, but to pathogenic bacteria invading from outside the body, notably the bacillus *Yersinia enterocolitica*.

In his classic book *The Wisdom of the Body*, written in the early 1930s before antibiotics were developed and before the vital function of gut flora was known, physiologist Professor Walter Cannon stated[38]: 'When disease-carrying bacteria get a foothold, they may do harm in one or more of three ways: they may attack locally, they may produce locally a poison which can enter the blood and injure the organism extensively, or they can enter the bloodstream and produce widespread damage.' It follows that anything liable to damage the gut walls makes us vulnerable to bacteria passing through into other vital organs.

What now makes so many people vulnerable to deep penetration by bacteria such as *K. pneumoniae, P. mirabilis* and *Y. enterocolitica*? One answer is a damaged gut lining: as with inflammatory bowel diseases, an intact gut lining, itself protected by the bacterial species that have evolved within the gut, is a natural shield against disease. And what damages the gut lining? One answer is antibiotics.

As with Dr John Hunter, the pioneering findings of Dr Alan Ebringer and his colleagues are significant but need to be confirmed by other well-designed research before they can be classed as solid evidence. Again, as with serious gut disorders, an association between antibiotics and some auto-immune diseases makes biological sense. If Dr Ebringer is right, it looks as if the more antibiotics you take, the greater your risk of some forms of arthritis.

14 Feeling Ill All Over

SUPERINFECTIOUS MOULD

Bacteria are not the only type of micro-organism that normally live harmlessly in the human body and which, after courses of antibiotics, are liable to multiply out of control into superinfections. So may moulds and fungi which, being eukaryotic, are unaffected by antibiotics designed to check or kill bacteria. As already stated, fungal superinfections are a common result of the heavy use of antibiotics.

Like mushrooms and toadstools, the microscopic moulds and fungi that live on or in the human body flourish in damp conditions. Common fungal infections of the skin are of the feet (athlete's foot) and the crutch (*tinea cruris*). Ringworm is a fungal infection commonly of the skin or nails.

Of the various moulds that infest humans, *Candida albicans* is the best known. This commonly invades the female genital organs as a result of repeated antibiotic treatment for urinary tract infections. In this form, candida superinfection is known as thrush; it is evident as a creamy, smelly ooze. Symptoms of thrush include an itching and painful vagina, likely to make sexual intercourse unpleasant or impossible. Thrush also occurs in the mouth and sometimes on the male genitals.[39]

Candida albicans and the other moulds and yeasts that live in the gut are potential parasites. Rather like the spores of dry rot that float about in every house, doing no good but also no harm until circumstances allow them to multiply and take root, candida is normally held in check by the gut's resident bacteria. But anybody given repeated doses especially of broad-spectrum antibiotics runs a risk of literally going mouldy.

The standard textbook *Antimicrobial Therapy*[40] says: 'In general, the worst culprits are broad-spectrum antibiotics such as the tetracyclines, ampicillin, and cephalosporins;' and goes on to say:

'Occasionally, this overgrowth may extend throughout the gut and produce a serious enterocolitis.' When candida and other fungi become superinfectious, they can be treated with anti-fungal drugs, of which nystatin is the best known.[41]

Fungal infections are now extremely common. Over a dozen brands of anti-fungal drugs are now available on prescription in the UK, designed as creams to be applied directly to the vaginal area. In the United States and the UK drug companies are persuading the regulatory authorities to make more anti-fungal creams available over the counter. A *Financial Times* report published in August 1992[42] predicted eventual sales worth $1 billion a year for such drugs.

CANDIDA: DRY ROT OF THE BODY

Like cystitis, thrush is unpleasant and often debilitating. It may wreck a sex life, and it is hard to eliminate. Candida superinfection in the vaginas of mothers may infect their newborn babies. Doctors and women often seem to think of thrush as a part of cystitis rather than a fungal infection, or else just as 'one of those things'.

As *Antimicrobial Therapy* says, candida infection does not always remain in the vagina; it can become systemic, spreading throughout the gut. Some scientists think that systemic candida infection is uncommon and anyway not usually serious. Others believe that it is now common and often dangerous.[43]

In the 1980s, the number of deaths officially attributed to systemic candidiasis (also known as candidosis) in the United States was around 200 annually. In Britain, a handful of people every year are registered as having died of the disease. As a killer, candidiasis rates comparably with salmonella poisoning; not major but not trivial either. Candidiasis is a controversial disease. Doctors don't understand it.

In 1986, the *Journal of the American Medical Association* carried a signed leading article entitled 'IS THERE AN EPIDEMIC OF CHRONIC CANDIDIASIS IN OUR MIDST?' It began:[44]

> There is a growing underground of public controversy surrounding the reputed presence of a 'new epidemic'. This epidemic involves chronic candidiasis, a condition in which there is an overgrowth of

> and systemic invasion by the yeast organism *Candida albicans*. The proponents indicate that non-specific symptoms such as fatigue, intestinal gas, depression, muscle aches, constipation, diarrhoea, loss of sexual desire and premenstrual syndrome are but a few of the signals that one may have chronic candidiasis.

How often do antibiotics cause candida superinfection in the gut? The textbook *Candida and Candidosis*[39] reviews a large number of human and animal studies. Those on hospital patients show that 'most antibiotics may enhance *Candida* carriage'. Those that work against the anaerobic friendly flora of the gut, such as metronidazole, 'are particularly effective in promoting candida overgrowth'.

Some antibiotics – aminoglycosides, chloramphenicol and cephalosporins – evidently cause candida superinfection at a rate of over 1 in 100 treatments. Penicillins and tetracyclines, with a rate of less than 1 in 200 treatments, are evidently not such a problem. Thirty-four animal studies are cited that show that superficial or invasive candidiasis can also be promoted by streptomycin, vancomycin, and combination antibiotics in animals. The textbook's conclusion is:

> Elimination of bacterial competition is almost certainly the important mechanism by which antibiotics affect *Candida* numbers . . . Certain antibiotics may have immunosuppressive properties that could reduce host resistance to *Candida*.[39]

People whose immune systems are exhausted or wrecked are most likely to suffer candida superinfection. Antifungal drugs are given as a routine to people on immunosuppressive drugs for cancer, and to AIDS patients. Old, weak, ill people sometimes die from candida invading their vital organs or blocking up their inner passages.

VAGINITIS: 'ABSOLUTELY DEVASTATING'

In a review of the scientific literature published back in 1966, Dr Mildred Seelig of the department of pharmacology at New York Medical College pointed out two sinister features of candida superinfection.[45] First, like dry rot, candida has two forms: as a mould, it infests surfaces on and in the body; but it can also grow into a fungus whose roots penetrate through the wall of the gut. Second, 'antibiotics enhance the invasiveness of *Candida albicans*, not wholly by a direct effect on the intestinal flora and on the candida itself, but also by depressing the host defence mechanism.'

Fungal roots are called mycelia. Autopsies of people who have died from candida overgrowth show 'massive mycelial invasion of the esophageal or intestinal wall'. And antibiotics can be a fungal fertiliser. When pieces of intestine were taken from the body of a woman with candida overgrowth,

> the candida in the gut obtained post-mortem proliferated and invaded the deeper tissues when segments of ileum [part of the small intestine] were immersed in penicillin solution, or streptomycin solution, or in chloramphenicol solution, but not when the segments were immersed in solutions free from antibiotics. In effect, candida feeds off antibiotics.

Dr Seelig's conclusion is that antibiotics lower immune resistance to candida which, in its fungal form, puts poisons into the bloodstream. This would explain why people infected with candida feel 'ill all over', with all sorts of symptoms that baffle doctors. As people get older, they become more vulnerable to penetration of the fungal form of candida through the gut wall.

Professor Steven Witkin of the immunology division of the department of obstetrics and gynaecology at the New York Hospital in Manhattan, specialises in diseases of the vagina. He agrees with Dr Seelig. He wrote in 1985: 'Antibiotics can interfere with the ability of the immune system to limit fungal infections.'[46] Interviewed in New York for this book, Dr Witkin said, referring to women suffering severe, invasive vaginal infections, or vaginitis: 'We do find in some women that their immune systems, normal in other respects, do not respond to candida. In most healthy people, if you take their white blood cells and incubate them with candida, the white blood cells proliferate. If you do the same thing in women with recurrent candida vaginitis, the white blood cells do not proliferate, showing that the women are immunosuppressed.'

Since antibiotics were originally discovered in mould and in the soil, it is not altogether surprising that they should have an affinity with moulds in the body. However, that does not explain why *Candida albicans* should be such an aggressive parasite, seemingly set on killing its host. Perhaps its function in the body's ecology is rather like that of vultures and hyenas in the outside world; if so, it would naturally multiply and invade a body sending out signals that it was dying and ready to be scavenged.

How big a part do antibiotics play in the growth and development of candida into its invasive, fungal form?

Dr Leo Galland, a physician in New York, has specialised in candidiasis for some years. Interviewed for this book, Dr Galland said:

> 'I have seen literally thousands of patients over the last ten years who have developed an illness following exposure to antibiotics which has responded to anti-fungal drugs. When I reviewed my patients, the commonest symptoms were fatigue, gastrointestinal complaints, constipation, diarrhoea, pain. Fatigue and food intolerances occur in the vast majority of patients. Most of the women have chronic vaginitis; a large minority complain of premenstrual symptoms. Anxiety, depression, headaches occur in about half the patients.

In his experience, vaginal thrush that develops into vaginitis caused by deeper penetration of candida can be a horrible disease. 'In about one in a hundred cases, women with vaginal thrush will go on to develop chronic vaginitis. The most anxious patients that I treat are women with this condition. The illness is absolutely devastating to them. It wrecks their sex lives, their marriages, their images of themselves as women.'

Finding out for sure how often candida mould develops into a fungal form that penetrates the gut wall depends on a large study of humans during surgery or at autopsy. This has not yet occurred.

In 1990, a leading article in the *New England Journal of Medicine* stated: 'Few illnesses have sparked so much hostility between the medical community and a segment of the lay public as the chronic candidiasis syndrome.'[48] Those who believe that candida superinfection is common and often dangerous 'have levelled a serious charge against the medical community, claiming that it is not fulfilling one of its most important obligations to its patients. The charge is simply put: you physicians are not listening to your patients.' The following year another review in the same journal stated: 'A disturbingly large number of [hospital] patients die with undiagnosed invasive candida infections.'[48]

THE CHRONIC FATIGUE ENIGMA

Another mystery illness that afflicts more women than men is chronic fatigue syndrome, also known as myalgic encephalomyelitis (ME) or else as post-viral fatigue syndrome. It seems to be infectious: the first known outbreak struck down 198 medical staff at the Los Angeles County Hospital in 1934. In the UK the best known incident was at the Royal Free Hospital, London, in 1955, when a total of 292 medical and nursing staff, 265 of whom were women, suffered symptoms of the disease, which includes loss of muscular strength, general exhaustion, inability to think, and loss of memory.[49]

For some time, the official line on 'Royal Free disease' treated it as some sort of one-off incident of mass hysteria. In the 1980s, when chronic fatigue syndrome became epidemic in Britain and North America, it was called 'yuppie flu' and often seen as sophisticated middle-class malingering. But now, although chronic fatigue syndrome is not yet listed in medical guides or textbooks, it has become accepted as a serious disease. Estimates of its incidence in the UK vary between 100,000 and 500,000 people.

One theory is that the disease is caused by a virus. At a conference organised at the Royal Society in August 1990, Dr Les Borysiewicz of Addenbrooke's Hospital, Cambridge, reported that many sufferers 'dated the start of their illness to a mild fever-like infection, and it was well known that viruses . . . could leave people feeling fatigued for long periods.'[50]

Professor James Mowbray of the Department of Pathology at St Mary's Hospital Medical School in London, in a study published in the *Lancet* in 1988, found evidence of invasive viruses in half of a group of 87 patients he examined.[51] The types of virus involved, enteroviruses, are found in the guts of healthy people; what makes them invasive? Professor Mowbray has suggested that research should focus on why the immunity of people who suffer the disease has evidently broken down.

In the USA Dr Carol Jessop reported data from 1100 patients with chronic fatigue syndrome, at a conference held in San Francisco in April 1989.[52] She stated:

> Past medical history of CFS patients is very enlightening and may represent the key to understanding this illness. Of 1000 patients the following was noted. First, 80 percent of the patients had recurrent

> antibiotic treatment as a child, adolescent and adult for ear, nose and throat infections, acne, and/or urinary tract infections. Second, 60 percent of patients developed sensitivity to many antibiotics over the years.

In common with other specialists, Dr Jessop thinks that the underlying cause of the disease may be the toxic effect of candida superinfection creating conditions in which a virus can invade and cause disease.

Many people with chronic fatigue syndrome also suffer from candida superinfection. (Likewise, AIDS: evidence of systemic candida overgrowth often prompts physicians to test for the presence of HIV.) But which comes first, the virus or the fungus? It may be that the damage done by penetrative candida overgrowth to the gut wall and its immune defences allows penetration by the types of virus identified by Professor Mowbray.

This theory of an underlying cause of chronic fatigue syndrome thus is as follows. Stage one is antibiotics: probably repeated courses. This causes stage two, candida superinfection, and its complication, spread of invasive fungal infection through the gut wall. In turn this causes stage three, penetration of goodness knows what micro-organisms, bacterial, fungal or viral, through the gut wall. And these directly cause general illness.

Once again, this is not to suggest that antibiotics are the invariable underlying cause of chronic fatigue syndrome. It is only recently that the disease was recognised as a real physical condition, and conventional scientists are sceptical about much of the data, pointing out that some is unpublished, or else anecdotal or carried out by enthusiasts. As far as I know, no epidemiologist has yet attempted to compare records of chronic fatigue syndrome with records of heavy and prolonged antibiotic use or with presence of candida. This and other research on the possible role of antibiotics in serious chronic fatigue states and other factors that make people (women, mostly) vulnerable to invasive fungal infections, should in my view be undertaken.

15 'Nature's Most Malicious Trick?'

REASONS TO BE CAREFUL

Once you know that you need the resident bacteria in your gut to protect your health, and that antibiotics especially when overused may eventually not only devastate these friendly flora but also may strip away the outer immune defences in your gut, it is easy to see that prolonged courses of antibiotics can in time lay you open to all sorts of infections and also non-infectious diseases.

Many diseases, some serious, have evidently become more common in countries like the UK and the USA in the last 50 years. They may in part be caused by medical treatment. Infants and children are vulnerable to repeated ear, nose and throat infections. Girls and women are vulnerable to repeated cystitis and to fungal superinfection, which can become invasive. Antibiotics are certainly one cause of these diseases, and may be one cause of a variety of bowel diseases and some forms of arthritis. And the serious general malaise known as chronic fatigue syndrome may be in part a complication of invasive fungal infection. Young children and old people are especially at risk, as are the chronically ill. This, in addition to the known immediate or acute ill-effects of antibiotics already described.

Once again, these are not reasons to always avoid antibiotics. To repeat, they are a precious resource: in cases of reliably diagnosed serious invasive bacterial infections their benefits far outweigh their risks. But risks there are: and many of the ill-effects of antibiotics are insidious, quite likely not to be linked with the drug either by victims or their doctors.

IMMUNOSUPPRESSION

Our resident gut flora have another vital function not mentioned so far. They stimulate the production of immunoglobulins, proteins in the blood integral to the body's inner immune defences. Experiments show that animals with all their gut flora removed, make only about one-fiftieth as much immunoglobulin as normal animals. Commenting on this finding, the standard textbook *Immunology*[53] states: 'If the commensal organisms of the gut are removed by antibiotics, pathogenic organisms can readily gain a foothold,' and emphasises the importance of not disturbing the relationship between the host and its indigenous flora.

Does this mean that antibiotics are immunosuppressant drugs? This is an explosive question. Drugs generally classified as immunosuppressants are very dangerous. They are used only on people with cancer, and also after organ transplants. They greatly increase the risk of serious bacterial and viral infection, and also of cancer, and are used only when patients are otherwise likely to die.

In ordinary circumstances, antibiotics are nothing like as dangerous as these drugs. As already stated, one course of antibiotics destroys the bacteria in the gut but not utterly, and a healthy balance of resident bacteria is usually restored soon after antibiotic therapy. The only class of antibiotic that is commonly identified as immunosuppressive is tetracycline[54], because of its profound destruction of so many species of resident gut flora. And in a sense allergic reactions are reassuring because, as mentioned, they show that the body's inner immune defences are being irritated, and therefore obviously in working order. Basically healthy people are very unlikely to disrupt their inner immune defences by taking just one course of antibiotics.

Nevertheless, antibiotics do have a suppressive effect on our defences against infection. Given that our outer defences, including resident bacteria and the mucosal lining of the body's inner passages, are an integral part of our immune system, it follows inescapably that all antibiotics are by their nature immunosuppressants – mildly so, no doubt, compared with the drugs used on cancer and organ-transplant patients, but immunosuppressive none the less.

How much this matters depends on the general state of the health of the individual, the type of antibiotic and the strength and length of the course. As ever, babies and little children, old people, hospital patients and anybody else who is generally weak or ill are at greatest risk, and this includes many, if not most, people on the antibiotic treadmill, taking more and more courses for recurrent infections.

Most vulnerable of all are people who are already immunosuppressed. But which came first; immunosuppression or antibiotics?

Here is the view of Professor Sandy Raeburn, head of the department of clinical genetics at Nottingham University, a specialist in disease of young children. In 1972 he wrote a paper for the *Lancet*, on 'Antibiotics and Immunodeficiency'.[55]

> Immunological-deficiency syndromes were not observed before 1952. A possible explanation is that some of these conditions are produced by administration of antibiotics to certain individuals at a critical point in the development of immune responses.

Dr Raeburn gave examples of immunodeficiency diseases suffered mostly by babies and young children. Combined immunodeficiency (CID) lays infants open to diarrhoea, thrush, pneumonia and other infections, and is treated by bone marrow transplants. Immunoglobulin deficiency (aglobulinaemias) lays babies open to all sorts of infection, and may increase the chance of cancer. Chronic granulomatous disease (CGD) also makes babies more vulnerable to bacterial infections.

'These diseases were not described before the antibiotic era,' said Dr Raeburn, 'and the usual view is that modern therapy has enabled affected patients to survive longer. An alternative explanation, however, is that antibiotics have actually led to immunodeficiency states – diseases which did not previously exist.'

He supports this proposal by three lines of argument. First, since one of the main purposes of the immune system (including the bacteria that have evolved with us) is to protect the body against invading micro-organisms, 'removal of bacteria by other means, such as rapidly effective antibacterial therapy, could have profound effects – for example, in infancy, during immunological development.' Later in life, antibiotics might provoke bacteria, even the friendly flora, into producing poisons that the immune system cannot handle. 'The rarest clinical effects will emerge sooner or later because antibiotics are so widely used.'

Second – and here Dr Raeburn draws on his own clinical experience – while antibiotics work well for previously healthy people with an acute infection, they usually don't work for patients who are immunodeficient.

> Failures of antibiotic therapy are often excused by an assumption that host resistance was impaired. Could it be that the infection

> persisted *because* the antibiotic interfered with host resistance in a susceptible patient? I have seen several patients whose infection progressed while they were receiving seemingly appropriate antibiotics.

Third, he cited the laboratory evidence showing that antibiotics make experimental animals more vulnerable to infection by suppressing their immune responses – some very much more than others. Those at greatest risk of immunodeficiency diseases caused by antibiotics will include: those born vulnerable; babies and young children; people who are suffering from other diseases; and anybody taking regular, heavy doses of antibiotics. He concluded: 'If this theory is substantiated, it follows that antibiotics should be reserved for life-threatening infections, until the risk of immunotoxicity is excluded in each patient.'

I wrote to Dr Raeburn asking him if, in the twenty years since he had published the *Lancet* paper, he had changed his view. He wrote back saying: 'Since I published that paper, there has been a vast amount of work on the interaction between antibiotics and the immune system. Much of it bears out my original hypothesis . . . When a patient receives antibiotic treatment, the beneficial effects due to antibacterial activity could be reduced or even negated by deleterious effects on the immune system.' Overall, he said, antibiotics are beneficial, 'but in my specialist area of medical genetics, we might well see patients in which the balance is set differently – for example, in cystic fibrosis.'

In 1984, a dozen years after Dr Raeburn's *Lancet* paper, Dr William Hauser of the Boston University Medical Center and Dr Jack Remington of the Palo Alto Medical Foundation, both specialists in infectious disease, published a review of the scientific literature on the 'Effect of Antimicrobial Agents on the Immune Response' in the textbook *Antimicrobial Therapy*.[56] Antibiotics listed as having ill-effects on the human immune response include: some aminoglycosides (gentamicin, tobramycin); a cephalosporin (cephalothin); chloramphenicol; a lincosamide (clindamycin); various sulphonamides, and co-trimoxazole; various tetracyclines; sodium fusidate; and a number of anti-fungal and anti-tubercular drugs. Penicillins are not included, and evidently do not have ill-effects on the body's inner immune defences.

Hauser and Remington comment:

> There is clearly a need for a better understanding of the potential beneficial and deleterious effects of antibiotic therapy on the host's immune defences, especially in the immunosuppressed patient.

Indeed there is. But when antibiotics suppress our immune defences against disease, as evidently they may do, then people given constant courses of antibiotics to drive out infection will be not so much on a drug treadmill as caught in a vortex pulling them down deeper into disease.

Here is an appalling prospect. A child suffers middle-ear inflammation, treated with antibiotics, which then recurs because of antibiotics. A woman suffers cystitis, which is cleared up with antibiotics, but which then recurs in a more invasive form because of antibiotics. These infections occurred in the first place because of antibiotics taken in infancy and childhood. Then people of all ages and both sexes suffer a cascade of diseases of the gut, each stage accelerated by antibiotics, which eventually cause irreversible infections carried by bacteria and by viruses that easily break through weakened immune defences. At some stage in this cascade, the victims become chronically immunosuppressed, vulnerable to invasion by any infectious agent around.

The idea that medicine can cure illness immediately and yet cause illness later may seem strange. But in other areas of life we know that gain now can mean loss later – this, after all, is one of the tenets of the Christian religion. Or, to take two familiar analogies, we know we can drive to destinations faster by breaking the speed limit, and we know we can spend our way out of immediate trouble by running up an overdraft. We also know we are running the risk of wrecking our car or our finances. A friendly garage mechanic or bank manager will advise us to be careful.

A LINK WITH AIDS?

When Professor Raeburn wrote his paper, chronic fatigue syndrome was obscure and AIDS was unknown. When Drs Hauser and Remington wrote their review, neither disease was common. While AIDS kills and CFS does not, the two diseases are in some ways rather similar. Both are new, epidemic, afflict young people, have no known cure, take many clinical forms, and cause profound debility. In the case of AIDS it is generally but not universally agreed that the infectious agent is the HIV retrovirus. In the case of CFS there is a growing belief that an enterovirus is involved.

As Professor James Mowbray has said of CFS, why has the immunity of people who suffer AIDS broken down? Why is it that some people who are exposed to the disease remain untouched while others become infected with HIV? Why is it that some people who test HIV positive remain in good health for many years, perhaps never suffering full-blown AIDS, while others die rapidly?

Because AIDS is a new disease, is deadly and is an accelerating epidemic, with in 1990 alone an estimated one million new cases of people worldwide infected with the HIV virus[57], other sexually transmitted diseases seem less important now. But at the end of 1990, the World Health Organisation announced that more than 250 million new cases of sexually transmitted diseases are reported every year. According to WHO Director-General Dr Hiroshi Nakajima, they 'have reached epidemic proportions globally, and if sexual behaviour is not modified and effective new prevention programmes are not implemented immediately, the resulting disease and mortality rates will be even more staggering.'

In 1990, 25 million new cases of gonorrhoea and 3.5 million new cases of syphilis were reported worldwide. Gonorrhoea is now often very resistant to penicillin, the original drug of choice, in which case, treatment is either with massive doses of penicillin, or other antibiotics including aminoglycosides, sulphonamides or co-trimoxazole. Penicillin usually still works for syphilis; an alternative drug is tetracycline. In the last half-century, other sexually transmitted diseases have become more common. These include: genital ulcers, treated with sulphonamides or tetracyclines; chlamydia, with tetracyclines; chancroid, with co-trimoxazole; trichomoniasis, with metronidazole; and genital herpes, a viral disease.

More than any other community, people whose lifestyle involves very many sexual partners are almost certain to suffer combinations and permutations of sexually transmitted diseases, which when bacterial are treated with constant courses of antibiotics, often broad-spectrum and/or in cocktails. Such treatment over time provokes superinfection and drug-resistant superbugs – so more antibiotics are used, often more toxic in their effect. On such a drug treadmill, people who have constantly quenched their sexually transmitted diseases with antimicrobial drugs are more vulnerable to any infection, whether bacterial, fungal, or viral, and, once infected, are more likely to be overwhelmed.

In his book *The Plague Makers*,[58] Dr Jeffrey Fisher states that Dr Luc Montagnier of the Pasteur Institute in Paris, co-discoverer of HIV, believes that gross overuse of antibiotics may be a co-factor with HIV in development of full-blown AIDS, and that HIV may by itself not cause AIDS. This theory, sensational if only because AIDS is the great deadly plague of our time, is also believed by some homoeopaths. Can it be true?

It makes microbiological sense: there is some experimental evidence suggesting that tetracycline has a side-effect of mutating mycoplasmas, including *M. pirium* and *M. fermentans*, into virus-type micro-organisms that can invade T-lymphocyte cells, whose function is crucial to the body's inner immunity against infectious diseases. The theory goes on to propose that if these cells are also already invaded by HIV, the mutated mycoplasmas effectively feed the HIV, activating them and enabling them to destroy T-lymphocyte function, thus laying the victim open to a great range of infections identified as full-blown AIDS.

On a separate point, Dr Fisher quotes other research scientists who confirm the findings of Drs Hauser and Remington, and who state that various antimicrobial drugs, including sulphonamides, cephalosporins, antifungals and antiparasitics, are directly immunosuppressive in different ways and, when overused, themselves increase vulnerability to infectious diseases.

If the mycoplasma theory is true, it would follow that people who test positive for presence for the HIV virus in their bodies, but whose lifestyles have not led them to gross overuse of antibiotics, will be less likely to develop full-blown AIDS. And indeed, haemophiliacs and others frequently show no signs of illness for ten or fifteen years after being accidentally treated or transfused with clotting factors or blood infected with HIV.[59]

If the mycoplasma theory turns out not to be supported by evidence from other researchers, it remains true that destruction of gut flora and damage to the body's immunological defences by continual courses of antibiotics lays the body open to all sorts of bacterial, fungal and viral infections, including those most commonly associated with AIDS.

For men, the dream of sexual liberation began in the 1940s. American GIs believed that because of penicillin they could go on the rampage with European and Asian women during World War II, and then during the Korean and Vietnam wars, without risk to themselves. The result is multi drug-resistant gonorrhoea. But antibiotics retained their reputation as magic bullets throughout the 1970s and 1980s, enabling increasingly wild lifestyles. In the USA and other rich countries, this is the context of AIDS. It can be said that AIDS is a disease that was waiting to happen.

INCREASING RISK OF COLON CANCER?

The proposal that antibiotics are one underlying cause of a number of gut diseases is in my opinion fairly convincing. I think there is also some reason to believe that antibiotics, when used in heavy prolonged doses, may increase the risk of colon cancer. Before going any further, I should make it clear that the argument put forward here is speculative and theoretical. But it does make sense.

It may at first seem fantastic to suggest any link between drugs used to treat infections and a deadly non-infectious disease – one which is common in all industrialised societies, and the second most common cause of cancer death in UK men (after lung cancer) and in women (after breast cancer). What possible connection could there be between a course of antibiotics and cancer?

But that is not the suggestion. Smoking is an established cause of lung cancer, and alcohol (with smoking) of throat cancer; but nobody has ever suggested that one packet of cigarettes or one bottle of wine put anybody at real risk. The people who increase their risk of cancer are regular smokers and heavy drinkers. Similarly, if antibiotics increase the risk of colon cancer the people in real danger will be the heavy antibiotic users.

With cancer, there are no simple causes and effects; it is a late stage in a long series of connected events. Even the most potent carcinogens, such as radioactive fallout, may take 20 years or more to cause an identifiable cancer. Likewise, it may take 40 years or more of regular smoking or heavy drinking before symptoms develop that are diagnosed as cancer. Also, not everybody exposed to a carcinogen develops cancer. Many smokers and drinkers eventually die of other causes, just as some Hiroshima victims survived into old age. What can be said is that regular smoking and heavy drinking increase the risk of specific cancers.

So are the millions of people throughout the world who from childhood take doses of antibiotics regularly, at greater risk of colon cancer? There is no hard evidence either way, of the type that impresses research scientists. No controlled trials of human beings over a long period of time, comparing heavy with light users of antibiotics – similar to the trials that strongly suggested that prolonged use of the contraceptive pill increases the risk of cancers of the breast and cervix – have been carried out. Nevertheless, there is some reason to believe that heavy use of at least some antibiotics may increase the risk of cancer of the colon.

First, ulcerative colitis increases the risk of colon cancer,[60] so if antibiotics are a cause of ulcerative colitis, they indirectly increase vulnerability to cancer. Second, it is generally agreed that a fatty diet is a cause of colon cancer, perhaps because it increases the concentration of bile acids in the colon, which in turn are converted by bacteria in the gut into carcinogens. But which bacteria? It may be that superinfectious bacteria are more dangerous than our resident friendly flora.[61]

The main argument suggesting that antibiotics may increase the risk of colon cancer follows from what you already now know about their effect on the gut. Cancer usually takes years to develop. It is often initiated by constant irritation of a vulnerable part of the body by a toxic substance, and the risk of cancer is increased if the irritation and toxicity causes wounds or ulcers. This is why sunburn increases the risk of skin cancer, and a very hot or spicy diet may cause cancer of the throat. The healthy body has strong immune defences against cancer, designed to nip cell mutations in the bud. But if the immune system is constantly weakened, constant damage to vulnerable parts of the body further increases the risk of cancers.

So a circumstantial case against antibiotics is evident. Antibiotics do irritate the gut lining, do allow the breeding of superinfectious toxic micro-organisms, can damage the gut wall and do disrupt both outer and inner immune defences. The textbook *Immunology*[53] states: 'The incidence of cancer in man is highest at the two extremes of life, and it is just at those times that the immune system is least efficient. All these observations point to the probable important role played by the intact mechanisms in keeping the body free of undesirable mutant neoplastic cells' – that is, cancers. And when superinfections spread from the colon to other parts of the body, then the load on the immune system is broader and heavier.

Systematic scientific research to check whether or not antibiotics evidently increase the risk of colon cancer has not been done, but the theory is worth investigation. Perhaps some antibiotics increase the risk, while others are in this respect harmless. Perhaps any increased risk is trivial unless specific antibiotics are taken above certain dosages for a long time. Perhaps any risk can be reduced or removed by special diet or therapy. It would be good to know. Indeed, it would be good to be really confident that antibiotics never increase the risk of colon cancer. But it seems to me that we cannot be so sure.

SUMMARY OF PART 4

While antibiotics are vital treatment against dangerous bacterial infection, they are overused and abused, and doctors tend to overlook the ill-effects of these potent drugs on the ecology of the human body. Continual use, especially of broad-spectrum antibiotics, makes us vulnerable not only to infectious but also to non-infectious diseases. Antibiotics may lay us open to many infections of the ear, nose and throat, diseases of the urinary and female reproductive tracts, and various disabling and even deadly gut disorders. Eventually they may also lower immunity to every kind of disease. How many diseases are caused in part by antibiotics is unknown.

Part Five

Superbug:
Nature's Revenge

Through a characteristically human combination of shortsightedness, greed, and ignorance, we are now well on the way to negating totally the usefulness of antibiotics . . . Antibiotics have been (and still are) given for everything from headaches to ingrown toenails; they are swallowed, sucked, injected and smeared; they are painted on cuts, dumped into wounds, fed to the chickens and pigs and sprayed on the floors of the hospital wards.

Dr Richard Novick
Director, Public Health Research Institute, New York; 1979

In the past twenty years we have witnessed a dramatic and frightening re-emergence of infectious diseases as a major force against which mankind must struggle for survival. Many of the old diseases which had appeared to be controlled, or even eliminated, have returned, and a host of new infectious diseases which were not even dreamed of fifteen years ago have made their appearance . . . Almost daily, new publications appear in the medical and scientific journals documenting life-threatening infection with organisms that were previously thought to be completely harmless . . . The horrifying possibility that subtle changes in genes of organisms of low virulence, may endow them with devastating new virulent properties, will almost certainly turn out to be a common explanation for the emergence of epidemics of new disease.

Professor Michael Levin
Darwin Lecture to the British Association for the Advancement of Science; 1993

16 The Bugs Bite Back

GETTING ILL IN HOSPITAL

The words 'hospital', 'hostel' and 'hotel' all have the same original root meaning: a safe place of refuge and succour. My own school, Christ's Hospital, was so called, on its foundation in the reign of the boy-king Edward VI in 1553, because it was meant to be a place where orphans and foundlings were sheltered, fed and educated.

What the word 'hospital' now means is an institution for the care and treatment of people who are injured or diseased or, for some other reason, in need of full-time medical attention. In this sense, hospitals have never really been seen as safe places. Indeed, the folk fear of hospitals as places you are liable to come out of feet first, is still with us. This is and always will be partly for obvious reasons: a proportion of people admitted to hospital are very ill and likely to die no matter what.

Another old fear of hospitals has receded: during the last 100 years, hospitals have become much cleaner; nurses, doctors and surgeons are highly skilled; and accidents, neglect or butchery of the kind that were commonplace in previous generations are now uncommon. If you develop a good relationship with your consultant and the nursing staff, as well as with your general practitioner, you are likely to be well looked after in hospital.

A third fear of hospitals is, though, still with us. Nineteenth-century pioneers such as Ignaz Semmelweis, Florence Nightingale and Joseph Lister realised that the hospitals of their day were all too often pest-holes: horribly dangerous places in which infections often became local epidemics, spread by inadequate sanitation and crowded beds, and by the doctors and surgeons themselves (often straight from the dissecting rooms), moving between patients, handling one, then another, and thereby carrying contagion. In the nineteenth and early twentieth century, the death rates from hospital infections – known medically as nosocomial infections – among surgical patients and women in childbirth were appalling. This dreadful era is over, but hospitals remain breeding grounds for disease. Hospital infections are common, and sometimes kill very weak, old or ill patients.

What is really fearsome, though, is the type of hospital infection caused by antibiotics, carried by bacteria that have evolved to become invulnerable to drugs. In hospitals, constant heavy use of antibiotics not only to treat infection but also as a precaution against infection is liable to cause microbiological havoc. Just as the healthy human gut is an ecosystem inhabited by balanced populations of many bacterial species, whose functions include protection of the body against takeover or invasion by dangerous species, so likewise a hospital is a larger and more complex ecosystem made up of its population of humans and other creatures living in a relatively closed environment. From a bug's point of view, a hospital is a bigger version of the human gut.

As you now know, in the gut, bacteria and other micro-organisms that are naturally drug-resistant are liable to multiply out of control after other species have been destroyed by antibiotics, causing super-infections which may be dangerous or on rare occasions even deadly, one example being *Clostridium difficile*, the microbiological cause of pseudomembranous colitis. In the same way, bacteria that are intrinsically resistant to antibiotics in the hospital environment are also liable to multiply out of control when the drugs have killed off normally dominant species, creating a microbiological void which they can fill. An example is the *Pseudomonas aeruginosa* bacillus, which in the age of antibiotics has become a menace in hospitals, a cause of appalling infections.

Patients whose flesh is exposed by surgery, who have indwelling tubes or who have burns, wounds or sores are especially at risk, as are those whose immunity to disease is especially weak. *P. aeruginosa* can cause vicious infections of the eyes, ears and urinary tract, and septicaemia involving gangrenous skin lesions.[1] It is a special threat to cancer patients undergoing chemotherapy. Another species in the same family, *Pseudomonas cepacia*, also now a danger in hospitals, is a cause of lung abscesses in patients suffering from cystic fibrosis.[2]

In response, a whole new family of drugs – the carboxypenicillins, also known as antipseudomonal penicillins – have been developed and marketed. These are all used intravenously for hospital patients, are expensive and, in high doses, can sometimes be very toxic.

Hospital infections now amount to a substantial public health problem. In the USA, Dr Theodore Cooper of the National Institutes of Health headed a special study group on the issue. Reporting in 1976, Dr Cooper and his colleagues reckoned that in the US alone, antibiotic-resistant bacteria caused anything between 70,000 and 140,000 new cases of infection every year, resulting in at least 18,000 deaths. Most of these deaths were caused by *P. aeruginosa* and *Proteus mirabilis* (another naturally resistant species) and by *E. coli*. As mentioned in the introduction to this book, in 1994 Professor Alexander Tomasz of Rockefeller University in New York reckoned that deaths from hospital infections in the USA, mostly involving drug resistant bacteria, totalled 65,000–70,000 a year.[3]

Statistics such as these should be put in perspective. It's worth repeating that hospitals in developed countries are now safer places than they were in the days before antibiotics. Most infections, including those carried by drug-resistant bacteria, can usually be successfully treated. And most people who die from hospital infections are already weak and ill; death from pneumonia is sometimes seen as a blessing in cases of AIDS or in senile patients who have no real life left. This said, though, the sense of apprehension that many people have when they are admitted to hospital has some justification.

In August 1992, British newspapers carried stories about two babies who were killed by bacterial infection at a major London teaching hospital. The *Independent* reported:[4]

> An intensive care unit at the hospital has been closed to new admissions since last week, after an outbreak of klebsiella which is resistant to most antibiotics. The bacteria can lead to pneumonia, blood poisoning and, in rare cases, meningitis in sick children.

Commenting, Dr Geoff Scott of the Hospital Infection Society said: 'It certainly is dangerous to go into hospital . . . Acquiring an infection in hospital is very common, but it's not serious unless the patient has some sort of wound, or is severely immunosuppressed.'[5] Dr Scott thought that the klebsiella – commensal flora in the healthy human gut, which thrive in warm moist environments such as those found in hospitals, and cause disease when they infect wounds and other vulnerable parts of the body – may have been passed from baby to baby on the hands of hospital staff. Dr Donal O'Sullivan of Lewisham and North Southwark Health Authority disagreed, saying there was no evidence to blame sloppy hygiene: 'This is a common problem in high technology or intensive care units where there are very sick children and powerful antibiotics are used, allowing the emergence of resistant strains of infection.'[4]

In 1982 The World Health Organisation published a report[6] stating that the spread of drug-resistant bacteria in hospitals could make the choice of antibiotic 'a gamble against worsening odds', adding:

> Many surgeons seek to compensate for poor hygienic conditions in their operating theatre or wards by employing prophylaxis [routine use of antibiotics on uninfected patients 'just in case'] . . . This results in excessive antibiotic use and is certainly counterproductive.

Following this result, a survey of hospital infections in fourteen countries and four continents was carried out for WHO, which concluded that 'hospital infection is a common and serious problem throughout the world.'[7]

The survey was carried out in Australia, China, Czechoslovakia, Denmark, Egypt, Greece, Kuwait, Malaysia, Nepal, the Netherlands, Singapore, Spain, Thailand and the United Kingdom, and involved a total of 28,861 patients of all ages. Roughly 1 in 12 patients (8.4 percent) suffered infections acquired in hospital. The highest rates were in intensive care units and surgical wards (over 1 in 8 patients). Infants and old people were also more at risk. The risk of infection after surgery varied enormously, from 1 in 30 to as many as 1 in 3 cases. The bacteria responsible for the infections in this survey were mostly *E. coli*, *Staphylococcus aureus* and *P. aeruginosa*. In Britain, as in other countries, the cost of hospital infection is enormous, in 1987 amounting to £115 million paid by the National Health Service, and 950,000 'bed days'.

Commenting, *Which? Way to Health*, published by the Consumers' Association, said:[8]

> The cost to patients and their families in pain and suffering cannot be estimated. At least 1 in 20 of all hospital patients will pick up an infection in hospital. But because these infections mean people spending longer in hospital, the number of hospital-infected patients on any one day will be higher – around 1 in 10.

Patients most at risk include babies and the elderly, the chronically ill, those severely injured or who have had open-body surgery, and those on immunosuppressive drugs for cancer, after transplants, or for other reasons. Large teaching hospitals can be among the most dangerous. Because they have a reputation for giving the best medical care, they treat very sick people and undertake 'heroic', very invasive surgery, and the more radical the procedure, the greater the danger of infection. The less time you spend in hospital, the less likely you are to suffer infection. Better still, if you can, stay at home. A study of elderly patients whose hips were fractured or needed replacement and who, after surgery, were cared for at home found that only 1 out of 150 suffered infection; they also recovered faster at home.[8]

SUPERSTAPH

Some years before the stories of the klebsiella outbreak at a London hospital surfaced, British newspapers carried a series of major features about what, at first reading, seemed to be a new epidemic of drug-resistant hospital infection. This was – and is – carried by a mutant strain of *Staphylococcus aureus* sometimes known as 'superstaph', because it has evolved so that almost all antibiotics are useless against it.

The headline in the *Observer* in August 1986 was: 'DEADLY "SUPER BUG" SPREADS THROUGH WARDS.'[9] Outbreaks of superstaph, amounting to an epidemic, had been identified in at least 32 London hospitals as well as ones in East Anglia, Nottinghamshire and Yorkshire. Dr Joan Bradley, who headed a working party considering the implications of superstaph in the North-East Thames Health Authority, was quoted as saying: 'It has caused deaths in people who were basically well before they came into hospital. They have had an operation and died from infection.'

In March 1986, *The Times* carried a three-part series of features, one of which, on superstaph, was headlined 'UNDER SIEGE FROM A SUPER-BUG'[10], and told the story of the havoc caused at a hospital in East London. The problem with *Staphylococcus aureus* is that most healthy people carry it in their noses, where it does no harm – to them.[1] So it flourishes in hospitals, spread by staff who may touch their noses and then patients. The old public health warning 'Coughs and sneezes spread diseases' certainly applies to *S. aureus* when it can enter vulnerable parts of people's bodies laid open by injury or by surgery or other invasive medical treatment.

S. aureus is the microbiological cause of most staphylococcal infections. On the surface of the body, it can cause boils, abscesses, conjunctivitis, and Lyell's syndrome, otherwise known as 'SSSS' or the staphylococcal scalded skin syndrome, in which the skin peels off in sheets. Once it has invaded the body, it can cause all sorts of dangerous infections, such as septicaemia, internal abscesses, pneumonia, endocarditis, meningitis and osteomyelitis (infection of the bone marrow). It also causes toxic shock, including the toxic shock syndrome that has killed a number of women using super-absorbent tampons during menstruation.[11,12]

The early, golden age of antibiotics created wonderful opportunities for surgeons. Open-body surgery and other massive 'heroic' procedures became feasible for the first time, because patients could be protected against what otherwise would be far too high a risk of dangerous or even deadly infections, by the use of antibiotics before, during and after operations. And, at first, penicillin worked against *S. aureus* and many other bacteria that had made major surgery such a hazard in the pre-antibiotic era.[13]

But the massive use of antibiotics in hospitals create the conditions in which bacteria become superbugs. *S. aureus* became resistant not only to penicillin but also to other early antibiotics such as streptomycin, tetracycline and erythromycin.[14] By the end of the 1950s, superstaph in hospitals had become resistant to all antibiotics known at that time. Interviewed for this book at the Royal Free Hospital in London, microbiologist Professor Jeremy Hamilton-Miller remembered: 'When I started to work, people were dying of infections because there was no antibiotic to treat them. In other words, we had gone back to the pre-antibiotic era.'

So for a while one dangerous bug had proved smarter than the drugs designed to kill it. But then, in the late 1950s, scientists working for Beecham designed a new generation of penicillins which became bestselling drugs specifically because they worked against drug-resistant *S. aureus*. Enthusiastic use of methicillin, the best-known of these betalactamase-resistant penicillins, predictably bred new strains of *S. aureus*, which came to be called MRSA, short for 'methicillin-resistant *Staphylococcus aureus*', which could, however, be killed by some antibiotics other than penicillins. But nature is never idle, and in the late 1970s and into the 1980s, hospitals in London were devastated by a new strain of MRSA – sometimes called EMRSA (the E' standing for 'epidemic') – which killed scores of patients. This superbug, which had probably spread from Australia, had evolved resistance to practically all antibiotics; only vancomycin and, sometimes, chloramphenicol worked against it.[15] In the early 1980s, outbreaks of EMRSA occurred in hospitals in the Middle East, the United States, South Africa, Continental Europe and the UK, where it was found at the London and many other major hospitals – hence, the *Observer* and *Times* stories.

Professor Hamilton-Miller said: 'The carrier state is an absolute menace, because if you have carrier patients, they have to be separated from other patients; and if you have a surgeon who is a carrier, you have to stop him operating, and that is extremely difficult. People are dying from MRSA but not,' he added, 'an inordinate number. It tends to attack the sickest patients; the mortality from MRSA is very much greater than the mortality from non-methicillin-resistant *S. aureus*.'

One London hospital, according to *The Times*, had 'suffered the most tenacious outbreak of resistant staphylococcus on record, disrupting surgery and jeopardising recovery. In 1982 and 1983 the superstaph outbreak was out of control, and an isolation ward was built, with a running cost estimated at £250,000 a year. This worked; cases of superstaph dropped. The ward was then closed to save money; cases increased again, and the ward had to be reopened.

Superstaph makes common operations like hip replacement surgery a hazardous procedure. *S. aureus* is a facultative aerobe – that is, it can live without air – and when it gets into surgical wounds that are then closed, it can cause internal infections that ruin the operation. Michael Freeman, consultant orthopaedic surgeon at the London hospital, said: 'If a resistant germ gets into the bone, the chances of success in an operation almost vanish.'

Vancomycin, now held in reserve in hospitals in order to kill EMRSA, is not a drug doctors like to use. It can damage hearing and affect kidney function; it is unpleasant to administer (it has to be given through a drip for an hour at a time, and can irritate patients' veins);[16] and it is very expensive. Paradoxically, these undesirable qualities are reasons why vancomycin was found to work against superstaph many years after it was first marketed: a safer, cheaper drug would have been used much more often, and would have induced resistance in the bug.

Just how much of a problem is superstaph in Britain? It's hard to say. In 1987, a total of 1891 cases were reported and 50 deaths were attributed solely to MRSA.[17] These figures are probably underestimates; patients who are infected with MRSA and then die are usually suffering from some other serious disease, the reason why they were in hospital in the first place; this disease will probably be stated formally as 'cause of death', with no reference to MRSA on the certificate.[18] And in the UK, sensitive statistics are secret: hospitals are required to collate details of patients suffering and dying from MRSA and send them to the Public Health Laboratory Service at Colindale, but these figures are available only to senior microbiologists.

One underpublicised result of hospital closures and mergers is that superbugs move from site to site, carried by hospital staff and patients. In July 1986, patients were transferred from a hospital in east London to a new building. According to a 'confidential interim report'[19] circulated the following month, a total of 35 Hackney patients carrying MRSA or actually suffering the infection were transferred and isolated in two wards at the new site, and the rest were classified as 'infected' in case the infection spread, with all staff and patients carefully screened. An 'MRSA steering group' was formed and met every day to check these procedures, in order to contain the infection and deal with any new outbreaks. An additional note included with the report said that, at that time, ten wards at another London hospital, were evidently 'clean', which is to say free of EMRSA, whereas another ten wards were contaminated.

Once it is established in a hospital, EMRSA cannot be eradicated, only contained.[20] Hospital administrators are anxious to play down its dangers, and patients are, typically, ignorant of the risk. At the time of writing, however, it seems that the epidemic outbreaks of MRSA in British hospitals have subsided. Countries whose hospitals have well-trained staff and well-stocked pharmacies can stop MRSA becoming rampant, albeit at great cost, of money, resources, suffering and an unknown number of deaths caused at least in part by antibiotic-resistant bacteria.

At any time, MRSA is liable to spread from hospital to hospital, town to town, country to country. 'People should not run away with the idea that hospitals are such hotbeds of infection that it is dangerous to enter them,' Dr Joan Bradley of North-East Thames Health Authority has said[10], and compared with the dangers of hospital infection in the pre-antibiotic era, this is a reasonable view.

But what if EMRSA develops resistance to vancomycin? 'The

potential is frightening,' Dr Richard Smith, now editor of the *British Medical Journal*, has said.[21] And microbiologist Professor Ken Harvey of the Royal Melbourne Hospital, who has seen the devastating effect of epidemic MRSA in Australia, has said: 'We may look back at the antibiotic era as just a passing phase in the history of medicine, an era in which a great natural resource was squandered, and where the bugs proved smarter than the scientist.'

THE DOOMSDAY SUPERBUG

Hospitals now harbour zoos of drug-resistant bacteria. MRSA is the best-known hospital superbug, along with *P. aeruginosa, E. coli* and other species already mentioned. But they are not all. In August 1992, *Time* magazine ran a feature entitled: 'ATTACK OF THE SUPERBUGS.'[22] It began: 'Using marvellous powers of mutation, some strains of bacteria are transforming themselves into new breeds of superbugs that are invulnerable to some or all antibiotics.' Examples cited included the superbugs that are the microbiological causes of drug-resistant malaria, tuberculosis and gonorrhoea.

The feature continued: 'Overuse of antibiotics has accelerated the evolution of superbugs, and hospitals, in particular, are major breeding grounds . . . Stubborn strains of bacteria resistant to many different antibiotics have taken up permanent residence in hospitals around the world.' Evidence for this conclusion had been provided the previous week, in a series of features published in *Science* magazine and, in particular, a major review, 'The crisis in antibiotic resistance'[2], written by Professor Harold Neu of the departments of medicine and pharmacology at Columbia University, New York.

A list of the 'Top ten drug-resistant microbes' included, as well as those already mentioned, the enterobacteriaceae family, the enterococci family, *Haemophilius influenzae, Shigella dysenteriae* and *Streptococcus pneumoniae*. Some of these are a menace in the community as well as in hospitals. *S. pneumoniae* is a major bacterial cause not only of pneumonia but also of middle-ear infections and meningitis in children and adults; in some countries, it is commonly resistant to penicillin. 'In 1941, 10,000 units of penicillin administered four times a day for four days cured patients of pneumococcal pneumonia,' wrote Professor Neu. 'Today, a patient could receive 24 million units of penicillin and die of pneumococcal meningitis.'[2]

Drug-resistant shigella dysentery is now common in American nursery schools and among homosexual men.[23] Resistant strains of *H. influenzae* – also a cause of bacterial pneumonia, middle-ear infections and meningitis, as well as serious nose and throat infections – are increasing. Enterobacteria intrinsically resistant to many antibiotics, such as *Serratia marcescens*, are a common cause of serious hospital infections, including septicaemia. According to Professor Neu, 'Serratia resistant to betalactams, aminoglycosides, fluoroquinolones, and even co-trimoxazole have been found in hospitals in the United States, Europe, and Japan.' And so on.

Professor Alexander Tomasz, writing in 1994[3] sees multi drug-resistant pneumococci as a potential global disaster. This family of bacteria are the microbiological cause of otitis media, meningitis and bacteremia (general infection of the blood) as well as pneumonia, and are reckoned to cause 40,000 deaths every year in the USA, and 3 to 5 million deaths worldwide.[24] Once readily treatable with penicillin, pneumococci are now commonly resistant not only to penicillin but also to erythromycin, tetracycline, chloramphenicol and co-trimoxazole. 'The patients at greatest risk of pneumococcal disease are young children and the elderly,' said Dr Tomasz.

Scientists, physicians and public health experts gathered at a 1993 conference held at Rockefeller University, New York, as reported by Dr Tomasz, recommended as a matter of urgency that doctors be formally requested to notify the US federal Centers for Disease Control and Prevention of cases and outbreaks of drug-resistant pneumococci and other major dangerous superbugs.[25]

In the late 1980s and early 1990s, there were signs of the emergence of drug-resistant bacteria with the potential to become doomsday superbugs, resistant to all antibiotics. These are enterococci, normally present in the guts of healthy people, but which may invade a vulnerable body, and which have become a cause of urinary tract infections, wound abscesses, septicaemia, endocarditis and meningitis.[26] Naturally resistant to various antibiotics, including some penicillins and cephalosporins, aminoglycosides, and co-trimoxazole, over time they have also acquired resistance to erythromycin, tetracyclines, chloramphenicol and other antibiotics.

In 1989, a report of enterococci also resistant to vancomycin and to teicoplanin (like vancomycin, a glycopeptide) appeared in the newsletter of the Alliance for the Prudent Use of Antibiotics.[27] Outbreaks in the USA, France and the UK were cited. Two species are involved: *Streptococcus faecalis* and to a lesser extent *Streptococcus faecium*. In 1992 and 1993, the *Lancet* carried reports of two outbreaks of infection caused by multiple-resistant enterococci, in London and New York City.[28] In the London cases, these bacteria had not only become resistant to vancomycin but, worse, this vancomycin resistance had evidently spread to other bacterial species. Therefore, 'there is a danger that the vancomycin-resistant gene may pass to other clinically important . . . bacteria such as methicillin-resistant *Staphylococcus aureus*.'

The New York cases, reported in July 1993, were rather more alarming. Dr Thomas Friedan and colleagues from the New York City Department of Health and elsewhere in the USA and Canada collected data on hospital patients infected with vancomycin-resistant enterococci, by then common enough to be referred to by the initials VRE. The number of hospitals in New York City reporting VRE increased from 1 in 1989 to 30 by October 1991. Most hospital patients infected with it were elderly and already seriously ill, and the great majority had been given vancomycin and/or cephalosporin antibiotics. The history of 100 such patients was reviewed. Of these, 42 had died, of whom five were judged to have been killed by VRE. In 19 cases, VRE was judged to have been a contributory cause of death. Commenting on the ability of enterococci to become immune to antibiotics, Dr Friedan and his colleagues concluded: 'These organisms, many resistant to all antimicrobials, present a unique challenge to infection control and clinical practice.'

The more vancomycin is used in hospitals, the more enterococci will become the ultimate superbugs. Dr Richard Novick of the New York Public Health Institute, who is a pioneer in MRSA research, told me that he is sure that VRE is indeed a peculiar menace. Effectively confirming Dr Friedan's findings, he said: 'I have had physicians say to me that they have watched people die in front of their eyes infected with *Enterococcus faecalis* resistant to every drug they had and could use against this organism, including vancomycin.' And the implications? 'It's a losing battle, in the long run. The bugs have proved smarter than the drugs, and the bugs have the advantage. What's particularly alarming to us, is that the vancomycin resistance is plasmid-carried, and the plasmids of *Enterococcus faecalis* are known to be able to transfer to *Staphylococcus aureus*.'

In developing countries, death from drug-resistant infections are common, simply because physicians often do not have access to newer, more expensive drugs to which bacteria such as enterococci are still vulnerable. In the UK, the USA and other developed countries, unless industry comes up with new drugs, it is conceivable that 'everything-resistant' enterococci will mark the beginning of the end of the antibiotic era.

THE DRUG-EATING SUPERBUG

Moulds can feed off antibiotics: this was mentioned in Part 4. So can mutant bacteria. In July 1994 a team of hospital doctors from Philadelphia reported that they had identified a new strain of everything-resistant *Enterococcus faecalis* in the urine of a 46-year-old woman in intensive care.[29] This had mutated not only to become resistant to vancomycin; it had mutated in another way too, to become dependent on vancomycin for growth. Also in 1994, vancomycin-eating *Enterococcus faecium* were in the faeces of two kidney patients in hospitals in Birmingham and Carshalton, in England.[30]

The ultimate superbug has been bred by systematic antibiotic use: the monster drug-eating superbug. 'Vancomycin dependence is an unusual clinical phenomenon,' commented the investigators dryly. It 'shows the remarkable ability of bacterial organisms to adapt to the intense antimicrobial pressure of the nosocomial environment'.

17 Infectious Drug Resistance

SURVIVAL OF THE FITTEST BUGS

How do bacteria become drug resistant so that antibiotics become useless? 'Very readily' is the short answer. Professor Tore Midtvedt, a man of quizzical humour, said to me as we talked in his laboratories at the Karolinska Institute in Stockholm, that drug resistance follows the use of antibiotics as inevitably as 'amen in church'.

A full answer to the question, though, involves looking again at the theories we have learned to accept about the origins and development of life on earth, for the means by which bacteria evolve so as to become invulnerable to drugs gives a new insight into evolution.

There are, it's said, more scientists alive today than ever previously lived throughout history, and modern science has transformed our world. Nevertheless, remarkably, we generally accept that the basic laws of the physical universe were identified some hundreds of years ago by such great scientists as Nicholaus Copernicus and Isaac Newton. Comparably, we are brought up to believe that the basic laws of the biological world, which explain our place and that of all living things in nature, were worked out in the nineteenth century, notably by Charles Darwin and Gregor Mendel, and that all subsequent discoveries in the biological sciences rest on the shoulders of giants such as these.

In particular, we are taught that the 'survival of the fittest' is a matter of chance. At my primary school, I learned that the boys who became dominant in the playground were those who happened to have the biggest fists or the sharpest sense of humour. This is a rough analogy with Darwin's theory of natural selection, which includes the view that living things evolve so as to survive and thrive in different and changing environments, as a result of random mutation.

Later at school, I was taught that the reason why giraffes have long necks is that they graze on the top branches of sparse trees growing on the African savannah; any short-necked giraffes die out. Human characteristics can also be explained in this way. Thus, it is supposed that, one day, millions of years ago, a primate was born with thumbs, and this freak grew up with a dexterity which gave it, and those of its descendants who inherited this trait, an advantage over others of the species, so that the primates with thumbs eventually became dominant.

Darwin's theory is also an elegant explanation of why some species die out and others multiply, in changing or new environments. Thus, it is generally agreed that the mammoths died out because they were unable to adapt to the Ice Ages; as vegetation became harder to find, they starved, while smaller creatures still had enough to eat. Environmental change exerts 'selective pressure'. Those species and variations of species able to withstand that pressure or adapt to it will effectively be the 'fittest' and thus survive and multiply. Darwin's theory evidently fits the facts. It has never been successfully challenged, and is central to the set of assumptions made about the living world by biological scientists and indeed by everybody who has been taught the fundamentals of biological science.

Given that all living things, including micro-organisms, evolve in the same way, by means of natural selection, the development of drug resistance in bacteria as a result of antibiotic treatment was predictable right from the start. Indeed, both of the pioneers of penicillin, Alexander Fleming and Howard Florey, were well aware that bacteria developed resistance to the drugs then in use for bacterial infections. In 1944, Florey noted that bacterial species such as *E. coli* might actually increase in number during a course of treatment; observed that in some cases relatively massive doses of penicillin were required to overcome resistant bacteria; and feared that, in time, penicillin might lose its effectiveness against bacterial infections.[31]

The assumption that Fleming and Florey made, as did all microbiologists in the 1940s and up to the late 1950s, is that bacteria evolve so as to become resistant to drugs strictly according to Darwinian principles, which (or so it was thought) govern the evolution of one-celled prokaryotic species in exactly the same way as with eukaryotic species made up of millions upon millions of cells, such as giraffes, mammoths and, indeed, *Homo sapiens*.

One obvious difference between us and bacteria is that they are very small; for every human, millions upon millions of bacteria can fit into any given space. Consequently, bacteria are comparatively very adaptable faced with a changed environment, simply because in any population of billions, some chance mutants will happen to be genetically suited to the new circumstances. Under selective pressure, large species like the mammoths may die out, or else take thousands of years to evolve suitable characteristics, such as light or dark human skin colour in different climates. But microscopic species can evolve adapted populations in a matter of days.

In his book *Chance and Necessity*[32] Professor Jacques Monod, then director of the Pasteur Institute in Paris, explains.

> Any mutation considered individually, is a very rare event. With bacteria . . . the probability of a given gene undergoing a mutation significantly affecting its functional properties, is of the order of between one in a million and one in a hundred million. But a population of several thousand million cells can develop in a few millilitres of water. In a population of that size, there will be maybe ten, or a hundred, or a thousand examples of any given mutation, and maybe a hundred thousand or a million mutants of all types . . . In so large a population, mutation is not the exception: it is the rule.

If only for this reason, the development of drug resistance in bacteria following the use of antibiotics is inevitable, as is superinfection. It seems that mammoths were unable to survive the Ice Ages.[33] But faced with a chemical cataclysm, the one bacterium that just happens to be naturally drug resistant – in a population of a million or hundred million bacteria in the species targeted by an antibiotic – will survive and multiply; and this mutant strain may then become the dominant species, just through force of circumstance.

SHOTGUN THERAPY

In the early 1940s, when penicillin was the only relatively safe antibiotic available, leading researchers such as Howard Florey were bound to wonder if drug-resistant bacteria would eventually make antibiotic therapy futile. But this apprehension dissolved into euphoria with the discovery and marketing of new antibiotics such as streptomycin, chloramphenicol and tetracycline, and then later with the development of successive generations of betalactams. According to the principles of random selection, the chance of resistance to one drug occurring as a mutation in a population of bacteria, and in time becoming dominant as a result of administration of that drug, is high. But the chance of random mutant strains of bacteria resistant to two different antibiotics is between a million and a hundred million times less likely; and the chance of random multiple resistance to three or more antibiotics is, for all practical purposes, zero.

So what became fixed in the minds of physicians in the 'golden age' of antibiotics is that, if one antibiotic doesn't work, try another; better still, try two at once, maybe in liberal quantities.[34] Dr Richard Novick recalled the recommended clinical practice he encountered in his early days as a doctor. 'When I was in medical school, antibiotics were new – this was in the late fifties. I was taught pharmacology by a very well-regarded microbial physiologist. He had a very clear-headed, rational view of pharmacology. And he taught us that resistance was going to be a problem with antibiotics, because bacteria could mutate, and that it had been shown recently that mutation was random – and he taught us that the clever rationale for using antibiotics was to use two, because then the chances of resistance occurring to both was infinitesimal, and you needn't worry about that. We all thought that was wonderful and enormously clever and intellectual, especially for second-year medical students, who'd never been exposed to anything like that before.'

Even in the days of greatest enthusiasm for antibiotics, physicians knew that giving two or more drugs to a patient at the same time was problematic. The greater the variety of drugs, the greater the chances of ill-effects, which might be difficult to trace. If you are suffering from an infection, are given two (or more) drugs, and remain ill afterwards, perhaps with symptoms similar to those you had before taking the drugs, what is causing your illness? The infection? The first drug? The second drug? The two drugs interacting with each other? And if it is the infection, does this mean you should be given a third drug? Polypharmacy – the administration of two or more drugs at the same time – can muddle physicians as well as patients. And when two or more antibiotics are given at the same time, the risk of superinfection increases, particularly if the total dose of the two or more drugs given is greater than that of one drug.

But polypharmacy did seem to be the answer to antibiotic resistance, which can be life-threatening when drugs are no longer effective against serious, invasive bacterial infection. And it is tempting to try a succession of drugs against any obstinate infection. Physicians want drugs to work, both for the sake of their patients' health, and because they do not want to be defeated.

Generations of medical students and young doctors – including those who have later become leaders of the medical profession – whose initial experience of medicine has involved antibiotics, have been trained to believe that although these potent drugs may not work in individual cases like magic bullets fired from a rifle, they should work if, in effect, fired from both barrels of a shotgun, with less discrimination. And this belief understandably persists, for of course it is true that, if two or more antibiotics are used simultaneously or in succession, as if from a shotgun, or a blunderbuss or a machine-gun, the chances that an obstinate infection will be blasted out of the body are increased.

Thus, the assumption that drug-resistant bacteria are solely the result of random mutation of bacteria is an important reason why antibiotics are often used aggressively by general practitioners and hospital doctors, as if weapons in an all-out war, without proper consideration of immediate and long-term ill-effects.

WHAT HAPPENED IN JAPAN

Bacteria do indeed become resistant to antibiotics as a result of random mutation. But bugs become superbugs characteristically by means of a biological 'intelligence' unknown and unimagined until the late 1950s, which astounded research scientists at the time, and which is quite amazing. Random mutation affects only one bacterial species, and almost certainly will result in resistance to only one drug. But bacteria do become resistant to two or more drugs, and sometimes to all available drugs, not normally, if ever, by random mutation. What actually happens is an altogether more fascinating phenomenon which contradicts conventional genetics, and which may one day encourage a new theory of the origin of species. Indeed, if Charles Darwin had been able to do his work with the aid of very powerful microscopes, he might himself have come to somewhat different conclusions.

The story of the discovery of multiple drug-resistant superbugs, and of how they have gained their power over antibiotics, begins in

Japan. After industrialisation, the Japanese people suffered successive epidemics of dysentery caused by *Shigella dysenteriae*. This species of shigella bacillus is the most virulent, and is most common in hot climates.[35] It may cause no more than mild or severe diarrhoea, but it can invade the body systemically, causing intense pain and fever. Adults usually recover from this 'bacillary' dysentery after anything between a few days and several weeks, but without prompt attention, it can cause severe fever, dehydration and even death in babies and young children, mostly in tropical countries.

After the Second World War, sulphonamides were introduced and widely used in Japan. They worked against bacillary dysentery: the epidemics were checked, and incidence of the disease dropped by four fifths in two years. But two years later, in 1949, the country was swept by new epidemics of bacillary dysentery caused by *S. dysenteriae* usually resistant to sulpha drugs; incidence of the disease rose higher than ever.[36] In the UK at the time, microbiologists feared that one day, drug resistance might eventually render penicillin useless. In Japan, physicians actually were becoming powerless, faced with sulphonamide-resistant bacteria.

But as elsewhere, streptomycin, chloramphenicol and tetracycline, all of which can be effective treatment for dysentery, were introduced in Japan and, by the early 1950s, had evidently given power back to the physicians. With the use of these drugs, the incidence of bacillary dysentery again dropped. It seemed that science was one step – or three steps – ahead of drug-resistant bacteria. Nobody worried about multiple drug resistance which, on the assumption of random selection, was practically impossible.

Well, almost nobody – for in 1952 the microbiologist Dr Tsutomo Watanabe found an example of *S. dysenteriae* which, against all the known odds, was resistant not to one drug, but to three: the sulpha drug sulphanilamide, streptomycin and tetracycline. Then in 1955, a woman returned from Hong Kong to Tokyo suffering from bacillary dysentery; and the hospital doctors called to treat her found that she was infected with a strain of *S. dysenteriae* resistant to all four drugs used to treat the disease: not only the ones already mentioned but also chloramphenicol. The seemingly impossible had happened.

The first findings of multiple drug resistance to bacillary dysentery were published in specialist journals little known to scientists outside Japan, and the first cases were thought to be freaks, in common with other inexplicable phenomena. But later in the 1950s, more waves of epidemic dysentery swept through Japan, which in many cases were resistant to all four drugs then used to treat the disease. What was happening? Then another microbiologist, Dr Tomoichiro Akiba of Tokyo University, made a discovery which made multiple drug resistance doubly mysterious. He examined samples of bacteria from the intestines of hospital patients suffering from bacillary dysentery. What he found was resistance to the four drugs of choice not only among *S. dysenteriae*, but also the same pattern of multiple drug resistance in an altogether different bacterial species present in the healthy gut, *E. coli*.[37]

There simply is no way that two different types of bacteria such as *S. dysenteriae* and *E. coli* could coincidentally both become resistant to the same four drugs as a result of random mutation. Consider the mathematics. Suppose the rate of mutation in bacterial cells is one in one million. The chance of coincidental mutations in two bacterial species making them each resistant to four drugs would be one million to the power of 8 – that is, one million million million million million million million million: vastly more cells than there are on earth. Multiple drug resistance cannot be random.

But if not random, what? Could bacteria in some senses *learn* to become drug resistant? The idea seemed incredible, but so it proved. The crucial experiment was done by a team led by Dr Kunitaro Ochai. Cultures of *E. coli* resistant to sulphanilamide, streptomycin, chloramphenicol and tetracycline were mixed with cultures of drug-sensitive *S. dysenteriae*, vulnerable to all four drugs. What then happened was that the *S. dysenteriae* changed in nature: they became multiply drug resistant too. There was only one possible explanation. Somehow, the *E. coli* superbug was able to transfer its powers of resistance to another bacterial species, turning the previously vulnerable *S. dysenteriae* into an untreatable and therefore potentially lethal superbug.[38]

At first, nobody knew how this happened. But the implications were staggering. Drug resistance caused by random mutation of specific bacterial species can always be overcome by use of a different antibiotic, just as Richard Novick had been taught in medical school. But drug resistance that is multiplied and transferred between bacteria, and from one bacterial species to another, is incalculably ominous. For there is no way of knowing how far or fast such drug resistance will spread, or when or where outbreaks or epidemics of bacterial infection will prove to be untreatable.

JUMPING GENES

Talking to Dr Novick in his office in downtown Manhattan, just by Bellevue Hospital, I asked him what impact the news from Japan had on him and other microbiologists in the field.

'Oh, it was devastating,' he said. 'But it was both devastating and fascinating. Everything we had been taught in medical school about antibiotics and resistance was tossed in the trash. It took a little while to sink in. For this was going to cause – and has caused – an incredible revolution in all of genetics, not just bacteriology and the treatment of bacterial infection. The idea that genes could be shuttled among bacteria, between species and between genera . . .' He paused, searching for a phrase. 'It was something that – that was so *radical*.' 'Unthinkable until it was proved?' I asked. 'It would never have occurred to anyone,' he replied. 'No one dreamed of its universality. The impact of that fact and that finding has matured only rather slowly, over the years.'

In the early 1960s, Dr Novick, working in Mill Hill, London, at the National Institute for Medical Research, realised that resistance transfer was not unique to *E. coli*, but also occurred in *Staphylococcus aureus*. Appalled by the implications, he wrote letters to the *Lancet* warning against the then common practice of surgeons in London hospitals, of 'spraying methicillin around the wards. I wrote saying this was outrageous, and would ruin the usefulness of the drug.' So it proved, with the emergence of MRSA – methicillin-resistant *S. aureus*. And as late as the 1960s, Dr Novick told me, he came across representatives of the pharmaceutical industry who refused to accept that drug resistance could transfer from one bacterial species to another, dismissing what was by then well-established fact as 'some figment of the scientific imagination'.

Dr Tsutomo Watanabe is credited with solving the mystery of what he himself aptly named 'infectious drug resistance', at the end of the 1950s.[36] He found that, while bacteria may have just one chromosome, they carry additional packages of genetic material within their cell walls, in the form of rings of nucleic acid now known as 'plasmids'.[39]

Like viruses, these sub-cellular organisms live and multiply only within the bacterial cell wall. But there are key differences between viruses and plasmids. While viruses are actually usually harmless or even beneficial to their bacterial hosts, bringing in new and sometimes useful genetic information, they can also destroy bacteria. By contrast, plasmids are always beneficial, and can be vital to bacterial health and survival.

Notably, plasmids can carry information not contained in bacterial chromosomes. This includes genes that protect their bacterial host against poisons in the environment – which now include antibiotics. And plasmids also enable bacteria to pass on genes by means of 'conjugation', or bacterial mating. These two qualities account for infectious drug resistance.

I asked Dr Novick to explain. 'Bacteria have fairly classical genes like you and me, and like cows, chickens, and so forth,' he said, 'although, interestingly, that was not realised until the 1940s or 1950s. They have genes organised as a single chromosome. As it turns out, bacteria have additional packages of genes outside the chromosome, and these are called plasmids. These are able to multiply inside the bacterial cell on their own; and remarkably, they contain the genetic information that enables them to be transferred from cell to cell, and not only from cell to cell but between different species and genera of bacteria.[40]

'What that means is that bacteria can actually mate, one with another, and during the mating of the cells, the DNA of a plasmid is passed from one cell to another. Not any other of the cell's genes are passed in that kind of mating; only the plasmids' genes are passed. The chromosomes of bacteria do not mate; only the plasmids do. And since most plasmids occur in more than one copy in any given cell, the original carrier retains its plasmid, and the new one gets its copy; so now both bacteria contain a plasmid – and so on. It's not an exchange like money; it's a multiplicative spread.'

So the reason why bacteria become multiply drug-resistant superbugs is that resistance is 'carried in packages in little sub-cellular vehicles that shuttle from bacteria to bacteria'. Dr Novick is inclined to think that plasmids are not just bacterial accessory gene packages, but are organisms in their own right, in this respect like viruses, working independently within and between host cells. From a bacterial point of view, whereas viruses may make war, plasmids always make love. Their evolutionary strategy is not to attack, but to defend individual bacteria and whole populations of bacteria, of the same and also of different species.

As a young researcher in the early 1960s, Dr Stuart Levy – now professor in the departments of microbiology and of medicine at

Tufts University in Boston – worked in Dr Watanabe's laboratories in Tokyo. The time 'was one of indescribable excitement,' he has said.[41] Infectious drug resistance transmitted by plasmids 'seemed almost unimaginable to us, since it flew in the face of so much accepted biology and genetics. It was completely new territory.'

But thc implications were truly frightening, as Dr Watanabe well knew. In 1967, he marked the end of the golden age of antibiotics, writing: 'Unless we put a halt to the prodigal use of antibiotics and synthetic drugs, we may soon be forced back into the pre-antibiotic era of medicine.'[42]

Whether or not plasmids are biologically separable from bacteria, it is known that bacteria contained plasmids before the antibiotic era. This has been established by research in remote communities in the world that, at the time, had not been exposed to antibiotics, and also by examination of bacteria from the pre-antibiotic age stored and sealed in test-tubes early this century, for the benefit of future scientists.[43,44] It is likely that bacteria and plasmids have evolved in harmony, as a mutually beneficial microbiological ecosystem.

Some but not all 'pre-antibiotic' plasmids have also been found to carry some drug-resistant genes.[45] Why? Probably because one benefit of plasmids to bacteria is protection against attack by microbiological predators in nature, whose chemical structure happens to be similar to that of antibiotics developed as human medicine. Since some antibiotics, such as penicillin, streptomycin and cephalosporin, were originally found in nature – in mould, soil or sewage – they no doubt had evolved as natural antimicrobials, against which bacteria in turn had evolved natural defences, by means of resistance genes.

In the pre-antibiotic world, bacteria could survive, multiply and retain their integral role in the perpetual renewal of life on earth with relatively few resistance genes; the risk of destruction was low. But the systematic worldwide use of antibiotics as human medicine, and also in the intensive rearing of animals, has put massive evolutionary pressure on bacteria to defend themselves. Bacteria now carry complex permutations and combinations of resistance to antibiotics, including to synthetic drugs with chemical structures not found in nature. In effect, bacterial plasmids have *learned* to become multiply drug resistant.

Writing in 1980, Richard Novick stated[40]:

> Today it is not uncommon to find a plasmid carrying genes for resistance to as many as ten antibiotics. The rather frightening

> clinical implication of this accumulation of resistance genes is that treating a patient with a single drug can promote the selection of an organism resistant to everything in sight.

That is, whenever you take an antibiotic, you run some risk of causing a cascade of drug resistance in the bacteria in your gut and elsewhere in your body, so that, in future, antibiotics won't work.

In the 1970s, another mystery of infectious drug resistance was solved. How is it that multiple drug resistance can and sometimes does spread explosively, as in Japan during the 1940s and 1950s? The answer is that the genes for drug resistance are carried on sections of plasmid now known as transposons, or 'jumping genes' because they behave like submicroscopic fleas. Transposons are able to jump out of one plasmid and into another, carrying drug resistance with them, and can also jump from plasmid to bacterial chromosome, and back again. By these means, plasmids accumulate resistance to an increasing number of antibiotics, which can then be transposed within and between bacterial species. It seems, for example, that enterococci such as VRE spread their immunity to antibiotics to other potentially lethal species such as *Staphylococcus aureus* by means of transposons.[26] In time, bacteria tend to become as protected against attack as they need to be: the more drugs, the more superbugs.

GLOBAL CONTAGION

Professor Thomas O'Brien is making a special study of antibiotic resistance worldwide, as head of the Centre for Surveillance of Antimicrobial Resistance supported with some funding from the World Health Organisation, called WHONET for short. After talking with Richard Novick in New York, I went to see Dr O'Brien in Boston. In common with other leading microbiologists interviewed for this book, he is concerned about the global spread of drug resistance and its implications for human health.

As a microbiologist, Dr O'Brien can readily see the world from a microbial point of view. The first thing to bear in mind, he said, is just how vast bacterial populations are. 'Bacteria are the most numerous living things on the planet – far and away. They exist in complex ecosystems of which each of us is one. The number of bacterial cells we carry in us and on us outnumber our own cells. If it came to a vote, we'd be in trouble!'

Second, he said, bacterial ecosystems are, by their nature, interconnected; the closer we and other living things live to each other, the faster the rate of bacterial interchange. 'The patients on an intensive care unit, for example: each one of them is an individual bacterial ecosystem, but the unit itself also is one.' And referring to an intensive system of rearing cattle common in the USA, he said: 'Certainly, an animal feedlot is itself an ecosystem; the bacteria will interchange at high rates there.' In the same way, schools, workplaces, villages, even whole towns and cities, as well as hospitals, function as bacterial ecosystems, within which vastly complex populations of bacterial species move around.

Third, bacteria have always been able to move fast, and the relatively very small number of species that are the microbiological cause of human disease can create explosive epidemics. 'This is not a new observation,' Dr O'Brien said. 'In the 1830s and 1840s, when cholera first left India, it travelled in the first great pandemic in a matter of months to Russia and then Europe, and then a year later was in the United States. The transmissibility of bacteria even before the jet age was impressive.'

When antibiotics were first introduced, scientists and physicians had no idea just how adaptable bacteria are, and just how fast they can resist drugs and share this resistance around. We humans may take thousands or millions of years to evolve significantly. What we gain in consciousness, we lose in genetic adaptability. Bacteria can evolve new characteristics, such as drug resistance, in minutes. Antibiotics have caused incalculable disruption to bacterial ecosystems worldwide. Dr O'Brien explained to me:

> Fifty years ago, there began the most massive intervention in population genetics imaginable on this planet, involving the most numerous forms of life – the bacteria. Suddenly, tons of sulphonamide were distributed and used all over the world, and then hundreds – thousands – of tons of penicillin. The experiment has been carried out; but the results have not been measured.

The purpose of Dr O'Brien's work with WHONET is to assess what effect antibiotics have had and are having on bacteria, and the implications for human health worldwide.

Before antibiotics, 'there were virtually no resistance genes around. Now there are more than a hundred that have been identified and named. The betalactamases are now quite an elaborate family of resistance genes, mutations with new generations emerging, which break the molecule of penicillin and inactivate it. And the different tricks they have!' He described the various mechanisms by which bacteria have learned to resist chloramphenicol, erythromycin, clindamycin, tetracycline, and other drugs.[46] 'We used to think of evolutionary changes happening over tens of millions of years. It's incredible to think that all these changes in these vast populations have happened since I was in the second grade at school.'

You do not have to be ill to harbour resistant bacteria. They are everywhere in the environment – in the air, in water, carried by other people and by animals, including those we eat, and in food and drink. In 1988, Professor Stuart Levy and co-workers published the results of a study of over 300 healthy people living in Boston who were not at the time taking antibiotics.[47] Over half carried bacteria resistant to at least one antibiotic, and around one third carried bacterial genes resistant to streptomycin, ampicillin, tetracycline and kanamycin (like streptomycin, an aminoglycoside). If these results are typical, it follows that, whereas half a century ago, bacterial resistance genes were rare, now over half of us carry mutant bacteria within our bodies; and this includes people who are not taking antibiotics.

While antibiotics are targeted against the bacterial species that carry disease, it is not only these pathogens that adapt and become drug resistant. Attacked by antibiotics, bacteria of all types evolve, develop and spread resistance genes. As already stated, these include commensal species normally present within the human gut, but which can cause serious or even dangerous infections when they invade elsewhere in the body, such as in wounds, or in vulnerable areas such as the vagina and urinary tract, which may have been laid open to infection by previous use of antibiotics.

Professor O'Brien said to me:[48]

> There is a lot of antibiotic resistance in the developed world, and it has the potential to get much worse. Resistance genes continue to encroach, and we physicians are losing our lead. In the 1980s, the drug companies got way ahead of resistance. They introduced third-generation cephalosporins: very expensive, but they worked. Later in the 1980s, the fluoroquinolones were introduced: oral drugs, very

> wide spectrum. But now, fifteen to twenty resistance genes have emerged that can destroy the third-generation cephalosporins. And we are now beginning to see resistance to the fluoroquinolones. But now, in the 1990s, there aren't a lot of new antibiotics being developed.

Drug resistance is contagious, but it is not itself a disease. Rather, a little like raised blood pressure or raised blood cholesterol, it is a danger sign, of vulnerability to disease.[49] If we carry drug-resistant superbugs, any bacterial infection may be hard to treat. For generally healthy adults living in rich countries with modern medical services, drug resistance is normally defeated, after an illness that may be prolonged with antibiotics that may be relatively expensive and/or toxic, but which do work. In developed countries, those most at risk from resistant bacteria include babies and young children, the elderly, and people of any age who are seriously ill. Ironically, it is such vulnerable people who are at high risk of illness from bacterial infection and therefore most likely to be on an antibiotic treadmill.

18 Chaos in the Third World

DEAD BABIES

In countries such as the USA and the UK, potent drugs such as antibiotics are controlled and generally available as prescribed by a physician, surgeon or dental surgeon. Nevertheless, overuse and abuse of antibiotics in the developed world amounts to an international crisis somewhat similar in its scale and implications to that caused by overuse and abuse of the world's energy resources.

By contrast, in countries within Africa, Asia, Latin America and elsewhere, drugs are often practically uncontrolled and may be available not only over the counter in pharmacies but in shops and markets; and the overuse and abuse of antibiotics in these nations amounts to a truly frightening crisis, which affects us all.

> As the boat drew in to the shore we heard a strange sound from the bank. A woman was crying. We found her with a dead baby in her arms, and a collection of medicine bottles beside her. She had spent all her money on these expensive drugs. She could not understand why they had not saved her baby. This Bangladeshi woman had never been told what was obvious to the doctor who found her. The baby had become severely dehydrated with diarrhoea. Her death could have been prevented with a simple home-made solution of water, salt and sugar. No amount of medicine could have kept her alive.

This is from the introduction of *Bitter Pills*[50] by Dianna Melrose of Oxfam, a book on the use and abuse of drugs in developing countries, published in 1982. This account of the Bangladeshi mother and child is one of scandal as well as tragedy; repeated countless times all over the developing world every year, it is the story of the wrong use of antibiotics to treat infant diarrhoea.

Diarrhoea is the biggest killer of children under the age of three, taking all countries in the world together. The younger the child and the poorer the country, the greater the risk of death. A task force of scientists set up to report to the US National Institutes of Health confirmed in 1987 that up to five million little children throughout the world die every year from diarrhoea, adding: 'This results in an enormous loss of potentially fruitful lives.'[51]

Just like tuberculosis, epidemic infant diarrhoea is a disease whose fundamental cause is squalor, specifically semi-starvation and wretched living conditions. The microbiological cause of diarrhoea can be either a viral or a bacterial infection. In developing countries, infant diarrhoea is not a great public health problem, simply because little children generally are better fed and live in a cleaner environment.

The most common simple infectious diarrhoeas are, in a sense, not so much diseases as dramatic signals that the body is trying to rid itself of a poisonous virus, or bacteria such as salmonella, campylobacter or (usually outside North America and Europe) shigella, a cause of dysentery. Just how toxic any micro-organism is in its effects depends not only on its strength (or 'virulence')[52] but also, and more importantly, on a person's strength. If I am strong and you are weak, and both of us are invaded by, say, *Salmonella enteritidis*, you are more likely to be overcome by the infection and show symptoms of poisoning, including general malaise, stomach cramps and diarrhoea; whereas I might feel only mild symptoms or none at all. Some people are immune to all but the most virulent micro-organisms. Others, including babies and young children, are vulnerable, and sickly babies are most vulnerable of all.

In the case of simple diarrhoea, no matter how explosive, just about the worst thing to do is dose the victim with antibiotics. First, diarrhoea is often caused by viruses, not bacteria, and, of course, antibiotics don't work against viruses. Second, many antibiotics, being themselves a cause of diarrhoea and therefore liable to make existing diarrhoea, more severe or prolonged. Third, what kills little children suffering from simple diarrhoea is typically not the infection, but the massive loss of water and salts in the diarrhoea. What the child needs is not drugs, but oral rehydration therapy, which can take the form of water, salt and sugar or, even simpler, rice water. As with the Bangladeshi girl witnessed by Dianna Melrose, any vulnerable little child with acute diarrhoea who is given drugs rather than fluids may die, if only because the drugs distract from proper treatment.

SWEETIES FOR DIARRHOEA

However, antibiotics for the treatment of diarrhoea are and remain a big industry, especially in poor countries. In the words of a drug industry representative speaking at a 'diarrhoea workshop' held in Frankfurt in 1983[53]:

> The market for anti-diarrhoeals is a huge market and certainly a challenge for the pharmaceutical industry. It is our sincere hope and trust that our initiatives, together with the programmes carried out by WHO, training programmes in universities, research activities, etc., will result in having better drugs and better means of treatment to control children's diarrhoea.

One company took an initiative in 1983, marketing an anti-diarrhoea drug containing chloramphenicol and tetracycline in the form of a chocolate-coloured and flavoured pill for children. The drug became a favourite in Third World countries, and was sometimes known as 'sweeties for diarrhoea'. It was later withdrawn.

Health Action International (HAI), a world network then supported by the International Organisation of Consumer Unions at its European headquarters in The Hague, made a count of anti-diarrhoeal drugs in 1986. Of the 398 brands identified on the world market, over three out of five – 64 per cent – contained antibiotics. 'More than 160 companies are involved in this trade,' the report said. These included many of the biggest multinationals, but also national and local firms turning out cheap replica drugs.[54]

Surveys of Third World countries in the mid-1980s quoted by HAI showed that four out of five anti-diarrhoea drugs sold in India contained antibiotics. In Bangladesh, Yemen and Sri Lanka, only one in five pharmacies recommended oral rehydration therapy rather than drugs for diarrhoea. In other countries, anti-diarrhoea drugs often contained antibiotics whose use is carefully restricted in the developed world. Examples were: streptomycin in nearly one in four antidiarrhoeals in India and Pakistan; chloramphenicol in over one in ten in India; sulphonamides in one in three in the Philippines; and neomycin (an aminoglycoside mainly restricted to use only on the skin in the UK, because of its toxicity), contained in nearly one in four antidiarrhoeals used in Africa, the Caribbean and Malaysia.

Infant diarrhoea is a top priority for the World Health Organisation, which is flatly opposed to the use of antibiotics for simple diarrhoea. A WHO manual for physicians issued in 1990[55] states that, every year, over 1.3 billion episodes of diarrhoea occur in children under the age of five in Asia (excluding China), Africa, and Latin America, and that babies and toddlers under the age of two are at greatest risk; four out of five of all deaths are in this age group. A note issued by the WHO Diarrhoeal Disease Control Programme in 1988[56] states: 'Oral rehydration therapy is the keystone of all national diarrhoeal disease control programmes because it is simple, highly effective, inexpensive, and technologically appropriate.'

And drugs? Tetracycline is recommended when the diarrhoea is due to cholera. Antibiotics are also recommended when the cause is shigella dysentery. Otherwise:

> No antibiotic or chemotherapeutic agent . . . has proven value for the routine treatment of acute diarrhoea: their use is inappropriate and possibly dangerous.

But in the 1980s, the world market for drugs used to treat diarrhoea more than doubled in value, and in 1989 was reckoned to be worth £300 million a year.

WHAT ABOUT WHO?

The key strategic decisions about drugs are taken not by national industries or by national governments, but by transnational companies with global policies. As *The Economist* stated in August 1990[57]:

> Companies are becoming stateless citizens independent of their original nationalities . . . The old 1960s model of the multinational, with a dominant parent company and an army of stand-alone clones in each overseas market, has been superseded by one in which firms locate production wherever the costs are lowest, and organise on a more equal, global scale.

Correspondingly, only the World Health Organisation, as an agency of the United Nations, is in a position to track the policies and practices of the world drug trade. Its role is, of course, advisory only.

In October 1989, the British TV current affairs programme *World in Action* broadcast a programme on infant diarrhoea, oral rehydration therapy and antidiarrhoeal drugs. One of the programme-makers wrote that the team[58]

> was fortunate in that we had a new World Health Organisation report to draw on. They told us that after ten years of hoping that the problem of anti-diarrhoeal drugs would go away, they had decided that they should go public with a detailed criticism of seven types of anti-diarrhoeal drugs 'at best inappropriate, at worst harmful'. Unless they attacked anti-diarrhoeal drugs they feared they would never succeed in effectively promoting oral replacement therapy.

Where was the WHO report? Eighteen months after the first draft had been circulated a WHO official told me: 'It's a hot issue. We're saying all anti-diarrhoeal drugs are not necessary.' Eventually the report was published, early in 1991, in a small edition designed for health policy makers, health educators and workers in the field.[59] Three of its sections, fully furnished with scientific references, state that streptomycins, neomycin and sulphonamides should not be used as treatment for infant diarrhoea.

The review of streptomycins states that these antibiotics are dangerous, often don't work and can make diarrhoea worse. It concludes:

> There is no evidence that streptomycin is effective in the treatment of diarrhoea . . . Streptomycin and dihydrostreptomycin preparations for oral administration are produced solely for the purpose of treating diarrhoea. Lacking any beneficial effect, however, they simply divert attention and resources from more important aspects of diarrhoea treatment, such as rehydration, proper nutrition, and appropriate antibiotics for the treatment of dysentery. 'Anti-diarrhoeal' agents containing streptomycin or dihydrostreptomycin should not be used in the treatment of diarrhoea, and the production and sale of these products cannot be justified.

The toxic effects of neomycin not only include permanent deafness and loss of balance but also, as stated in the WHO report, destruction of the inner surface of the gut wall. Taken under careful medical supervision, such disasters should be rare. However, drugs are taken in Third World countries often with little or no supervision. The section on neomycin concludes:

> There is no good evidence to support the use of neomycin in the routine treatment of diarrhoea ... Widespread use of neomycin promotes resistance to anti-microbials, and the gastrointestinal toxicity of this antibiotic may actually increase the severity or duration of diarrhoea ... The production and sale of these antidiarrhoeals cannot be justified.

Of sulphonamides the WHO report concludes:

> Adverse reactions to sulphonamides can involve almost every organ system and may be life-threatening. There is no justification for the use of non-absorbable sulphonamides ... to treat diarrhoea or dysentery.

In its introduction, the report says: 'Antibiotics should *only* be used for dysentery and suspected cholera. Otherwise they are ineffective and should *not* be given . . . Antidiarrhoeal drugs . . . should never be used. None have proven practical value. Some are dangerous.' But, it continues, 'unfortunately, appropriate treatment of diarrhoea oftèn remains the exception rather than the rule.'

What this means is that drugs whose use in North America and Europe is usually carefully restricted because of their toxicity, are made and freely sold in Asia, Africa, Latin America and other developing countries. Without effective regulation, and with a free market economy, it is hard to say who can be held to account, or to see what can be done. All over the world, people believe in modern medicine, including drugs. If transnational companies do not make drugs, national or local firms will. If drugs are banned in developing countries, they will turn up on the black market. As it is, though, much of the developing world is wide open to drugs.

TRANSNATIONAL GERMS

Few babies and young children die of diarrhoea in the Western world, and you the reader may now be experiencing feelings of both sympathy and relief. You may now believe that infant diarrhoea, along with other bacterial infections that are rampant and often deadly in the Third World, amount to just another item on the list of calamities that afflict people in faraway countries – disasters and scandals such as floods, earthquakes, starvation, massacres and torture, which we see on our television screens but rarely if ever touch us. It's understandable if you are now thinking: 'How horrible. How fortunate we are in the West, to be spared.'

Sorry; not altogether true. The overuse and abuse of antibiotics in developing countries, and the consequent breeding and spread of resistant genes, threatens us, too.

Just as the dreadful living conditions of the newly industrialised nineteenth-century European working classes were breeding grounds for the tuberculosis that then spread and became an epidemic killer of the middle classes (and so could, not altogether fancifully, be seen as a revenge of the masses on their masters), similarly, the dreadful living conditions that so many people in the Third World now suffer breed diseases that are liable to infect us, too. And there now is a new threat: infectious drug resistance.

For example, of the 300 million or so people who cross international boundaries every year, many millions – and between one fifth and one half of travellers to Africa, southern Asia and Latin America – suffer from 'traveller's diarrhoea', an acutely painful and often temporarily disabling infection of which the main single cause is infection by variations of *E. coli* to which the guts of travellers in foreign lands are not accustomed.[60] The mismanagement of infection in Third World countries by the gross overuse and abuse of antibiotics has induced drug resistance in such 'enterotoxic' *E. coli* and in other bacteria that cause traveller's diarrhoea.

In 1990, many Americans travelled to Saudi Arabia for unusual business: Operation Desert Shield, in preparation for the war against Saddam Hussein's Iraq. By the end of that short conflict, over half the American troops suffered from diarrhoea, and a fifth were at some time unfit to fight. Of those suffering from diarrhoea caused by enterotoxic *E. coli* infections, two fifths were resistant to co-trimoxazole, just under a half to ampicillin, and over three fifths to tetracycline, the antibiotics of choice likely to be used to treat acute diarrhoea in special circumstances, such as war. A report in the *New England Journal of Medicine* concluded: 'Gastroenteritis caused by enterotoxic *E. coli* and shigella resistant to a number of drugs was a major problem that frequently interfered with the duties of American troops during Operation Desert Shield.'[61] Here is an irony: whereas sulphonamides and penicillin fortified troops in previous wars, drugs of choice against pathogenic bacteria common in the Third World now frequently do not work. If the opposing armies in Iraq had been more equally matched, the outcome of the war might have been somewhat different.

For the reasons already given, it is usually best to avoid antibiotics for diarrhoea in adults as well as in children, although war is perhaps a special case. The worry is that drug-resistant *E. coli*, once in the gut, can spread drug resistance to other bacterial species, infecting not only soldiers but also ordinary travellers in foreign lands with toxic time-bombs.[62]

Like drug companies, germs have become transnationals. Professor Stuart Levy is now chairman of the Alliance for the Prudent Use of Antibiotics (APUA), a world network of scientists concerned about antibiotic overuse and abuse. 'We're caught in a global web,' he has said.[41] 'Bacteria don't pay attention to international borders and customs . . . They're moving around! That's their evolutionary imperative.' Africa and Asia are now just a few hours away from Europe and North America. The 'jumbo jet syndrome' speeds up – from months and years to days – the potential for intercontinental infection with drug-resistant bacteria.

If infectious diseases are uncommon they are likely to remain vulnerable to antibiotics. The strains of bubonic and pneumonic plague that became epidemic in India in the second half of 1994 for the first time in 28 years responded to tetracycline.[63] But other killer infectious diseases are more common and so have become resistant to drugs. Typhoid fever is endemic in Asia, Africa and Latin America. In the early 1970s an epidemic of typhoid resistant to chloramphenicol killed hundreds of people in Mexico.[64] Mindful of the long border Mexico shares with the United States, a US Senate Committee was set up to investigate this disaster.

Professor Philip Lee, then US Assistant Secretary for Health, stated in his evidence that *Salmonella typhi*, the microbiological cause of typhoid, had mutated into a superbug because the drug industry promoted chloramphenicol for all sorts of infections in Mexico and other developing countries. This, he said, 'can affect not only the residents of the countries involved and all those that visit there as well, but people who have never travelled in Latin America.'[65]

Since the late 1980s typhoid has become commonly untreatable not only by chloramphenicol but also by the three alternative drugs used to treat the disease: co-trimoxazole and amoxycillin or ampicillin. Multi drug-resistant strains of typhoid are now epidemic in India, Pakistan and China, have spread to South Africa and the Middle East, and now are also found in Europe. These superbugs can be especially virulent and invasive. In 1994 newer drugs, quinolones such as ciprofloxacin, or else third-generation cephalosporins, worked against superbug strains of *S. typhi*, but quinolone resistance has already been reported in India and in one case in the UK. Other problems with ciprofloxacin include possible risk of cartilage injury in growing children and pregnant women; and new drugs protected by patent are expensive and therefore sometimes not available in poor countries.[66,67]

In the UK chloramphenicol has been the drug of first choice for typhoid, once again the ironical reason being that because it is so comparatively toxic, it is rarely used, therefore remains an effective drug, and in the case of typhoid is judged less dangerous than the disease. However, in 1991 scientists from the Public Health Laboratory Service reported that in the previous year, of the 248 cases of typhoid in the UK, 50 had turned out to be superbug strains resistant to chloramphenicol, and that in almost all cases the drugs of second choice in the UK, ampicillin and trimethoprim, did not work either.[68] Victims were almost without exception people who had returned from Pakistan and India, where common use of chloramphenicol has bred *S. typhi* superbugs. The investigators concluded that chloramphenicol should therefore no longer be the drug of first choice for typhoid in the UK.

Cholera is also endemic in Asia, Africa and Latin America. An outbreak caused by a multi drug-resistant version of *Vibrio cholerae* (the strain known as El Tor), occurred in Tanzania in 1977, then in Bangladesh in 1980 and 1981. El Tor cholera appeared in Peru in 1991 and by late 1992 had caused illness in about half a million people, with around 3000 deaths. The epidemic then spread to other Latin American countries. A study in Ecuador in 1992 showed that of twelve El Tor strains, two were resistant to sulphonamides, chloramphenicol, the aminoglycoside kanamycin, tetracyclines, ampicillin, and trimethoprim.[69]

Epidemics of cholera are common in Pakistan and Bangladesh. A new, virulent strain of cholera now known as Bengal, resistant to co-trimoxazole while vulnerable to tetracycline, emerged in

December 1992 in Pakistan; four months later over 100,000 cases and nearly 1500 deaths had been reported.[70] 'The strain seems to have pandemic potential,' reported the investigators. 'It is important that other countries in south-east Asia are aware of the strain's potential to cause severe morbidity and mortality.'

As with the thinning of the ozone layer in Antarctica and the burning of the rain forest in Brazil, both of which contribute to the 'greenhouse effect' or global warming, we in the developed world are vulnerable to contagion rippling out from the developing world.

THE GLOBAL MICROBIAL VILLAGE

No scientist cited in this book believes that antibiotics should never be used. On the contrary: they are a precious medical resource – and 'precious' is the key word. Concern about drug resistance underlines the fact that antibiotics are a vital treatment for serious, invasive bacterial infection. One reason why it is wrong to use bacteria for trivial or self-limiting bacterial infections is that the greater the use, the greater the risk of breeding infectious drug resistance that may create superbugs that cause dangerous and even deadly infection in you, your family or your community.

And now the global village is also a global microbial ecosystem. We are not quarantined against the wrong use of antibiotics in other countries and continents. In November 1985, the World Health Organisation called a five-day meeting in Nairobi to discuss 'The Rational Use of Drugs'.[71] Two advisors to the conference published the following composite story of how antibiotics may become available to people in developing countries, based on a compilation of evidence from health workers in the field.[72]

> Reports of shortages of essential drugs (obtained in bulk through a non-profitmaking agency) led to the discovery that the freight van in which half the year's supply is shipped is still in the customs warehouse because of a dispute with the Ministry of Finance over clearance and demurrage charges. Once cleared, a crate of drums of bulk tetracycline powder falls off a central stores truck during a rainstorm. Some drums are recovered, soaked through, and others are later found in bazaars, the contents being sold as anti-diarrhoeal powder in glassine envelopes to individuals. Meanwhile someone

> measures the interior temperature of the vans transporting the drugs to remote health centres, a three-day journey in a tropical area, and finds it to be 82°C. No one asks which drugs are spoiled or rendered toxic. Pilferage at the docks and along the way decimates the stock, drugs being a valuable commodity.

The advisers to the WHO conference who compiled this report commented:

> Subtle and pervasive harm comes from the excessive use of ostensibly useful antimicrobials with the result that pathogenic bacteria are now commonly resistant to multiple antimicrobials worldwide (and susceptible only to second-line, highly expensive antimicrobials). When an antibiotic is given to which a pathogen is resistant, the illness frequently becomes worse.

They added:

> The population explosion in the developing world promises a bonanza for pharmaceutical manufacturers, drug sellers and medical practitioners. Three billion people with more than their fair share of illness have discovered modern drugs, and sales curves are rising exponentially; even while (paradoxically) the poorest, sickest and most remote people have virtually no access to good therapy.

In 1988, the World Health Organisation published a further report on 'The World Drug Situation'.[73] This states that in Europe, just over one eighth of the total market for drugs used on humans is for antibiotics. The market in the developing world is relatively much bigger, amounting to a fifth or even a quarter of the total drugs market. In many if not most developing countries, antibiotics are the bestselling drugs, and the bestselling antibiotics often include those now generally restricted in North America and Europe because of their toxicity.

Evidence of the dramatic spread of drug resistance, especially in developing countries, was given by Dr O'Brien and co-workers in 1990.[49] Children between the ages of five months and six years were studied in Boston, Venezuela and China. To qualify for the study, the children had to have been free of antibiotics for the previous four months. In each centre, of those screened, less than one in ten children qualified – that is, more than 90 per cent of babies and young children in these centres had been given antibiotics in the previous four months.

The antibiotic-free children were then screened for drug-resistant *E. coli*. In Boston, just over half the children (21 of 39) carried bacteria harbouring resistance genes. But in Venezuela, of 41 children screened, 40 (98 percent) were infected with drug-resistant *E. coli*. In China, of 53 children screened, 51 (96 percent) were infected. In Boston – where, in common with other places in the developed world, antibiotic use is relatively careful – only two children (6 percent) carried *E. coli* that were resistant to three or more drugs. But in Venezuela, three out of ten children, and in China, over four out of ten children, were so infected, notably with *E. coli* resistant to combinations of sulphamethoxazole, streptomycin, tetracycline, trimethoprim and ampicillin. Yet nine children in Venezuela (over a fifth of the total) and 15 in China (over a quarter) who had qualified for the study had never taken an antibiotic drug. This is a bad start in life.

IT HEALS EVERYTHING

Research for this book included correspondence with health workers in the developing world, who sent testimony, comments and other evidence that antibiotic toxicity and infectious drug-resistant superbugs are a major threat to public health in many countries.

Here is an account given by Pierre Pradervand to Health Action International, of tetracycline sales in Ougadougou, Upper Volta.[74] He purchased '*tupaye*' in the central market, and found it available in markets everywhere in the country. '*Tupaye*' is the name given by the people to antibiotics, especially tetracycline; the word means 'it heals everything.' Antibiotics are illegally imported from Ghana, Nigeria and Togo, stolen from hospitals and pharmacies, and distributed as free samples by industry salesmen. Doctors, nurses, chemists, drug company representatives and ordinary people all confirmed that *tupaye*

> is used for absolutely everything: from stomach ache to backaches, from toothaches to open wounds, headaches to malaria, diarrhoea, and so on . . . Capsules are opened and poured into open wounds, emptied into cavities in the teeth, diluted in all sorts of liquid.

The case of a boy aged 11–12 is cited:

> He informed me that when he had a problem, he took five capsules (1250 mg) which he emptied into a glass of lemonade . . . The case of *tupaye* is typical of the use of Western drugs in many parts of Africa. The only adequate description of this use is total anarchy.

Michael Tan of Health Action International sent me his book *Dying for Drugs* published in 1988[75], which includes a description of chemists' shops in Bangkok. Bestselling lines over the counter included co-trimoxazole, and chloramphenicol, streptomycin and tetracycline were also freely available without prescription. Michael Tan commented: 'With the emergence of antibiotic resistance, we face potential catastrophies for infections when the antibiotics are needed.'

Tetracyclines – urgent control needed on sale and use is the title of a report published in 1989, sent by the Consumers' Association of Penang.[76] This lists 37 brands of tetracycline available in Malaysia. A survey of 4500 Malaysians found that 1 in 50 had teeth permanently discoloured by tetracycline. The report cited examples of branded tetracycline products which failed to mention side-effects.

Tetracyclines and chloramphenicol are a problem in Indonesia. The Management Sciences for Health Group based in Boston, Massachusetts, sent their report *Where does the tetracycline go?*, published in 1988.[77] In Indonesia at that time, the top-selling drug of any type was tetracycline, with ampicillin second (and aspirin third). Six of the eight bestselling drugs were antibiotics, including two branded chloramphenicols. Like the children elsewhere in the world studied by Dr O'Brien and his co-workers, nine out of ten Indonesian children under the age of five had been given antibiotics at some time.

The grey and black markets in antibiotics were condemned by Nigerian microbiologists in papers published in the *Journal of Antimicrobial Chemotherapy* in 1987 and 1989.[78] A survey of 500 people showed that all adults in Nigeria use antibiotics without consulting a physician. 'About 400 (80 percent) went for laboratory examination only after repeated self-medication for sexually transmitted diseases.' The most abused antibiotic at that time was ampicillin (used by four out of five people to dose themselves), followed by tetracycline (three out of every five people), co-trimoxazole (two of every five) and chloramphenicol (one of every three). A separate survey of students showed that nearly three quarters dose themselves with antibiotics, for all sorts of ailments.

In its spring 1989 issue, the newsletter of the Alliance for the Prudent use of Antibiotics carried the following report:[79]

> Brazil has one of the highest rates in the world of resistance . . . to almost all therapeutically useful antibiotics. It is believed that this situation has developed as a result of overuse of antibiotics in and outside hospitals and free access to almost all antibiotics in public pharmacies.
>
> The problem is so severe that it is sometimes difficult to find antibiotics to treat life-threatening hospital-acquired infections. In 1980, 15 per cent of all hospital admissions, about 1.7 million patients, had nosocomial [hospital] infections. It cost US$1.2 billion to treat them, and 30,000 patients died of the infections.

Everywhere in the world, drug-resistant bacteria mean trouble. Dr Scott Holmberg and colleagues from the US Centers for Disease Control and Prevention, investigated 175 reports of outbreaks of bacterial infection in American hospitals and communities in the USA. The conclusion was: 'In almost every outbreak investigation and published study we could find, infections with antimicrobial-resistant organisms were associated with substantially worse health and economic effects than were infections with antimicrobial-susceptible organisms.'[80] Both in hospital and in the community, people infected with superbugs were twice as likely to need hospital treatment, stayed in hospital at least twice as long, and were more than twice as likely to die.

19 Animal Pharm

GOING FOR GROWTH

Antibiotics are not only used to treat human disease. They work on animals, too. Modern intensive animal farming methods, which make chicken, beef, pork and their products cheap everyday food, depend on antibiotics. Before the antibiotic era, chickens were free-range, pigs were reared outdoors, and cattle had plenty of space. Most animal farms were small family businesses, needing a lot of human labour. The reality of farming up to the 1930s and 1940s was somewhat like its depiction now in advertisements for processed food products: hedged fields, some with animals, some for crops; tractors and harvesters supporting the work of horses and men; feed stored on the land on haystacks; farmhouses integrated into the landscape; and farmers dependent on the quality of the soil and the nature of the climate. The work was hard and the rewards sometimes meagre – farmers do not always have romantic feelings about their business. But well-cultivated land produced plenty of good food, although countries with big cities also needed to import some. Meat was relatively expensive to produce: on family farms not using modern technology, animals need a lot of care as well as a lot of food.[81]

Within industrialised countries, farming has been transformed in the second half of the twentieth century. The systematic use of chemical fertilisers and pesticides has dramatically increased productivity. And amenable animals are now almost always reared intensively. Sheep still graze in open country, but chickens and pigs are usually reared in sheds that may house thousands or tens of thousands of animals, and cattle spend more and more time out of the fields, grazing off concrete floors. River and sea fish such as trout and salmon, once 'wild' food, are now usually bred on farms in great tanks boiling with countless thousands of fish.

The more intensive the method of production, the cheaper the finished product. Poultry, once eaten only occasionally, is now a staple food because chickens are factory-farmed. In the United States, the hamburger is now a national icon because cattle there and in other countries are raised in feedlots, fenced enclosures in which thousands and tens of thousands of beef cattle are factory-farmed. If what you want is cheap meat and plenty of it, factory farming is what you get – and that means antibiotics. Modern farming depends on drugs.

When humans are crushed together in camps, slums and other grossly overcrowded and insanitary places, infection is inevitable, and can be controlled only by systematic use of drugs; likewise, animals. Traditional farmers, including those who now use sustainable 'organic' methods and avoid drugs, give animals plenty of space not out of ignorance, but because they know that overcrowding breeds and spreads diseases. 'Modern' farmers see things differently; without antibiotics, the mass production and distribution of animals would be impossible. Crops may also be sprayed with mixtures including antibiotics.

In the USA, the total tonnage of antibiotics used on farms nearly equals that used as human medicine. In Britain, where the use of drugs by farmers is subject to more control, the proportion is lower.[82]

Antibiotics are used by farmers on animals for all or any one of four reasons. First, to treat illness believed to be a bacterial infection. This use, termed 'therapeutic', is comparable with the use of antibiotics as human medicine, except that it is generally less controlled. Best practice is when veterinary surgeons administer the drugs and check their effects; in practice, though, supplies of antibiotics are often obtained and used by farmers themselves, who may sometimes give heavy doses 'to be on the safe side'.

Second, antibiotics are used on animals 'subtherapeutically' in cases where the farmer, preferably with support from a vet, believes that an animal is not doing well because it is suffering a 'subclinical' infection without any obvious symptoms. This is comparable to people taking antibiotics not because they are ill but because they feel 'a bit under the weather'. When farmers feel under pressure to produce animals in the best possible marketable condition, as they often do, they may use antibiotics subtherapeutically as a sort of tonic. Such doses should be much lower than therapeutic doses.

The third use of antibiotics for animals is 'prophylactic', which is to say preventive. In human medicine, surgeons use antibiotics as prophylactic 'cover' before, during and after open-body surgery on individuals; also, physicians. Physicians working with armies or other groups of people liable to contract sexually transmitted diseases may also use antibiotics prophylactically on whole groups or select populations of people. Similarly, healthy animals may be given antibiotics because they may become infected in future. A vet may prescribe antibiotics for an entire herd or flock when some of the animals are becoming diseased, or when those on a neighbouring farm are suffering an outbreak of infection. But mass production of animals itself greatly increases the risk of infection, to the point that epidemics are at least occasionally inevitable unless drugs are used. So partly for this reason, animal feed commonly contains small amounts of antibiotics.[83]

The fourth, economically imperative reason for farmers to give antibiotics to mass-produced animals is for growth promotion. Why antibiotics should make animals grow faster is still not known for sure, but they do. The discovery was made in 1949 by Dr Thomas Jukes, who at the time was a research director working for Lederle, one of the drug companies who were then developing new versions of tetracycline.[84] Dr Jukes was looking for a cheap source of vitamin B_{12} for use in animal feed, and found it in waste products left over from the fermentation process used to produce chlortetracycline. He included this mash in feed for chickens and found, to his great surprise, that they gained weight up to 20 percent faster than usual. He tried the same mash on piglets, with even more impressive results, and established that it is not the vitamin B_{12} but the antibiotic residues in the feed that worked this wonder.

Antibiotics promote the growth of young farm animals. Dr Jukes described his discovery as 'a unique phenomenon, perhaps without precedent in medical history', but its significance was chiefly economic. Manufacture of antibiotics for use in feed as growth promoters rocketed into a multi-million dollar industry. Speed of growth of animals reared for food can make the difference between prosperity and bankruptcy for farmers, who were bound to step on this accelerator.

Animals react badly to being crushed together, and it may be that antibiotics have the effect of preventing stunting as well as disease. There is some evidence that animals reared traditionally without drugs grow as well as mass-produced animals given them.[85] Certainly, drugs seem to be specially effective when used on animals stressed by crowding. 'It was the discovery of the effectiveness of drugs as feed additives in these conditions that led to the concentration of the meat industry,' Dr Jukes has said.[41] 'For the first time, farmers could confine a large number of animals and still keep them healthy.'

By 1979, Dr Richard Novick reckoned that[86]

> Some 40 per cent of all the antibiotics currently produced in this country [the US] are added directly to the feeds of livestock. Most of the animals raised under these conditions receive antibiotic supplementation from birth to death, and the entire chain of supply, from manufacturer to animal, proceeds without veterinary supervision.

In the United States, farmers are relatively free to use whichever antibiotics work best in animal growth promotion; regulations in the UK are somewhat tighter.

Dr Novick cited industry estimates that the use of antibiotics in animal feed was then worth around US$2 billion a year to American meat producers. In the 1990s, this figure would certainly be double. The use of antibiotics is intrinsic to modern intensive agribusiness. In the UK, the UK Veterinary Association does not dispute this[87]: 'Antibiotics are vital for the health and welfare of animals [and] for the efficient production of farm animals which is necessary for producing cheap food, adding, We are not sitting on top of a "super bug" time bomb.'

A RESIDUAL WORRY

Is the use of antibiotics on animals a significant threat to public health? My impression is that more people are concerned about the ill-effects of antibiotics used in animal husbandry than about their ill-effects when used as human medicine. Certainly, the issue of the overuse and abuse of antibiotics and other drugs used by farmers is debated regularly and energetically not only by scientists, but also in the broadcast and print media. On being told that I was preparing a book on antibiotics, acquaintances as often as not assumed that its subject would be agriculture.

Those who defend the use of antibiotics have a strong interest in doing so. It is understandable that manufacturers should speak up on behalf of their products, and the agrichemical industry – which, in the case of antibiotics, includes the pharmaceutical industry – is a powerful lobby in any country as well as globally. In addition, though, almost all national governments, together with international agencies such as the Food and Agriculture Organisation (FAO) and the World Bank, are committed to a free trade policy and to the further development of intensive agriculture to produce cheap food to feed an increasing hungry global population. Antibiotics, together with other chemical inputs, are defended as an essential means to this end. In such a context, any ill-effects of antibiotics as used on animals are liable to be minimised as trivial or, at most, incidental.

On the other hand, campaigns against the use of antibiotics in agriculture may well exaggerate their ill-effects. Some campaigners are not so much concerned about the impact of antibiotics on human health as with animal rights. Others are vegetarians or vegans, or else opposed to the regular consumption of meat and dairy products because of their high saturated fat content. Others are environmentalists or advocates of farming by sustainable methods, who are therefore opposed on principle to intensive agriculture. And still others object to any contamination of the food supply with chemical residues, just as some people are opposed on principle to the addition of fluoride to the water supply, irrespective of the evidence on safety or danger.[88]

For these and other reasons, much of what is published about the effects on human health of antibiotics used in agriculture generates more heat than light. One example is what became known as the 'sulphadimidine scandal' in the late 1980s. Sulphadimidine is a sulphonamide commonly given to pigs. In the UK, as in other countries, the use of antibiotics on animals is subject to guidelines on withdrawal periods – that is, the number of days before slaughter during which the drug should not be given – and on maximum residue levels of drugs in meat, above which it should not be sold.

In the UK, the official government advisory Veterinary Products Committee has specified a maximum residue level of 0.1 milligram per kilogram, or one part in ten million, for any sulphonamide in meat. In 1987, the UK Ministry of Agriculture published a report prepared by another official advisory body, the Working Party on Veterinary Residues in Animal Products, which acknowledged that, in over one fifth of samples analysed, sulphadimidine was turning up in pigs' kidneys at levels, on average, fifteen times higher than the specified maximum residue levels. 'This suggests that withdrawal periods for pigs were commonly being abused, that dosing instructions were not being followed or, more likely, a combination of several factors including these two.'[89] Farmers were urged by the Ministry not to exceed the stated dose of sulphadimidine for their pigs, and to withdraw the drug well ahead of slaughter, in which case 'we hope . . . that the problem will diminish'.

However, there turned out to be a special problem with sulphadimidine. Tests on experimental rats and mice revealed that at doses well over 10,000 times the maximum residue level, and 1000 times or more above the high levels sometimes found in pigs' kidneys in Britain, sulphadimidine could be a cause of thyroid cancer, as is the case with other sulphonamides when given in massive doses.[90] In the USA, the so-called Delaney Clause, an amendment written into the Food, Drug and Cosmetic Act of 1958, specifies that 'no food additive shall be deemed safe if it is found to induce cancer when ingested by man or animal.' This law is often criticised as unrealistic, but there it is, on the US statute books.

Consequently, in late 1989, the US Food and Drug Administration announced its intention to ban the animal use of sulphadimidine. However, no ban was introduced in the UK and, meanwhile, further analyses showed that high levels of sulphadimidine residues in pigs' kidneys had become less common. In 1992, the Ministry agreed to maintain surveillance of sulphonamide residues in the kidneys of pigs, sheep and cows, and the flesh and livers of poultry.[91]

It is very unlikely that sulphonamides as used on animals are a detectable cause of human cancer. The doses required to induce cancer in animals are vastly higher than the amounts sometimes found in pig meat. It is true that prolonged courses of sulphonamides can affect thyroid hormone levels in humans, which could possibly increase thyroid cancer risk. But a World Health Organisation expert committee set up to evaluate drug residues in food concluded in 1989 that 'thyroid effects were unlikely to occur in humans except at (and above) therapeutic levels.'[90] Which is to say, worry about the toxicity of sulphonamides should not be so much about their use on animals, as their use direct on humans, as medicine.

Organisations working in the public interest in the USA, the UK and elsewhere are also concerned about antibiotic residues in milk. The antibiotics given to dairy cows include penicillin, administered to treat or prevent inflammation of the udder (mastitis), which affects one in three milking cows every year in the UK.[92] Inevitably, therefore, traces of penicillin can sometimes be found in milk. The position of the British Veterinary Association[87] is:

> The quantity of antibiotic which a person might drink in cows' milk is minute. In the virtually impossible situation that all the milk contained antibiotic, the maximum exposure of the consumer in the case of penicillin will be 0.7 mg/person/year [which] should be compared with the average annual consumption of 2.4 g penicillin/person/year in human medicine.

In other words, even in a 'worst case' scenario, the average person takes in over 3000 times as much penicillin from drugs as from milk.[93]

Farmers are also concerned: penicillin is potent stuff, and residues in milk are liable to kill the bacterial cultures used in the making of cheese and yoghurt. In Britain, the milk industry carries out regular random tests of milk for contamination with antibiotics. Some farmers who fear their milk may contain detectable residues are said to kill off the penicillin by adding penicillinase to the milk tank before inspection.[94]

Could penicillin in milk be a hazard to human health? There is no evidence that people have suffered serious illness directly and solely as a result of consuming traces of penicillin in milk. Given the widespread use of this antibiotic as human medicine, such evidence would be hard to find; besides which, penicillin is a relatively non-toxic drug.

There is evidence, though, that people who have already become allergic to penicillin after using it as a medicine may then suffer allergic reactions as a result of drinking milk containing penicillin residues.[87] Illicit use of penicillinase by farmers may make matters worse. According to Dr Joe Collier, editor of the independent UK journal *Drugs and Therapeutics Bulletin*[94]

> Penicillinase may well destroy the potency of the penicillin – resistant strains of bacteria prove that by staying alive and multiplying. But the enzyme does not destroy the allergic fragments of the penicillin which cause adverse reactions in sensitive people. In fact, there is evidence that the enzyme can actually enhance the allergic reaction.

People who are 'exquisitely' sensitive to penicillin residues in milk are advised to stop drinking it.[87]

Allergic reactions can be very unpleasant – even more so when their cause is difficult, if not impossible, to trace. And any evidence that a food contaminant could conceivably be a cause of human cancer is worrying, even when the indications from animal tests are that ill-effects might occur only at levels vastly above those present in food. All in all, though, it's hard to believe that the amount of antibiotics we may consume in meat and meat products, in milk and dairy products or in fish[95] are a major direct cause of human disease. Commonly, hostility to antibiotic residues in food springs from an instinctive dislike of any chemical contamination of food. And those who remain worried do have choices: they can go vegetarian or only eat meat and other foods of animal origin produced to recognised 'organic' standards by farmers using traditional, sustainable methods with low or no chemical inputs.

REVENGE OF THE ANIMALS?

Most scientists are relatively unconcerned about the direct toxic effects of antibiotics used on animals, apart from special situations where people – farm workers, for example – are exposed to high levels of drug residues in their immediate environment.[96]

As with antibiotics used as human medicine, the main worry about antibiotics used on animals is their longer-term ill-effects. What does greatly worry microbiologists is that the systematic use of antibiotics in any crowded environment breeds drug-resistant superbugs liable to spread and cause outbreaks or even epidemics of untreatable infection. As with armies and hospitals, and some developing countries, so with modern farms.

Intensive farming breeds disease in animals; the use of antibiotics to treat or prevent disease or as animal growth promoters breeds drug-resistant bacteria; and these superbugs spread from animals and infect humans. There's no doubt about this sequence of events; the only argument is about the scale of the problem.

In 1984, Professor Stuart Levy estimated that around 15,000 tons of antibiotics were manufactured in the United States, of which nearly half were used on animals, mostly in feed. In an editorial published by the *New England Journal of Medicine*, he wrote[97]:

> Every animal or person taking an antibiotic (therapeutically or subtherapeutically) becomes a factory producing resistant strains [of bacteria] . . . Since there are two or three times more livestock than people in the United States, the number of animals fed antibiotics at subtherapeutic levels (almost all poultry, pigs and calves) is enormously greater than the number of people taking antibiotics.

Large animals can void anything between 400 and 500 times the volume of faeces excreted by humans, and the disposal of animal excrement, containing residues of all sorts of chemicals including antibiotics, is haphazard. Professor Levy concluded: 'Many consider the use of antibiotics in animals to be a more important contributor to the environmental pool of resistant strains than their use in human beings.'

Dr Novick is characteristically more outspoken. He has said[41]:

> I think that the evidence is overwhelming that what we have been doing with antibiotics in both animal and human use is very dangerous and entirely self-defeating . . . We can't keep spewing biologically active substances into the environment without paying a high price in undesirable modifications of the biosphere. What is happening to animals on antibiotic feed is having an effect on levels of resistance in human beings, because of the plasmid trade-around.

A major report of the US National Academy of Sciences on the effects on human health of penicillin and tetracyclines as used by American farmers, published in 1988, was more circumspect. It concluded[98]: 'There is indirect evidence implicating subtherapeutic use of antimicrobials in producing resistance in infectious bacteria that causes a potential human health hazard.'

The two superbugs evidently most likely to be bred and spread by the use of antibiotics on the farm are salmonella species and *E. coli.*

Many of the bacterial infections that afflict animals do not affect humans. Other animal infections, known as zoonoses, are also a hazard to human health. One of the two most common zoonoses is diarrhoeal disease caused by various species of salmonella bacteria. In the USA, the UK and other industrialised countries, salmonella infection is now principally spread from animals to humans and, in the 1980s, became epidemic. A World Health Organisation report published in 1988[99] accepted that 'salmonellosis is a real or potential problem in all areas of the world.' In the mid-1980s, around 40,000 cases of salmonella poisoning were reported by physicians in the US every year. However, most people with diarrhoeal disease do not go to the doctor, and epidemiologists reckon that, for every case reported, between 10 and 100 people are infected and suffer some symptoms. This means that between 400,000 and 4 million Americans are afflicted with salmonellosis every year. A study by scientists working for the Centers for Disease Control and Prevention published in 1986[100] estimated that in the US, 'more than 18,000 hospitalisations and 500 deaths are associated with salmonellosis annually', and 'when the total costs of the unreported cases and the costs to industry and business are included, salmonellosis may cost billions of dollars each year.'

The root cause of most cases of salmonella infection is the factory farming of animals. By 1990, the main single infective organism in the US was *Salmonella typhimurium* from beef; in the UK, it is *Salmonella enteritidis* from chicken. In a sense, antibiotics are implicated in most cases of salmonella infection in developed countries, simply because the factory farming of animals is only possible with the systematic use of antibiotics and other antimicrobial drugs. In grossly overcrowded conditions, when feed itself may be contaminated and animals are unable to escape their own wastes, the closed circles of contagion thus created, can be broken only temporarily with drugs; and salmonella and other zoonotic bacteria inevitably spill and spread into the human food supply, causing outbreaks and epidemics of infection. If we want factory farming, we will also have to accept widespread diarrhoeal diseases, as a kind of revenge of the animals.

We will also get drug-resistant bacteria as an inevitable result of constant use of antibiotics. In December 1987, Dr John Threlfall of the UK Public Health Laboratory Service addressed the Royal Society of Medicine's Forum on Food and Health, in London.[101] In the eleven years between 1976 and 1987, PHLS data showed that drug resistance in cattle bacteria to chloramphenicol had increased from 1 to 88 percent, to ampicillin from 3 to 82 percent, to tetracyclines from 10 to 95 percent, and to trimethoprim from less than 1 to 83 percent. This staggering and very rapid increase in drug resistance 'has been brought about by repeated unsuccessful attempts to combat calf salmonella with an ever-increasing range of antibiotics ... multiple drug resistance to four or more antibiotics is the norm in cattle.' Correspondingly, by 1987, 60 percent of *Salmonella typhimurium* infections analysed in the UK in humans had become resistant to three or more antibiotics. Dr Threlfall's conclusion was: 'There is little doubt that the use of antibiotics in calf husbandry is responsible for the appearance of the majority of multi-resistant strains of *S. typhimurium* which have caused infection in humans in recent years.'

The *S. typhimurium* infection now most common in cattle, and thus humans, in the UK is a very specific strain known as 'phage type 204'. The *S. enteritidis* infection that became epidemic in chickens, and thus in humans, in the UK in the late 1980s is another very specific strain known as 'phage type 4'. Why did this latter strain suddenly become epidemic? Dr Anita Rampling, then working at the UK Public Health Laboratory Service in Cambridge, has suggested an imaginative and alarming theory. With colleagues, she found that *S. enteritidis* phage 4 infection is generally vulnerable to antibiotics, but with one highly significant exception: nitrofurans, which are used in human medicine for urinary tract infections, and in intensively reared chickens for protozoal infections of the gut.[102] Dr Rampling has suggested that the use of nitrofurans on poultry may have, by selective pressure, in effect *created* the new phage 4 strain of salmonella to which chickens and humans have turned out to be vulnerable; in which case, *S. enteritidis* phage 4 is a superbug.

This theory is speculative. What is sure is that drug-resistant salmonella infection is a special menace to human health. People in general good health ordinarily should not be given antibiotics for diarrhoeal diseases of the type caused by *S. typhimurium* and *S. enteritidis*, in which case the disease process itself will not be affected by drug resistance. But hospital infection is another story. As stated by the World Health Organisation[99], this

> often causes explosive outbreaks of salmonellosis in hospitals, particularly in maternity, paediatric, and geriatric units and among chronically sick and immunosuppressed patients. These outbreaks often cause high mortality, are difficult to control, and can persist for long periods of time.

When hospital patients are generally very ill, salmonella (and other bacterial infections) are dangerous, and more likely to become invasive, in which case antibiotics are needed. If the infection is multiply drug resistant, the patient may die.

Dr Scott Holmberg of the US Centers for Disease Control and

Prevention, published, with colleagues, an analysis of 52 outbreaks of salmonella food poisoning in the United States during a thirteen-year period up to 1983[103]. A total of 19 outbreaks were known to have been caused by drug-sensitive salmonella: these infected 1912 people, of whom 4 died. By contrast, 17 outbreaks were caused by drug-resistant salmonella: these infected 312 people, 13 of whom died. 'The case fatality rate for patients with identified infections with multiply-resistant salmonella was 4.2 percent, 21 times higher than the case fatality rate associated with antibiotic-sensitive salmonella infections.'

Why this massive difference? One explanation suggested by Dr Holmberg[97] and by other CDC investigators[100], is that salmonella superbugs are especially dangerous when they infect people who are already being treated with antibiotics for some other bacterial disease. In these cases, the drug-resistant bacteria can flourish and become dominant in the guts of victims because other normally competitive bacterial species have been wiped out. The result is liable to be very severe acute illness, unresponsive to antibiotics, which can kill already weakened people.

SILENT INFESTATION

With infections, as with non-infectious diseases, prevention is better than treatment. Maybe the single most important protection against disease caused by bacterial infection is the closed sewer. In developed countries, human wastes, once liable to spread epidemics of infectious diseases, are now contained and carried out to sea, or else made safe in sewage treatment plants.

Not so animal wastes. The intestinal contents of animals bred for meat, milk and dairy products are splattered everywhere. Every year, countless millions upon millions of tons of animal faeces and urine soak into the soil or run off into rivers in countries all over the world. At slaughter, bodies of animals are smeared with faecal matter, and more pours out of their intestines on the disassembly lines; although most of this will be washed away and run off, some may remain to contaminate meat and cause food poisoning. Insects and birds pick up faecal fragments in fields or from untreated sewage, and fly off with it. We cannot avoid animal gut bacteria; they are everywhere.

If the bacteria that cause animal diseases were different from those responsible for human disease, this would not matter much, except to the animals themselves. But a number of bacterial infections are zoonotic and salmonella are not the only zoonotic superbugs causing infection in animals which then spreads to humans in drug-resistant form. As time goes on, and antibiotics remain an integral part of intensive farming, more and more animal bacteria capable of causing diarrhoeal and other diseases in humans become multiply drug resistant. These now include various species of shigella, *Clostridium perfringens* (a cause of gas gangrene if it penetrates wounds), *Yersinia enterocolitica* (a cause of septicaemia), *Staphylococcus aureus*[104], various species of campylobacter (notably *C. jejuni*, an even more common cause of food poisoning than salmonella in the US and UK[105], and *Listeria monocytogenes.*[106]

Intensive farming, itself feasible only with the systematic use of antibiotics, is arguably one of the main underlying causes of food poisoning in developed countries, where diarrhoeal and other diseases are now commonly caused by bacterial species and strains that a generation ago were insignificant as human pathogens. Some of these, notably *Salmonella enteritidis* and *Campylobacter jejuni*, have caused mass epidemics since the 1980s. It is theoretically possible, as may be the case with *S. enteritidis* phage 4, that the use of antibiotics on animals is creating new zoonotic disease entities, subtly but crucially different from previous strains, to which humans are at least initially vulnerable.

How much of a threat are pathogenic zoonotic superbugs to human health? Nobody really knows. In the 1988 report of the National Academy of Sciences,[98] there is an estimate that deaths from salmonellosis attributable to the use of antibiotics on animals might amount to 70 a year in the US, a tiny proportion of the total number of cases. It is probably fair to guess that zoonotic superbugs are the direct cause of human death only rarely.

It may well be, though, that the greatest hazard to human health caused by the use of antibiotics in agriculture is a silent one, without direct evidence of disease, carried out by bacterial species that are usually harmless commensals in the guts of animals and also of humans – in particular, the ubiquitous *Escherichia coli*. Like other enterobacteria (also known as coliforms), *E. coli* tend to become drug resistant as a result of antibiotics directed against other, more pathogenic species of bacteria. The more drugs, the more superbugs. Analyses of cattle and pigs performed in the UK between 1981 and 1983 found that the *E. coli* in over four fifths of healthy animals were resistant to at least one antibiotic[107], and other analyses of pigs and chickens[108] showed that resistance to specific drugs can persist in populations of pigs and chickens up to a decade after those drugs have been withdrawn from use.

Can drug-resistant *E. coli* transfer from animals to humans? Certainly. This was originally proved by two classic experiments in the mid-1970s. The first, carried out by Professor Stuart Levy and co-workers, took place on an American farm.[109] Chickens were given feed supplemented with tetracycline. Within two weeks, over nine out of ten *E. coli* excreted by the birds were tetracycline resistant, and after two months, over one fifth were multiply resistant – to streptomycin and to ampicillin or sulphonamides as well as tetracycline. Within five to six months, nearly one third of the faeces of the 11 people on the farm were mostly tetracycline resistant, and multiply-resistant patterns like those in the birds were emerging in the humans. During the period of study, nobody on the farm became ill. The fear, though, is that the resistant *E. coli*, transferred from animals to humans, could then themselves transfer their drug resistance to other, harmful species of bacteria. 'The resistant intestinal bacteria represent a reservoir of transferable resistance genes . . . The possible transfer of these plasmids from non-pathogenic to pathogenic bacteria or from animal to man must be considered a possible consequence.'[101]

The second experiment was carried out earlier among British volunteers. Professor Alan Linton of the department of microbiology at Bristol University purchased fifteen frozen chickens over a three-month period from randomly selected shops. The samples of *E. coli* that he collected from the birds was tested for drug resistance; he then gave the meat to five colleagues to prepare and eat. In due course, one of the volunteers became colonised by drug-resistant *E. coli* from the chicken meat. Dr Linton concluded[110]: 'It is probable that substantial numbers of antibiotic-resistant *E. coli* reach man by way of the food chain and, under certain circumstances, are able to colonise the human alimentary tract for significant periods of time.' In 1975, 300 million chickens were eaten in the UK; in 1992, 600 million.

The World Health Organisation report on drug resistance published in 1982[6] confirmed the validity of experiments such as those carried out by Professors Levy and Linton, stating:

> Resistant strains reach man via the food chain. The most definitive work has been done with *Escherichia coli*. The highest incidence of

> antibiotic-resistant *E. coli* is found in calves, pigs and poultry species in which antibiotics have been widely used. Under commercial slaughter conditions, contamination of carcasses on the slaughter line regularly occurs with strains of *E. coli* of the same serotypes and antibiotic-resistance patterns as those found in the guts of the animals being slaughtered. These strains reach the kitchen on meat and meat products [and] subsequently colonise the gut of man.

The fear is as follows. Superbugs bred in animals by the systematic use of antibiotics, and which then infect humans, will, once in the human gut, transfer their drug resistance to other species of bug. In which case, the use of antibiotics on intensively reared animals could become a silent source of epidemic human disease.

In practice, does this happen? Industry says no. The UK National Office of Animal Health (NOAH), representing the animal drug industry, has said[111]: 'There has not been a single recorded case of any human being suffering from antibiotic residues in meat or animal products in more than 30 years of feed additive use.' Dr Richard Novick takes a different view. Writing about the possibility that superbugs will transfer their drug resistance to other, more dangerous bacterial species, he has said[104]: 'It is a virtual certainty that this will happen, and probably fairly soon, if the massive overuse of antibiotics in animal husbandry and human medicine continues unabated.'

SUMMARY OF PART 5

Drug-resistant bacteria, otherwise known as superbugs, are bred in over-crowded environments like hospitals, the developing world, and farms. From there, they can spread everywhere. Modern hospitals can become pest-holes, infested with mutant bacteria resistant to most or practically all drugs. Chaotic overuse and abuse of antibiotics jeopardises the health of people living in developing countries. Factory farming depends on antibiotics to check epidemics of infection otherwise inevitable in any grossly overcrowded environment, and the superbugs thus bred are also a threat to human health. Time and again, microbiologists have warned against the dangers of overusing and abusing antibiotics. These warnings have not yet been heeded.

Conclusion

Democracy, whether in medicine or any other area, remains our best, indeed only hope for achieving lasting social change . . . Something new must be tried if we are to stem the haemorrhage of public expenditures on high-cost technologies of questionable benefit, the denial of care to those in greatest need, the over-reliance on drugs and techniques that endanger patients while leaving the underlying causes of disease untouched, the unabashed pursuit of private profits at public expense, and the indefensible discrepancies between stated public wishes and governmental actions. It is time for lay citizens to heal some of society's wounds.

Diana Dutton
Worse Than The Disease: Pitfalls of Medical Progress; 1988

A new scientific truth does not triumph by convincing its opponents and making them see the light, but rather because its opponents eventually die, and a new generation grows up that is familiar with it.

Professor Max Planck
Scientific Autobiography and Other Papers; 1949

20 How to Live with Antibiotics

BALANCE BETWEEN BENEFIT AND RISK

Fifty years ago, scientists believed they could conquer nature with chemicals. Biocides would create a new agriculture and thus a world of plenty. Antibiotics would create a new medicine and thus a world free from infection. But things have not worked out like that. When attacked, nature fights back. Agriculture and medicine have indeed been transformed, the global population has greatly increased, and the material circumstances of most people in rich countries have greatly improved. But starvation and disease have not been generally diminished, and in some countries and continents, continue to devastate whole populations. And for all their benefits, the chemical agriculture and the chemical medicine we live with have created new plagues.

It is a mistake to refuse an antibiotic cautiously prescribed by a trusted and knowledgeable physician for an identified bacterial infection that has invaded a vital organ of the body, or may well do so. But it is also a mistake to accept antibiotics casually prescribed as 'protection' against the possibility of bacterial infection, or for an infection that is relatively trivial, and/or likely to clear up by itself, or one that can be treated by safer means. The responsible use of antibiotics involves assessment of the balance between benefit and risk, which can never be entirely known in advance. One purpose of this book is to encourage both awareness of the power of antibiotics and informed partnerships between patients and physicians.

When should you or members of your family use antibiotics? No book can make such a judgement. The only reliable individual advice can come from qualified practitioners with good knowledge not only of diseases and drugs but also of the people who consult them. That said, there is reason to believe that most common simple infections of the skin, ears, mouth and throat, bronchial passages, vagina, urinary tract and gut are usually better not treated with antibiotics. But when is an infection simple and when is it complicated or liable to become invasive and really dangerous? Again, any such judgement can only be made case by case. The first advice this book can give you and your family is to sustain a trusting relationship with your general practitioner.

One reason why antibiotics are overused and abused is that they usually seem to work, as quick fixes. They make us feel better. They are drugs of choice for societies whose motto might be: 'I want it now.' Their benefits are obvious, their risks intangible. But when people evade responsibility for their own health and expect a pill for every ill, it is no wonder that physicians choose to save their breath and their time and reach for the prescription pad.

It is also usually better not to use antibiotics in an attempt to prevent infection, unless the risk of dangerous disease is really very high, as in major open-body surgery. As one example, travellers may be tempted to take antibiotics to avoid diarrhoea, notably when in tropical countries. A review article in the *New England Journal of Medicine* published in 1993[1] listed the risks of such prophylactic use of drugs:

> The side-effects of antimicrobial drugs include skin rashes and vaginal candidiasis, which occur in about 3 per cent of persons; photosensitivity reactions, bone marrow hypoplasia or aplasia, dental staining in young children, and antibiotic-associated colitis; and severe reactions, including the Stevens-Johnson syndrome and anaphylaxis, which occur in perhaps as many as 1 in 10,000 exposed persons. Travelers choosing antimicrobial prophylaxis therefore risk a potentially fatal reaction to prevent a disease that is self-limited.

And such immediate and longer-term toxicity is not of course all; as with all other uses, there is also the risk of superinfection and of drug-resistant superbugs.

> Antimicrobial resistance or microbial overgrowth may develop during the administration of the prophylactic drug, resulting in resistant intestinal flora, antimicrobial-associated colitis induced by *Clostridium difficile*, intestinal salmonellosis or campylobacteriosis, or candida vaginitis. Prophylactic therapy also gives a false sense of security to a traveler who would otherwise exercise caution in selecting food.

It would indeed be wonderful if antibiotics were harmless. But right from the start, over half a century ago, physicians who observed their effects on patients became aware that they are mixed blessings, that they do harm as well as good, and that the more they are used, the greater their ill-effects are liable to be. However, modern medicine and modern agriculture as now practised throughout the world could not function without antibiotics. Like nuclear power – another awesome but problematic scientific development – antibiotics are here to stay, whatever our misgivings. They will remain an inescapable fact of life as we approach and move into the new millennium, and we will do well to learn how to live with them as best we can.

The analogy with nuclear power is a fairly good one. Both are spectacular attempts to shape and control the natural world for the benefit of humankind which, once sanctioned, generated colossal industries and thus became important sources of employment and capital. Both may be immeasurably valuable when all goes according to plan, but they challenge human knowledge and wisdom, and their effects on the environment are incalculable. Scientists are not omniscient; they cannot foresee all the implications of their inventions which, once made part of national and international policies by legislators for persuasive economic or political reasons, may become monsters. And there is no way to ensure that the most potent scientific and technological developments remain in safe hands. Indeed, whose hands are completely safe?

There comes a point, however, when the analogy breaks down. We all know that nuclear power, and also planned genetic engineering, are fearful. Their dangers are acknowledged by governments, and means of controlling them remain items on national agendas throughout the world, reflected in the broadcast and print media. They have been and will remain publicly debated, as issues we need to think about, as consumers and as citizens.

By contrast, although we care more about our health and that of our families than about any other issue[2], we tend to leave the thinking about drugs, including antibiotics, to the experts – that is, to the medical profession and the pharmaceutical industry. But as long as we do not know or do not care about the impact of antibiotics, the damage their overuse and abuse may do to our health, and does do to public health, can only get worse.

On the other hand, when antibiotics are used appropriately,

cautiously, thoughtfully and sparingly, with a view not only to their effect on the individual but also on the community and the environment, their benefits can and should outweigh their risks. And the chance that drugs including antibiotics will be used rationally, is increased when both physicians and consumers are knowledgeable and prepared to enter into dialogue rather than to rely on blind faith.

What can be done to regain the benefit of antibiotics as a precious resource, to be used only when they are really needed? On a personal level, quite a lot – and more of that below. On a national and international level, perhaps not very much, for tough regulations are the only sure way to restrict the use of drugs, and in the 1990s we have all become subject to the ideology of the free market, which involves abandoning restrictions on industry and trade, and limits the authority of any national government to act on behalf of its own citizens.

However, here in conclusion are fifteen proposals designed to reduce the risk and increase the benefits of antibiotics, in the public interest. Although some may meet obstruction, they are not revolutionary; and it is not proposed that all or most antibiotics be prohibited or even severely restricted. Much change for the better can come simply as a result of increased awareness of the potency and thus the dangers of antibiotics. Some of the proposals here can be applied to drugs generally, as well as to antibiotics specifically. They are designed to work internationally and globally; some have particular application to the UK but can be adapted for use in other countries.

The proposals are divided into five sections, each including three proposals: for government (and international agencies such as the World Health Organisation); for industry (including its regulatory interface with government); for the medical profession (from research science to general practice); for public interest organisations; and for ourselves (as citizens as well as consumers).

GOVERNMENT: VIGILANCE

Traditionally, governments have exercised their power to protect the interests of their citizens by means of laws. Lately, the legislative process has become increasingly international, and the development of 'harmonisation' of regulations designed to protect health and to ensure safety within the European Union discourages national initiatives. Inasmuch as the proposals here can be made to work effectively only by means of statutory authority, they will need to be incorporated into European law. But meanwhile the British government can set an example simply by encouraging industry, the medical profession and consumers to become more prudent in the use of antibiotics.

1: Publish an annual list of essential antibiotics

In 1977 the World Health Organisation first published a list of essential drugs.[3] Secretary of the expert committee responsible for the list was Dr Hiroshi Nakajima, who by the 1990s had become WHO Director-General. One purpose of the list was (and is) to bring some order into the increasing chaos of drug supply and use: 'In recent years, there has been a tremendous increase in the number of pharmaceutical products marketed; however, there has not been a proportionate improvement in health.' Another purpose was to guide physicians and protect the public: 'Adoption of a list of essential drugs is part of a national health policy. This implies that priority is given to achieving the widest possible coverage of the population with drugs of proven efficacy and safety.' Essential drugs should meet the needs of the great majority, but all countries should adapt the list for their own circumstances: 'Each country should appoint a committee to establish a list of essential drugs. The committee should include individuals competent in the fields of clinical medicine, pharmacology and pharmacy, as well as peripheral health workers.' The 1977 WHO list included twelve drugs designed to treat bacterial infections and identified as 'essential'; another four were identified as 'complementary', useful as treatment for drug-resistant or rare infections.[4]

The UK government should not only welcome this WHO initiative but should itself publish a list of essential and reserve antibiotics, to be included in the British National Formulary[5], updated every year, allowing for changing circumstances in the UK and in Europe. The drugs to be included in the list, wherever possible, to be relatively safe, effective and cheap. Details of toxicity, drug resistance and price to be appended to the list. The work of compilation and approval of the list to be given to a Department of Health expert advisory committee whose members are all independent of industry, and who include medical microbiologists already responsible for the antibiotic guidelines used in hospital practice, together with physicians and pharmacists.[6] When published, the list to be well publicised, circulated to all doctors, and produced in the form of notices to be posted in waiting rooms and other public places. In due course, the UK list to be amalgamated with other such lists produced in Europe.

It is not proposed that doctors be obliged to use only those drugs on an essential and reserve list; they will be free to prescribe any antibiotic on the market that they consider to be in the best interests of their patients. That said, they and their patients will be guided towards those antibiotics that are generally the best choices, and public awareness of the benefits and risks of antibiotics will be raised.

2: Make invasive drug-resistant bacterial infections notifiable

Starting over a century ago, British doctors have been required to notify an appropriate authority (who now may be their local consultant in communicable diseases) of certain infections that could become a serious threat to public health and thus need to be watched. When considered necessary, somebody with a notifiable disease may be carefully examined and asked to list their contacts, and may even be isolated at home or in hospital. Notifiable diseases now include bacterial infections such as cholera, dysentery, tuberculosis and typhoid. This system of notification has done much to protect public health in Britain.

Given the scale of drug resistance, the fact that it is itself infectious and is able to spread from drug to drug and bacterial species to bacterial species, and the emergence not only of multiply drug-resistant superbugs but now also of the ultimate 'everything-resistant' enterococci, all drug-resistant invasive (and therefore potentially deadly) bacterial infections should now be made notifiable. Serious drug-resistant infections to be treated not only as separate disease entities, which effectively they are, but also as an intrinsic threat to public health. The information about drug resistance to be collected by the Public Health Laboratory Service, published, and circulated locally, regionally and nationally, to physicians, health authorities, the Department of Health and the media. A publicly funded unit concerned with drug resistance to be set up within a scientific centre of excellence designated as a World Health

Organisation collaborating centre and, as such, the British input to WHONET, the WHO global drug-resistance surveillance programme.[7]

Reliable information about drug-resistant bacterial infections throughout Britain will require substantial funding. This could come from the Department of Health, or from a body charged with allocating public funds such as the Medical Research Council, or else be raised from a charge on the pharmaceutical industry, levied from firms according to the tonnage of antibiotics they manufacture. Perhaps the most important use of what would effectively be a national map of drug resistance would be the identification of local 'hot-spots' where high levels of resistance should lead to unusually careful use of antibiotics.

3: Ensure that antibiotics are available only on prescription

The original mistaken belief that any ill-effects of antibiotics are trivial, has resulted in them being made too easily obtainable. In the UK, some antimicrobial drugs are now beginning to become available without prescription, over the counter (OTC) at chemists.[8] In some other European countries, broad-spectrum antibiotics are already available OTC. Farmers are free to use antibiotics not only under veterinary supervision as treatment for animal infections, but also without supervision to promote the growth of intensively reared animals. In some regions of the developing world, supply of antibiotics is subject to little effective regulation, with relatively toxic drugs on sale not only in chemists but also in street markets.

The UK government to ensure that, as potent drugs, antibiotics are used only for medical purposes, and only on prescription. This requires legislation. Antibiotics never to be made available OTC as such, or as part of any drug or cleansing agent. Comparably, the use of antibiotics as animal growth promoters to be prohibited, and a veterinary prescription or at least supervision to be required before antibiotics could be used on farms. In the short term, fair international trade to be ensured, if necessary, by paying farmers compensation to allow for any price differences between home and imported meat, and/or by taxing and labelling imported meat from animals fed growth promoters. In the longer term, the UK to seek agreement to a European and then worldwide withdrawal of antibiotics for the purpose of animal growth promotion.

The industry is likely to oppose this initiative. So may consumers, unable to buy any antimicrobials over the counter, and faced with more expensive meat. Government to therefore give a clear and well-documented account of its actions, to be prepared also to crack down on black markets in drugs for use on farms, and to warn the public against the use of OTC antibiotics when travelling abroad.

INDUSTRY: RESPONSIBILITY

For many years now, the pharmaceutical industry has been carefully regulated in developed countries such as the UK and the USA. At the same time, regulators are bound to place almost total reliance on research carried out by an industry that is eager to market new products; in addition, the key information on drugs available to physicians is produced by industry. The right balance between commercial interests and the public interest is not yet achieved, and in any case, it is not always reasonable to expect industry to produce objective information. Some responsibility for drug regulation and information to be removed from industry and given to independent bodies, funded either with public money or from a levy on industry.

4: Create an independent drug regulatory agency

In the UK, the agency responsible for the supervision of drugs is the Committee on Safety of Medicines (CSM).

Responsibility for the approval and withdrawal of drug licences, and for surveillance of the safety of drugs in use, to be given to a new regulatory agency, modelled on the US Food and Drugs Administration (FDA). The agency to be given statutory powers and be accountable directly to Parliament. Its staff to have the resources to undertake independent research and any industry connections as a matter of public record to be disclosed. As one of its first tasks, the agency to assess the safety in the use of antibiotics, and then withdraw licences from antibiotics either because they are unacceptably toxic or because there is no longer need for them, and to require the restriction of other antibiotics because of their toxicity or to guard against multiply drug-resistant bacteria. The agency to be publicly accountable: agenda and minutes of its meetings, and its decisions and their rationale, to be released to the media, and some of its meetings to be held in public.

The CSM cannot be expected to cope with the vast number of drugs now on the market, and will be distrusted as long as its decisions are made in secret. Industry may resist the establishment of a strong regulatory agency, but would be wise to accept it, as increased protection against drug scandals. The main issue is: who will pay? Again, the agency to be funded with public money, or else from a levy on industry.

5: Distribute independent data on drugs to all doctors
One main source of information about drugs used by UK physicians is the *ABPI Data Sheet Compendium*, compiled and published by industry. Some of the information in the *Compendium*, which is updated every year, is detailed and useful (and has been used as a source for the appendix to this book). But industry should not be expected always to be frank in giving details about the disadvantages of its products. Data in the *Compendium* is an unsatisfactory blend of information and promotion. Advertisements for drugs in the medical press are also problematic: while subject to regulations requiring details of adverse effects to be included, these details can be too summary and printed in a style that is hard to read.

The industry is, of course, entitled to publish information and advertisements about its products, subject to regulations designed to protect physicians and the public. These regulations to be strengthened – for example, warnings of adverse effects to be printed in easily readable type and to use clear, precise language. But the regularly updated data on drugs, their uses and their effects, on which physicians rely, to be supplied by industry to an independent publisher. Once an independent drug regulatory agency is set up, the publishing of this information to be part of its work; meanwhile, the work to be done by another appropriate body.

Physicians should welcome such a relatively independent source of objective information about drugs which, as with an independent regulatory agency, should protect industry as well as the public. Again, funding to be with public money or else from an industry levy.

6: Encourage industry to market drugs consistently, worldwide
The claims that industry make for drugs in its marketing and advertising varies in different countries. In those where such information is carefully regulated, claims are correspondingly circumspect. In

countries with little effective regulation, claims are often exaggerated, and sometimes can be misleading.[9] Antibiotics are a case in point. In the UK, relatively toxic drugs are marketed with clear warnings about their ill-effects. In developing countries, such drugs may be marketed as cure-alls. Drug resistance means that the indiscriminate use of antibiotics in one country is a global health hazard.

There is no way that industry can be forced to market its products consistently in different countries, and in developing countries, firms manufacturing pirated products will remain a problem. But considerable pressure can be put on industry, not only by networks working in the public interest (such as Health Action International) but also by international agencies, notably the World Health Organisation. The UK government should play a leading part in encouraging WHO to publish detailed codes for the marketing of antibiotics and other drugs, and in encouraging industry to accept these codes. Such encouragement when possible to take positive forms – for example, industry should publicise where its marketing follows the WHO code.

International initiatives such as this will take time to succeed, but a start can readily be made if the UK government takes a lead, initially in Europe in collaboration with the WHO European Region office, and then in English-speaking developing countries. It should not be assumed that industry will necessarily oppose such a programme; rational regulations as well as well observed codes of practice are in the interests not only of the public but also of responsible drug manufacturers.

THE MEDICAL PROFESSION: PRUDENCE

Generally speaking, physicians and surgeons do not take much interest in the ill-effects of antibiotics unless these are immediate and obvious. This is understandable: whether in general practice or hospital, busy doctors deal with patients and the symptoms in front of them there and then, and often have neither the time nor the means to look for subtler harm. All too often, antibiotic toxicity, superinfection and multiply drug-resistant superbugs are dismissed as 'one of those things', and not identified as the result of drug treatment. At present, microbiology is no longer an important subject in the curriculum for medical students, and investigation into the ill-effects of antibiotics is a low research priority.

7: Look for possible links between antibiotics and disease

A substantial number of diseases are identified in textbooks as of 'unknown aetiology' – meaning, their causes are unknown. Others are identified as in part the ill-effects of antimicrobial drugs. These include a number of diseases of the skin and the gut, or else affecting the nervous or immune systems. Some have become common and even serious diseases only during the last half-century. Some have symptoms known to be similar to the ill-effects of antimicrobial drugs. Yet other diseases are known to be caused by antibiotics – including superinfections and drug-resistant infections – but their incidence is unknown.

The Medical Research Council therefore to fund a series of epidemiological and clinical trials designed to determine the extent to which antimicrobial drugs themselves cause disease. Surveys within the UK, and comparing the UK with other countries, to identify diseases whose incidence is coincident with use of antimicrobial drugs. Animal trials to be carried out to establish which animal diseases are evidently caused by administration of antimicrobials, and to test specific antibiotics and other antimicrobials. Clinical trials to follow this epidemiological and animal work when evident links between antimicrobials and disease are identified. Further investigations to be done into the possible biological mechanisms whereby antimicrobials may cause disease. As these trials produce results, national antimicrobial policy to be reviewed, and relevant drugs issued with new warnings of ill-effects, or else withdrawn.

These trials will be very expensive, and it is likely that they will be opposed by industry, who may say that their own clinical trials establish the safety-in-use of drugs, which are then licensed. But this is not altogether so. There is an urgent need for independent trials designed to investigate possible links between antimicrobial drugs and many diseases not so far agreed to have drugs as a cause, but where circumstantial evidence to that effect exists.

8: Publicise information about drug-resistant infections

The reason that little is publicly known about superbugs, notably those in hospitals, is that outbreaks of multiply drug-resistant diseases are kept quiet. Hospital administrators do not advertise the fact that superstaph or 'everything-resistant' *Enterococcus faecalis* is lurking in their wards, just as industry executives do not encourage television programmes explaining the hazards of their products. The transformation of many British hospitals into independent trusts, which are anxious to work on business lines, will, if anything, create even more secrecy.

The public has a right to be fully informed about outbreaks of drug-resistant bacterial infections both in hospitals and in the community. Making invasive, resistant infections notifiable diseases is a means to that end. The Department of Health to require all hospitals and general practices not only to inform the public health authorities about the incidence of notifiable diseases, but also require them to publish this information in public places such as hospital and general practice waiting-rooms, and to release it to the local press. Correspondingly, the Public Health Laboratory Service regularly (say, every three months) to publish national figures with regional and local details, together with comparisons over time, with a clear commentary. This information also to be released to the media.

Hospital administrators may well resist this initiative at first, but letting the public know about drug-resistant infections is in the spirit of internal health service competition, and will also encourage hospitals to 'clean up their act'. Specifically, it is likely that superbug outbreaks will sharply decrease after their existence is disclosed, simply because hospital administrators will then have an extra incentive to approve antibiotic guideline policies that will reduce the rate of drug resistance.

9: Give microbiology a higher priority in medical education

Modern medicine teaches doctors about disease rather than health. As part of this bias, doctors learn about those micro-organisms that may cause infectious disease, and therefore they are unlikely to gain a good understanding of microbial ecology. Specifically, physicians and surgeons are likely not to perceive the vital role of bacteria in the protection of human health, unless they happen to have a special interest in the subject. Medical and surgical practice still operates as if the germ theory of disease is valid, notwithstanding the fact that, today, most major diseases in developed countries are not infectious.

Microbiology to be given a much higher priority on the syllabus for medical students, and young doctors to be taught the value of preserving the body's microbial ecology. All major hospitals to include a well-set-up department of medical microbiology, and accept antibiotic guidelines designed to encourage prudent use of antimicrobial drugs. In addition, general practitioners to be given refresher courses in microbiology as it is now understood. By these means, physicians in general practice and in hospitals will be encouraged to use antibiotics cautiously, and surgeons will use antibiotic prophylaxis only in special situations. In particular, general practitioners to be encouraged to avoid prescribing antibiotics for trivial infections or, when practical, for infections not yet definitely identified as bacterial.

Deans of medical schools may have some objection to this proposal, because the syllabus for medical students is already very full. But it is just as important to prevent infectious diseases as it is to prevent non-infectious diseases such as heart disease and cancers. The reputation of the medical profession, and the effectiveness of medical practitioners, will be enhanced when good practice involves protection of the body's own natural defences against infection.

PUBLIC INTEREST ORGANISATIONS: EMPOWERMENT

Consumer organisations in the UK have generally not been very effective in seeking to protect the public against the ill-effects of dangerous drugs, or against the overuse and abuse of drugs such as antibiotics. Both government and industry are secretive, and drugs are very big business. The exception to this lack of effectiveness is the Consumers' Association, which for many years has given support to the newsletter *Drugs and Therapeutics Bulletin* and the small public-interest group Social Audit. Other small groups representing drug victims have campaigned with some success against the abuse of barbiturates and tranquillisers, but there is no watchdog organisation concerned to scrutinise the use of antibiotics.

10: Establish a national group to audit antibiotics

When consumers act as citizens, they can work wonders. More and more in developed democracies, public policy is shaped by special-interest groups outside government. If citizens want their voices to be heard, they must work as effectively as industry does. Large public-interest organisations, ranging from the National Trust to Friends of the Earth, are influential forces; and small knowledgeable, well-connected specialist organisations committed to specific causes may also be heard with respect by legislators and civil servants.

It is therefore time to set up a new national organisation in the public interest, committed to the rational use of antibiotics. It should not be 'anti-drug'. Such a body can start small, as long as its founding members are energetic and able to raise enough money to set up an office. A large part of its work should be to gather reliable information about the benefits and risks of antibiotics and circulate this information to members, the press and policy-makers. Although strengthened by scientific advisers, it should always be controlled by its lay membership. It should network with organisations monitoring other types of drugs, and be prepared to enter into dialogue with industry, to give testimony at public hearings, to propose legislation, regulation and codes of practice, and to campaign fearlessly when drugs should be restricted or withdrawn.

But how will such an organisation be funded? Where there's a will, there's a way. Initially it may be sufficient to establish a database of, say, a thousand people convinced that the rational use of antibiotics is vital to protect public health. Some of these will subscribe money; others will have relevant skills, such as word-processing, facility on the Internet, journalism or a knowledge of law or medicine. Of all the proposals listed here, this is perhaps the simplest and potentially the most effective. Certainly, public policy towards antibiotics in Britain will not change unless and until there is an effective antibiotic watchdog organisation.

11: Develop this public interest group internationally

Any national group committed to the rational use of antibiotics will have a limited value. Science is by its nature international; so is bacterial infection. To get a complete picture of the beneficial effects and ill-effects of antibiotics and of the spread of drug resistance, it is necessary to accumulate international and global information. This will be of immediate benefit to members of the group who are travelling abroad.

Therefore, as soon as the UK group is set up, it should seek to find similar groups in other countries. In some cases, these may be part of a consumer network – for example, the Consumers' Association of Penang in Malaysia campaigns vigorously on a broad range of issues including drugs.[10] In other cases, these may be scientifically based – for example, the Alliance for the Prudent Use of Antibiotics, originally set up by Professor Stuart Levy and based at Boston, Massachusetts.[11] It may be that the global organisation should be concerned not only with antibiotics but also with the rational use of medical drugs generally, in which case it could be called 'DrugNet'. As with any national organisation, the international network should be well advised scientifically and technically, but should always be controlled by lay people.

Setting up international networks nowadays is far less daunting than it used to be. Computers and faxes greatly simplify communication. An international network should have the resources to plug into relevant computerised scientific and medical databases. It can also work with other sympathetic global organisations, such as the International Organisation of Consumer Unions (IOCU).[12]

12: Publish a newsletter on antibiotics

People without experience of the media may suppose that journalists seek and find stories 'out there', using their contacts, skills and special knowledge. In fact, there are not many fearless newshounds around, and probably never were. Most of the items you read in newspapers or see on television are there because somebody packaged these stories for journalists. Many, perhaps most news and features stories in newspapers are repackaged from press releases prepared by interested parties. One sufficient reason why medical drugs in general and antibiotics in particular are rarely on news editors' agenda is that they are not being fed interesting information.

Therefore, one of the first tasks of the national (and later the global) organisation concerned with antibiotics should be to publish a newsletter. This should draw on any data distributed to physicians but should not be confined to medical information. It should have a news sense. It could include interviews with leading scientists in the context of important new developments – say, the spread of drug-resistant tuberculosis in London, the establishment of new antibiotic policies in specific hospitals, new evidence that good nutrition reduces the incidence of infection, or results of scientific trials on antibiotics. It should also draw on information compiled by the Public Health Laboratory Service and other reliable sources, and explain the significance of such data. The newsletter might at first appear only quarterly but, as soon as resources allow, should be published monthly or more frequently. It should be press-released and, of course, distributed to all members of the organisation. It should also be published electronically on the Internet.

Perhaps the most valuable resource of any public interest organisation is a regular newsletter. It creates a sense of community among the membership, keeps the organisation in the public eye, and is a key means of communication with policy-makers and the media. Again, it should not have an 'anti-drug' editorial policy; its commitment should be to the rational use of antibiotics.

CITIZENS: SELF-DETERMINATION

This means you! Never forget that antibiotics are a precious resource and that one day your life or that of a member of your family may be saved by antibiotics. They are drugs to be used carefully against dangerous, invasive bacterial infections. Otherwise it is best to avoid them; common simple infections should be allowed to run their course, and the infected person looked after, if necessary in bed with relief for pain or fever plus some tender loving care. Your best defence against infectious disease is your body's own immune defences, which you can strengthen. Your best friend if you are considering using antibiotics, is a sympathetic physician.

13: Protect yourself against infection

The modern medical profession and pharmaceutical industry is founded on the germ theory of disease, according to which, disease is 'out there', a visitation that invades us 'out of the blue', by chance. If this is true, disease has nothing much to do with us: we are not responsible for our own health, and when we are ill, we go to the doctor who we think will make us better. However, the germ theory of disease has misled us, and the main responsibility for the protection of our health is ours. Specifically, infectious disease is usually a sign that the body's defences are fragile, which is of course why vulnerable groups such as babies and the elderly are more likely to suffer infections.

There are a number of ways in which you can strengthen your defences against infection (viral as well as bacterial). First and perhaps foremost, eat wholefood. Developments in the science of nutrition in the last few years have shown that wholefoods – especially fresh vegetables and fruit, and wholegrain bread and cereals – contain natural anti-infective chemicals designed to protect the plant, which may protect us, too.[13] In any case, a wholefood diet also protects against non-infectious diseases. There is some evidence that fermented foods rich in lactobacilli – live yoghurt, notably – may be beneficial if eaten regularly. Various herbs have powerful anti-infective qualities; the best researched is garlic.

Second, pay attention to hygiene. This is usually easily done in developed countries, but holiday-makers should take special care. The sea at many resorts is now heavily contaminated, and it is prudent when travelling abroad in hot climates to avoid food of animal origin, to prefer well-cooked food, and to drink only bottled water.

Third, be aware that overcrowding breeds infection. Most infections contracted by children at school, by workers in crowded offices, or by those who eat meat from intensively reared animals, are relatively trivial. But mothers of babies and young children, and those who care for weak ill people in hospital, should take special care: easier said than done sometimes, of course.

Fourth, accept that suffering and recovery from infection is a natural process, as a result of which the body's defences against future infection are strengthened. If you can hold out without drugs, and wait for the infection to run its course, you should as a result have increased your resistance to disease. This does not mean that you need not consult a doctor when you or a member of your family, notably the young, the already ill, and the old, are suffering infection. But let the doctor know that you would prefer to avoid antibiotics if at all possible.

14: Find a sympathetic physician

General practitioners and hospital doctors have different attitudes towards the use of antibiotics. Medicine is not an exact science, and general practitioners often prescribe antibiotics 'just to be on the safe side'. It is up to you to find a physician who prefers to prescribe antibiotics only for serious bacterial infections. As one check, you could ask your physician to read this book and see what he or she thinks of it.

When you do consult your physician, be helpful. Say that you prefer to avoid antibiotics, and that if your infection is not serious, you would rather do without them. If the physician nevertheless proposes to prescribe antibiotics, ask if he or she is quite sure the infection is bacterial and in case of any doubt, you would rather wait for the results of a test. If the physician is quite sure your infection is bacterial and serious, or potentially so, ask for the chemical as well as the trade name of the drug prescribed so you can note it down in your drugs diary (*see below*), and ask for the minimum effective dose. Also ask about the most common ill-effects of the drug, so that you know what to look out for.

These questions apply to anybody in your care, such as a child or other relative or friend. If your physician refuses to be questioned courteously in the way indicated here, change your physician: you are entitled to do so.

15: Keep a drugs diary

When you take antibiotics and other drugs, notice what happens. The more observant you are, the more your physician will be guided. Remember, antibiotics are powerful medicines, and reactions vary from person to person. Your physician may not realise that an antibiotic is hazardous to your health unless you report ill-effects precisely.

Keep a drugs diary for yourself and for all members of your family. Among other medicines, list full details of all antibiotics prescribed and taken. Details to include chemical and trade name, dose, length of treatment. The diary also to give details of non-prescription drugs (aspirin, cough mixtures, etc.), and of substances liable to interact with drugs such as alcohol. Use the diary to list symptoms and possible ill-effects of drugs, rating symptoms on a scale from 1 to 10, 1 being very mild indeed, 5–6 being bad enough to interfere with daily life, 10 being intolerable (in which case somebody else will be noting your symptoms . . .). Remember to include details of drugs prescribed by practitioners other than your own doctor – for example, by your dentist, or when you have been in hospital, or by a foreign doctor when you have travelled abroad. The only way you and your doctor can make really accurate judgements is if your drug history is complete. Nobody else will do this for you. Take the diary with you whenever you consult your doctor.

USING ANTIBIOTICS WISELY

Antibiotics are valuable drugs – there is no doubt about that. But taking the evidence all together, from scientific textbooks and journals, from medical research, and from the testimony of scientists and health workers in the community, of the benefits and risks of antibiotics, and of the short-term and long-term effects of their use, overuse and abuse on human health worldwide, it seems to me that, like other mixed blessings, antibiotics now do more harm than good. That is, as now used, they cause or contribute to more disease than they cure.

If you take your health into your own hands and choose to use antibiotics prudently, you will be making your own contribution to a safer world, in which, on balance, antibiotics do more good than harm to the community, your family and yourself.

Afterword

by Professor Richard Lacey

Antibiotics are prescribed too often, and the result of their overuse and abuse is bad not only for public health but also bad for the health of the individual patient.

All drugs are prescribed on the basis of balancing estimated likely benefit with possible risk. In practice, busy doctors and anxious patients both tend to overestimate the benefits of antibiotics and underestimate their immediate and longer term risks. This bias is exacerbated by the fact that appropriately prescribed antibiotics are effective and their adverse effects often less obvious; by energetic pharmaceutical industry promotion to the medical profession; and by the common misperception that bacteria are generally harmful and better eliminated.

In my judgement, evidence from modern medical and microbiological science indicates that in countries like the UK antibiotics are grossly overused, and that they are appropriate only in one in ten or less of the cases where they are now prescribed. Translated to individual patients this implies on average a course of antibiotics not at the current rate of once or twice a year, mostly for trivial illness, but once or twice every ten years, or less often, for serious bacterial infections.

This guide to the use of antibiotics is adapted from those issued to general and hospital practitioners by the Health Authorities in the Leeds region, following recommendations made by an expert panel of microbiologists, physicians and other health professionals of which I am chairman. It is a practical guide and it works in general and hospital practice in a large area of northern England as a means to encourage rational and prudent use of these potent drugs. Similar guides are used elsewhere in the UK and in other countries.

In any individual case reliable diagnosis and prescription can be made only by a medical practitioner. The purpose of this guide is to enable patients to increase their understanding of the benefits and risks of antibiotics and to ask for them only when advisable, and to discourage doctors from what I call the CAP (Compulsive Antibiotic Prescribing) syndrome.

GENERAL GUIDELINES

Here are seven general guidelines, for patients (and parents of patients) to bear in mind, and for medical practitioners. In any individual case the needs of the individual patient and the judgement of the medical practitioner must take precedence and a guide like this cannot of course replace doctors' advice. Perhaps the best general guidance for patients is to seek out community and hospital doctors sympathetic with the points made here.

1 *Most illnesses are not infections*
Most serious diseases and disorders in countries such as the UK are not infections. The majority of people in developed countries die from diseases of the circulation system, such as heart attacks and strokes, or else from cancers of the lung, breast, colon and other sites that have nothing to do with infectious agents. Likewise diabetes, multiple sclerosis, hypertension, gall stones and kidney stones. Common disorders such as constipation, indigestion, obesity, backache, migraine, hernia and depression are of course not infections. Drugs have only a limited role as treatment of any of these conditions and antibiotics are irrelevant. The best approach to such diseases and disorders is preventive: a healthy lifestyle encouraged by effective public health policies.

2 *Many infections are viral and so cannot be treated*
Many common infections, notably colds and flu, are caused by viruses, and most common infections of the skin, ear, nose and throat are often not bacterial but viral in origin. Antibiotics are useless as treatment of virtually all viral infections. In cases of doubt as to whether an illness is bacterial or viral (or whether it is an infection of any kind), it is always best whenever practicable to take a sample for laboratory analysis before considering antibiotics as treatment. If an infection is bacterial in origin such analysis will also identify the species, and so enable precise use of the most effective antibiotic. It is however prudent to use antibiotics before laboratory testing on a 'best guess' basis if an undiagnosed infection is evidently serious.

3 Many simple bacterial infections are best left to clear up by themselves

Many common infections such as those mentioned above, and of the gut and urinary tract, while often acutely unpleasant, are likely to clear up by themselves without prescription drugs in otherwise healthy people. They are usually best left alone or treated with remedies obtained over the counter in chemists, such as dressings, mild painkillers or antiseptics. Taking it easy and resting in bed is often sensible. The body's own powers of healing are strengthened when diseases take their natural course. Simple gastroenteritis, colitis and/or diarrhoea caused by infection should never be treated with antibiotics, which themselves may cause diarrhoea and may make matters worse. Complicated or invasive bacterial infections are likely to need antibiotic treatment, but complications are fairly likely to follow the treatment itself.

4 Infections can be the result of antibiotic use

Properly prescribed, antibiotics should usually be effective treatment of bacterial infections. But after-effects of antibiotic use are to make the patient more vulnerable to infection by other bacterial species and by other microbes such as fungi, and also to promote drug resistance in both commensal and pathogenic bacteria. The stronger the dose, the longer the course and the broader the spectrum of the antibiotic, the greater the degree of disruption of the beneficial bacteria in our bodies, and the risk of recurrent infection. Drug resistance in hospitals is very troublesome. Most hospital infections now are caused by species of bacteria that before systematic use of antibiotics were harmless or readily treated, but which have become multi drug-resistant 'superbugs'. Most antibiotics now used in hospital are designed to treat these new major pathogens.

5 Avoid antibiotics as a means to prevent infections

It is tempting to use antibiotics not to treat but to prevent bacterial infection. Sometimes this is the right thing to do. For example, children in contact with a case of known bacterial meningitis at a nursery school should be prescribed antibiotics prophylactically, as should patients facing major surgery in which vital organs are opened. But contrary to common practice, I believe it is usually better not to prescribe antibiotics to guard against invasive bacterial infection in general or in dental practice where there is no direct evidence of such infection; in such cases I believe that the risks generally outbalance the benefits. Certainly, it is usually wrong to use antibiotics in cases of simple infection 'just in case' they become invasive.

6 *Prefer cheap, safe, simple antibiotics*
The benefits and risks of drugs that have been on the market for a long time are well known. Such well-established drugs will be out of patent and normally available in cheap generic versions. Newer drugs, such as later generation cephalosporins and the quinolones, should normally be avoided in general practice for two reasons: first, their adverse effects and interactions with other drugs and environmental agents will be not well known; second, they should be held in reserve for use against drug-resistant bacteria. Avoid combination drugs, notably penicillin mixtures and co-trimoxazole: these have a wider spectrum than single agents and so are more likely to breed superinfection, and are more toxic. Also avoid superseded relatively toxic drugs, notably the aminoglycosides, the lincosamides, the sulphonamides and the tetracyclines, with the exceptions listed below.

7 *Use antibiotics precisely, briefly and cautiously*
Laboratory analysis should be used when practicable to identify the microbial cause of an infection which, if bacterial, can then be treated with a narrow spectrum drug with as little as possible additional, irrelevant activity. The drug selected should be used in the lowest dose and the shortest time appropriate. Generally, five days for respiratory tract infections and three days for urinary tract infections is adequate. As a rule, antibiotics should be stopped when the patient feels better. The doctrine of 'complete the course' is generally mistaken, and applies only in cases of embedded bacterial infections treated in hospital, such as brucellosis or tuberculosis. Patients should be advised of side-effects of drugs when they are prescribed, and doctors should take special care to monitor patients taking drugs with known serious adverse effects.

WHAT TO DO IN CASE OF BACTERIAL INFECTION

Antibiotics are of course absolutely essential in cases of serious invasive bacterial infections, such as meningitis, pneumonia, typhoid, syphilis and deep wound infections. In general, symptoms of overall systemic illness are a sign that drug treatment may be necessary.

Suspected cases of serious infection should be referred to special clinics or treated in hospital, and positive diagnosis of bacterial origin urgently made by laboratory analysis before treatment. In hospital there is a somewhat greater case for carefully monitored drug treatment for patients who are very young, very old, or very ill, even though the risks of treatment are greater too.

The infections listed below are among the most common found in the community. Patients, parents of patients and doctors should be aware that antibiotics are generally not the first treatment of choice for these and other common conditions, unless otherwise stated below.

EYES: Conjunctivitis Most cases of red, sticky or sore eyes are viral in origin. Whether viral or bacterial, use eye drops from the chemist as treatment. Exception: in newborn babies bacterial conjunctivitis may be dangerous and need antibiotic treatment in hospital. It is bad practice to use chloramphenicol eye drops or ointment, which may be absorbed into the body causing serious adverse effects, and also could breed drug resistance in the bacteria naturally present in the throat, which when invasive can cause meningitis.

EARS: Otitis media Otherwise known as middle ear infection, this is usually viral in origin. Earache caused by build-up of microbial and other debris inside the ear can be very painful and should be treated with painkillers.

MOUTH: Abscesses Abscesses of the gums or under teeth that are bacterial in origin are treated by drainage (lancing, root canal therapy, extraction) and with antiseptics. Dentists recommend antibiotics for more invasive procedures (scaling, extraction) not to treat local bacterial infection, but in case it spreads through the blood into the area of the heart, causing bacterial endocarditis. If a dental patient is known to have a history of heart problems such as rheumatic fever this may be appropriate, but otherwise in my opinion antibiotics are rarely justified in dentistry.

SKIN: Acne Usually acne eventually clears up by itself. Antiseptics can help. If antibiotics are chosen in cases of severe acne, use a low dose and review after three months. It is best not to use antibiotics in cases of simple teenage acne. Oxytetracycline is effective but problematic: it often works only if used over long periods of time, and has many side-effects that may well prove more troublesome, if less visible, than acne. It must not be used for pre-teenage children or if there is any possibility of pregnancy.

SKIN: Cuts, ulcers Broken skin often becomes infected with bacteria, leading to 'weeping' and pus, which may smell unpleasant. Keep the skin clean, and use dressings and antiseptics. Do not use topical antibiotics. In cases of cellulitis, when infection has invaded deeper tissues causing swelling and pain, antibiotics may be appropriate and laboratory blood tests should identify the bacteria involved to check that appropriate antibiotics are being used.

RESPIRATORY TRACT: Tonsillitis, laryngitis, tracheitis Most sore throats are viral in origin. Most of the rest (about one fifth) are bacterial, typically caused by *S. pyogenes*. It is usually not possible to distinguish between viral and bacterial sore throats simply by examination of the patient. Antibiotics of course have no effect on viral sore throats, and usually will make little, if any, difference to the natural course of those that are bacterial in origin. As with mouth disease, above, a rationale for antibiotics is not to treat the infection itself, but in order to prevent it invading the area of the heart and causing rheumatic fever. However, rheumatic fever is now very rare indeed in the UK, and so the risk of this complication is insignificant. In my view it is almost always best not to treat sore throats with antibiotics, and instead let them clear up by themselves, if necessary with painkillers.

RESPIRATORY TRACT: Bronchitis Most cases of bronchitis (soreness and pain lower down the throat and in the chest) are caused by toxic irritation such as smoking or fumes, or else are viral. A common cold accompanied by a cough should not be treated with antibiotics. In relatively severe cases when a bacterial infection is superimposed on underlying bronchitic disease and pus is coughed up, it can be useful to use antibiotics for a few days, but only after laboratory tests have specified the bacteria involved. Otherwise as above.

GASTROINTESTINAL TRACT: Gastroenteritis Cramps and diarrhoea often referred to as food poisoning may be viral in origin.

They are commonly caused by bacteria such as salmonella and campylobacter species, but in such cases antibiotics are not helpful, may make matters worse, and should not be used; the body should be left to rid itself of the infection. Food poisoning is only rarely helped by antibiotics; exceptions are severe cases in generally vulnerable or very ill hospital patients, and protozoal amoebic dysentery. Copious diarrhoea notably in children should be treated with fluid replacement.

URINARY TRACT: Cystitis Inflammation of the urinary tract, more common in women, is usually bacterial in origin, but is liable to recur after treatment with antibiotics and may recur in drug-resistant form. Simple cases may resolve by themselves, and if not are best treated by drinking large amounts of water and then being careful to empty the bladder, thus flushing the bacteria out, and also with alkaline agents. In acutely painful cases use narrow-spectrum antibiotics in a short course, perhaps of three days. If antibiotics are advisable then appropriate laboratory tests should identify the bacterial species involved, particularly if these have invaded the upper urinary tract. Try to avoid antibiotics if pregnancy is possible or within pregnancy until after 16 weeks. Note: bacteria may be present in urine without causing symptoms. This is only rarely a problem needing any treatment.

PELVIS: Pelvic inflammatory disease If positively identified as bacterial in origin this should be treated with antibiotics.

SEXUAL ORGANS: Gonorrhoea, syphilis, chlamydial infection These and other microbial diseases of the sexual organs, once positively diagnosed, require prompt antibiotic treatment in specialist clinics.

SEXUAL ORGANS: Vaginal discharge If positively identified as caused by moulds (candida) or by protozoa (trichomonas) this also needs antibiotic treatment.

VIRAL INFECTIONS: Colds, flu, measles, mumps, chickenpox, herpes and shingles These are all examples of common viral infections. Antibiotics are useless in these cases.

ESSENTIAL ANTIBIOTICS

Most common simple bacterial infections can be successfully treated by one of a relatively small number of antibiotics. The general purpose of a list of essential antibiotics is to make best use of the most effective, least toxic and cheapest drugs and to preserve their value.

Careful and sparing use of antibiotics will reduce the incidence of adverse effects, trivial and dangerous, and of drug resistance in the individual patient, in the community, and in hospital. When possible always prefer the generic (non-proprietory) version of a drug, indicated below as (n/p).

There are many antibiotics on the market that are not included in any of the lists below. These generally, in my view, are not the best first treatment of choice, but some may be options in case of drug allergy or resistance, unavailability of the first choice drug (unlikely in the UK), complicated chronic infections, or in special circumstances as judged by the medical practitioner, preferably with guidance from a microbiological service.

The lists of essential and reserve drugs below apply in the UK in the mid 1990s. They are not 'written in tablets of stone': they may need some variation elsewhere or at other times as patterns of disease and of drug resistance vary. Other such lists published and used in the UK may be somewhat different but usually apply the same general principles.

Antibiotics should usually not be prescribed until after an illness has not responded to simple non-antibiotic treatment (cleaning, dressings, irrigation, antiseptics, etc.) and also, if practicable, the illness has been positively identified as of specified bacterial origin by means of laboratory analysis. It is however, appropriate to use antibiotics immediately for undiagnosed illness that may be an invasive, dangerous bacterial infection. Examples of essential antibiotics (in alphabetical order of family name):

FAMILY NAME	GENERIC NAME	TRADE NAME
Cephalosporins	**Cephradine**	*Velosef*

Hospital use. Effective against a wide range of hospital infections; flexible, cheap. When necessary a good choice for surgical prophylaxis. Drug resistance may oblige use of newer cephalosporins. Option for osteomyelitis and septic arthritis, notably caused by *S. aureus* or *S. pyogenes*. Option for severe persistent urinary tract infection in pregnancy (but only after 16 weeks).

FUSIDANES **SODIUM FUSIDATE** *FUCIDIN*

Community and hospital use. May be needed in combination with cephradine or erythromycin or flucloxacillin.

IMIDAZOLES **METRONIDAZOLE** *METRONIDAZOLE (N/P)*

Community and hospital use. For diagnosed fungal or protozoal vaginal or gastrointestinal infections.

MACROLIDES **ERYTHROMYCIN** *ERYTHROMYCIN (N/P)*

Community and hospital use. Relatively safe, cheap. Effective against a range of infections. Options for severe pharyngitis and tonsillitis (notably when caused by *S. pyogenes*), and sinusitis, middle ear infection, bronchitis and pneumonia (notably when caused by streptococci or *H. influenzae* and legionella infections. Option for skin and soft tissue infections, pelvic inflammatory disease, and for osteomyelitis and septic arthritis, notably caused by *S. aureus* or *S. pyogenes*. Watch for severe gastrointestinal ill-effects.

NITROFURANS **NITROFURANTOIN** *NITROFURANTOIN (N/P)*

Community and hospital use. Option for urinary tract infections caused by *E. coli* or proteus.

PENICILLINS **AMPICILLIN** *AMPICILLIN (N/P)*

Community and hospital use. Good standard antibiotic; flexible, cheap. Often the first choice for severe ear, nose, throat, respiratory tract infections and pneumonia (notably when caused by streptococci or *H. influenzae*) and severe persistent urinary tract infection in pregnancy (but only after 16 weeks). Avoid overuse: resistance, including multi drug-resistance transfer to other bacterial species, is now a major problem.

PENICILLINS	**BENZYLPENICILLIN** (AKA PENICILLIN G)	*CRYSTAPEN*

Hospital use only. Good standard drug, effective against many bacterial infections.

PENICILLINS	**PHENOXYMETHYL-PENICILLIN** (AKA PENICILLIN V)	*PHENOXYMETHYL (N/P)*

Community and hospital use. Good standard drug, effective against many bacterial infections, flexible. Option for bacterial pharyngitis and tonsillitis (notably when caused by *S. pyogenes*), pneumonia (notably when caused by *S. pneumoniae* or *H. influenzae*) and severe surface ulcers.

PENICILLINS	**FLUCLOXACILLIN**	*FLUCLOXACILLIN (N/P)*

Community and hospital use. Option for skin and soft tissue infections. Can be effective against *S. aureus*. Option for osteomyelitis and septic arthritis, notably caused by *S. aureus* or *S. pyogenes*.

QUINOLONE RELATED	**NALIDIXIC ACID**	*NALIDIXIC ACID (N/P)*

Community and hospital use. Option for severe persistent urinary tract infection in pregnancy (but only after 16 weeks).

TETRACYCLINES	**OXYTETRACYCLINE**	*OXYTETRACYCLINE (N/P)*

Community and hospital use. Option for pelvic inflammatory disease, chlamydial or mycoplasma infections, severe acne, severe sinusitis. Not to be used on women if any possibility of pregnancy. Note: minocycline may be a possible alternative.

Trimethoprim	**Trimethoprim**	*Trimethoprim (N/P)*

Community and hospital use. Option for severe bacterial bronchitis, sinusitis and middle ear infection (notably when caused by streptococci or *H. influenzae*). First choice for urinary tract infection caused by *E. coli* or proteus. Always preferable to co-trimoxazole.

RESERVE ANTIBIOTICS

Some relatively toxic or expensive or specialist antibiotics are valuable but should be held in reserve and used only in special circumstances, almost always only in hospital practice, and after positive identification of specific bacterial origin. Typically these are used to treat severe infections caused by hospital pathogens: or as treatment of complicated chronic infections where previous antibiotic treatment is itself a factor (for example chloramphenicol) or as emergency treatment of specific life-threatening acute infections. Ironically, toxicity can give antibacterial drugs special value when dangerous bacterial infections are resistant to less toxic and therefore more commonly used drugs. Patients must be monitored with special care. Examples:

FAMILY NAME	GENERIC NAME	TRADE NAMES
Aminoglycosides	**Gentamicin**	*Cidomycin* *Genticin*

For drug-resistant hospital septicaemias caused by *P. aeruginosa, S. aureus* and other pathogens. Other aminoglycosides probably more toxic, or more expensive. Watch for damage to cranial nerves or kidneys.

Betalactams	**Imipenem/Cilastatin**	*Primaxin*

New very expensive thienamycin betalactam. Very broad spectrum, only for massive multi-bacterial hospital infections.

Cephalosporins	**Cefaclor**	*Distaclor*

Alternative in respiratory infections including pneumonia if ampicillin fails.

CEPHALOSORIN	**CEFOTAXIME**	*CLAFORAN*

Expensive but perhaps less toxic alternative to gentamicin.

CHLORAMPHENICOL	**CHLORAMPHENICOL**	*CHLOROMYCETIN* *KEMICETINE*

Comparatively toxic option for meningitis caused by *S. pneumoniae, N. meningitidis* or *H. influenzae* (not babies), typhoid fever and cerebral abscess. Watch for severe blood disorders.

GLYCOPEPTIDES	**VANCOMYCIN**	*VANCOCIN*

Comparatively toxic, expensive. For severe multi drug-resistant hospital septicaemias, notably those caused by *S. aureus* (also known as MRSA or EMRSA) and *C. difficile*.

PENICILLINS	**PIPERACILLIN**	*PIPRIL*

Effective against drug-resistant hospital infections (including those caused by *P. aeruginosa*). Best choice among antipseudomonal penicillins. May be used together with gentamicin.

QUINOLONES	**CIPROFLOXACIN**	*CIPROXIN*

Effective against drug-resistant hospital infections (including those caused by *P. aeruginosa*) and also a choice for vulnerable patients with dangerous salmonella or campylobacter infections. Best choice among quinolones. Above all reserve antibiotics its use should be exceedingly limited in general practice to protect its value in treatment of serious hospital infections.

SULPHONAMIDE MIXTURES	**CO-TRIMOXAZOLE**	*CO-TRIMOXAZOLE (N/P)* *SEPTRIN* *BACTRIM*

All the ill-effects of sulphonamides, no advantage over trimethoprim alone. One exception: may be useful in hospital only for patients with *Pneumocystis carinii* infections (usually AIDS patients). Trials may in time show that trimethoprim is equally effective in these unusual cases, making co-trimoxazole altogether redundant.

REDUNDANT ANTIBIOTICS

There is in my view practically no justification in countries such as the UK for the use of a number of antibiotics currently on the market, some of which are now commonly prescribed and may have once been useful therapy when better drugs had not been identified and marketed. These redundant drugs are usually best avoided. Let me say again that this is my personal view as a medical microbiologist with considerable experience in these matters, and of course when put into effect it would be more restrictive than common practice elsewhere.

Compared with better choices that should be readily available in community and hospital pharmacies in developed countries, redundant drugs are either relatively toxic, and so increase the risk of acute adverse effects; or else very broad spectrum, and so increase the risk of superinfection and drug resistance; or else have no advantage over options likely to be more effective. They should therefore be used only when there really is no alternative available. Examples:

FAMILY NAME	GENERIC NAME	TRADE NAMES
AMINOGLYCOSIDES ALL EXCEPT GENTAMICIN	**AMIKICIN**	*AMIKIN*
	KANAMYCIN	*KANNASYN*
	NEOMYCIN SULPHATE	*MYCIFRADIN*
		NIVEMYCIN
		POLYBACTRIN
	NETILMICIN	*NETILLIN*
	SPECTINOMYCIN	*TROBICIN*
	STREPTOMYCIN	*STREPTOMYCIN SULPHATE*
	TOBRAMYCIN	*NEBCIN*

Relatively toxic, never preferable to safer drugs. Neomycin may sometimes be useful topically.

LINCOSAMIDES (ALL)	CLINDAMYCIN LINCOMYCIN	*DALACIN* *LINCOCIN*

Avoid all lincosamides. Relatively toxic; erythromycin or metronidazole better choices.

PENICILLINS	AMOXYCILLIN	*AMOXYCILLIN (N/P)* *ALMODAN* *AMOXIL*

Amoxycillin is not a specially problematic drug, but I believe ampicillin generally to be the better choice.

PENICILLINS	CARBENICILLIN	*PYOPEN*

Very expensive. More toxic than other carboxypenicillins.

PENICILLIN COMBINATIONS (ALL)	AMPICILLIN/ CLOXACILLIN	*AMPICLOX*
	AMPICILLIN/ FLUCLOXACILLIN	*CO-FLUAMPICIL (N/P)* *FLU-AMP* *MAGNAPEN*
	AMPICILLIN/ SULBACTAM	*DICAPEN*
	AMOXYCILLIN/ CLAVULANIC ACID	*AUGMENTIN*
	AMOXYCILLIN/ CLAVULINIC ACID	*CO-AMOXYCLAV*
	PENICILLIN G/ PROCAINE PENICILLIN	*BICILLIN*
	PENICILLIN G/ PROCAINE PENICILLIN/ BENETHAMINE PENICILLIN	*TRIPLOPEN*

	PIVAMPICILLIN/ PIVMECILLINAM	*MIRAXID*
		PONDOCILLIN PLUS
	TICARCILLIN/ CLAVULANIC ACID	*TIMENTIN*

It is better to avoid all penicillin combinations. Broad spectrum. Single agents better choices.

SULPHONAMIDES (ALL)	SULFAMETOPYRAZINE	*KELFIZINE*
	SULPHADIAZINE	*SULPHADIAZINE (N/P)*
	SULPHADIMIDINE	*SULPHADIMIDINE (N/P)*
		SULPHAMEZATHINE
	DAPSONE	*DAPSONE (N/P)*
		MALOPRIM

Avoid all sulphonamides (except co-trimoxazole in one special situation: see pages 258–9). Relatively toxic (many ill-effects); obsolete. Better restricted for use in agriculture, as long as resultant meat and other human food contain no residues.

TETRACYCLINES (ALL BAR TWO)	TETRACYCLINE	*TETRACYCLINE (N/P)*
		ACHROMYCIN
		PANMYCIN
		SUSTAMYCIN
		TETRABID
		TETRACHEL
		TETREX
		DETECLO
		MYSTECLIN
	CHLORTETRACYCLINE	*AUREOMYCIN*
	CLOMOCYCELINE SODIUM	*MEGACLVA*
	DEMECLOCYCLINE HYDROCHLORIDE	
		LEDERMYCIN
	DOXYCYCLINE	*DOXYCYCLINE (N/P)*
		NORDOX
		VIBRAMYCIN
	LIMECYCLINE	*TETRALYSAL*

All except oxytetracycline and perhaps also minocycline. Relatively toxic, very broad spectrum, no advantage over erythromycin. Generally better restricted to use in agriculture, as long as resultant meat and other human food contain no residues, and in horticulture.

Richard W Lacey MA MD PhD FRCPath DCH
Professor of Medical Microbiology, University of Leeds

Appendix

THE A-Z OF ANTIBIOTICS

The aim of this comprehensive guide to all antibiotics now available in the UK for human use is to give you the information necessary to have an informed discussion with your doctor about the use of antibiotics in the management of bacterial infections. It is taken from the standard formularies issued to doctors and includes lists of the main current uses of all antibiotics. The antibiotics listed include antibacterial and antifungal drugs currently used to treat human disease in Britain. Antiparasitic drugs are not listed. Details current as of January 1995.

CONTENTS OF APPENDIX

HOW TO USE THIS APPENDIX

If you want to find out more about an antibiotic that has been prescribed for you, look on your prescription sheet or on the label of your medicine for the name and then look for this name in the index that starts on page 265. The index will refer you to the appropriate page of the appendix. (It is sometimes necessary to peel off the chemist's own label to see the name of the particular preparation you have been given.) You will see that some of the names of drugs in the appendix are in *ITALIC SMALL CAPS* while others are in SMALL CAPS. The names in *ITALIC SMALL CAPS* are those given to the drugs by their manufacturers. In other words, they are trade names. The same drug is often produced by several different companies, each of which gives it a different name and price. To try to avoid confusion, the medical profession tries nowadays to refer to drugs only by their generic (chemical) names. These generic names are listed in SMALL CAPS.

Resistance. Overuse and abuse of antibiotics has accelerated the development of resistant strains of many types of bacteria: these are often known as 'superbugs'. If an organism is resistant to a particular antibiotic, there is no point in using that antibiotic for an infection caused by that organism. The way to avoid this problem is for the doctor to take a swab or sample for laboratory testing before prescribing an antibiotic. If an infection fails to respond to antibiotic treatment, it is always worth considering the possibility of resistance.

Antibiotic formulations. Antibiotics for internal use can be given as tablets, capsules, liquids and also by injection. The types of formulation available for each drug are shown in brackets after the name (T for tablets, C for capsules, L for liquids and I for injections).

Lotions, creams, ointments and sprays for external use are referred to as topical preparations.

The sources used for this appendix include:
BNF, British National Formulary, Number 28, September 1994
ABPI Data Sheet Compendium, 1994

New drugs are being introduced all the time. For up-to-date information, please refer to the current edition of the *British National Formulary*.

INDEX OF MANUFACTURERS' TRADE NAMES

1 AMINOGLYCOSIDES

Historical. Streptomycin was the first important antibiotic to be discovered after penicillin. Several other aminoglycosides have been developed subsequently. They resemble each other in their mode of action and toxicity. The differences in their use reflect variations in their antibacterial activity.

Common features. The main use of the group is the hospital treatment of serious acute bacterial infections. They are not absorbed from the gut and are therefore given by injection to treat systemic infections. They are bactericidal (kill bacteria) and are effective against staphylococci and a wide range of Gram-negative organisms. Streptomycin is now used mainly in the treatment of tuberculosis. Spectinomycin is reserved for penicillin-resistant gonorrhoea infection.

Mode of action. Interfere with protein synthesis in bacteria.

Resistance. Variable. 'Cross-resistance' within this group is becoming an increasing problem. Bacterial resistance can develop quickly and is transferable between different species of bacteria. There are variations in resistance patterns both between and within hospitals.

GENERIC NAME	TRADE NAME	MAIN USES
AMIKICIN	*AMIKIN (I)*	Short-term treament of serious infections.
GENTAMICIN	*CIDOMYCIN (I)* *GENTICIN (I)* *ISOTONIC GENTICIN (I)*	Serious infections / septicaemia. Also bacterial endocarditis.
KANAMYCIN	*KANNASYN (I)*	Serious infections due to organisms that have proved resistant to other antibiotics.

GENERIC NAME	TRADE NAME	MAIN USES
NEOMYCIN SULPHATE	*MYCIFRADIN (T)* *NIVEMYCIN (TL)*	Gut sterilisation.
with polymyxin	*POLYBACTRIN (L)*	For bladder irrigation only.
NETILMICIN	*NETILLIN (I)*	Serious infections.
SPECTINOMYCIN	*TROBICIN (I)*	Gonorrhoea caused by penicillin-resistant organisms.
STREPTOMYCIN	*STREPTOMYCIN SULPHATE (I)*	Tuberculosis. Brucellosis. Infective endocarditis. (Now rarely used.)
TOBRAMYCIN	*NEBCIN (I)*	Infections of the nervous system, bowel, urinary tract, lungs, skin, bone and soft tissues.

2 BETALACTAMS

Historical. The largest group of antibiotics. The group is divided into **penicillins** (names often end in -cillin), the **cephalosporins** and **cephamycins** (recognised by a 'cef' or 'ceph' in their names) and the newer **monobactams** and **thienamycin betalactams.**

Common features. See individual groups. For clarity (and because this group is enormous) the betalactam group has been divided in this appendix, with the cephalosporins and penicillins considered as individual groups.

Mode of action. All betalactams work by interfering with bacterial cell wall synthesis. They are 'bactericidal' (kill bacteria).

Precautions. Cephalosporins produce 'cross-reactions' in about 10 per cent of penicillin-sensitive patients.

Resistance. Bacteria build up resistance to betalactams by producing enzymes called 'betalactamases' (also known as 'penicillinases') which are capable of antagonising the bactericidal action of betalactams. Resistance may also be caused by reduced binding at or penetration of site of action.

Some penicillins (and many of the newer cephalosporins) are resistant to the betalactamases.

MONOBACTAMS

GENERIC NAME	TRADE NAME	MAIN USES
AZTREONAM	*Azactam (I)*	Respiratory tract infections, urinary tract infections, gonorrhoea, bone and joint, skin, soft tissue, intra-abdominal and gynaecological infections. Septicaemia and meningitis. Resistant to betalactamases.

THIENAMYCIN BETALACTAMS

GENERIC NAME	TRADE NAME	MAIN USES
IMIPENEM / CILASTATIN	*PRIMAXIN (I)*	Very broad spectrum.

3 CEPHALOSPORINS

Historical. First obtained from a fungus cultured from the sea near a Sardinian sewage outfall in 1945. Until recently, they were rarely considered as antibiotics of first choice but now are worldwide best-sellers. Relatively infrequently used in the UK. They are divided into orally active, first, second and third generations. The early versions (first generation) have, to a large extent, been replaced by other antibiotics which are less expensive and easier to administer. The second generation are less sensitive to betalactamases and more effective than the first generation. Late versions (third generation) are less toxic, less sensitive to betalactamases and have a broader range of activity, but are very expensive.

Common features. Closely related to penicillins. Bactericidal (kill bacteria). Wide spectrum of activity but low toxicity. They are used for infections related to the gall-bladder and bile duct, before surgery, for urinary tract infection caused by multiply-resistant bacteria and to treat penicillin-resistant gonorrhoea.

First, second and third generation are given by injection because they are not absorbed after oral administration. Orally active cephalosporins are used to treat urinary tract infections which do not respond to other antibiotics. They can also be used in the treatment of bronchitis.

First generation. Largely superseded by newer cephalosporins or other types of antibiotics which are less expensive and easier to administer.

Second generation Less susceptible to inactivation by betalactamases than the first generation.

Third generation May cause 'superinfection' with resistant bacteria or fungi.

Resistance See BETALACTAMS (p. 270).

GENERIC NAME	TRADE NAME	MAIN USES
Oral		
CEFACLOR	*DISTACLOR (CL)*	Urinary and respiratory tract infections, middle ear infections, skin and soft tissue infections, kidney infections and gonorrhoea. Also used before surgery.
CEFADROXIL	*BAXAN (CL)*	
CEFIXIME	*SUPRAX*	
CEFPODOXIME PROXETIL	*ORELEX (T)*	
CEFTIBUTEN	*CEDAX (C)*	
CEFUROXIME AXETIL	*ZINNAT (T)*	
CEPHALEXIN	*CEPHALEXIN (TC)* *CEPOREX (TCL)* *KEFLEX (TCL)*	
CEPHRADINE	*VELOSEF (CLI)*	
***First generation** (INJECTABLE)*		
CEPHALOTHIN	*KEFLIN (I)*	Before surgery.
CEPHAZOLIN	*KEFZOL (I)*	Before surgery.
CEPHRADINE	*VELOSEF (I)*	See *Oral* above.
***Second generation** (INJECTABLE)*		
CEFODIZIME	*TIMECEF (I)*	Urinary and lower respiratory tract infections.
CEFOXITIN	*MEFOXIN (I)*	Abdominal infections such as peritonitis.
CEFTRIAXONE	*ROCEPHIN (I)*	Used before surgery.

GENERIC NAME	TRADE NAME	MAIN USES
CEFUROXIME	*ZINACEF (I)*	Before surgery. Meningitis, penicillin-resistant infections, gonorrhoea.
CEPHAMANDOLE	*KEFADOL (I)*	Before surgery. Serious and life-threatening infections.

Third generation (INJECTABLE)

GENERIC NAME	TRADE NAME	MAIN USES
CEFOTAXIME	*CLAFORAN (I)*	Before surgery. As cefaclor.
CEFSULODIN SODIUM	*MONASPOR (I)*	Before surgery. Respiratory tract, urinary tract, soft tissue and bone infections.
CEFTAZIDIME	*FORTUM (I)* *KEFADIM (I)*	As cefaclor.
CEFTIZOXIME	*CEFIZOX (I)*	As cefaclor.

4 CHLORAMPHENICOL

Historical. Chloramphenicol was one of the first broad-spectrum antibiotics to be discovered and is now used throughout the world. It was originally produced from a culture of a soil organism *(Streptomyces venezuelae)* but is now made synthetically.

Main features. Wide spectrum of antibacterial activity. Chloramphenicol should only be used for serious infections where other drugs have failed and is particularly useful in the treatment of enteric fevers (such as typhoid and paratyphoid fever). It is used to treat meningitis and epiglottitis in children and is also widely used to treat eye infections (as ointment or drops).

Mode of action. Bacteriostatic and bactericidal. Inhibits bacterial protein synthesis.

Resistance. Some bacterial resistance to chloramphenicol is now common.

GENERIC NAME	TRADE NAME	MAIN USES
CHLORAMPHENICOL	*CHLOROMYCETIN (CLI)* *KEMICETINE (I)*	Severe (life-threatening) infections, meningitis, typhoid fever, other salmonella infections and cholera.

5 GLYCOPEPTIDES

Historical. The glycopeptides include vancomycin and teicoplanin. Vancomycin has been available for many years while teicoplanin is a new drug.

Common features. Glycopeptides are natural antibiotics. They are similar but teicoplanin is longer acting than vancomycin.

Mode of action. Penetrates the cell wall of Gram-positive bacteria. Bactericidal (kills bacteria). Not absorbed by the gut and must therefore be given by injection. Vancomycin is given by mouth in the management of pseudomembraneous colitis.

Resistance. Resistance pattern has changed little since vancomycin was introduced 30 years ago; some enterococci are vancomycin-resistant. There is no cross resistance with other drugs.

GENERIC NAME	TRADE NAME	MAIN USES
TEICOPLANIN	*TARGOCID (I)*	For serious infections (e.g. endocarditis, peritonitis and infections caused by *Staph. aureus).*
VANCOMYCIN	*VANCOCIN (I)*	Potentially life-threatening infections. Often used combined with aminoglycosides. Used in the treatment of MRSA (methicillin-resistant *Staph. aureus)* infection; and pseudomembranous colitis associated with antibiotic treatment.

6 IMIDAZOLES

Historical. Metronidazole and tinidazole both belong to a group of antimicrobials called imidazoles. They are active only against anaerobic bacteria and protozoa. A number of very toxic organisms are anaerobic. The use of imidazoles against anaerobic infections was first discovered by a dentist whose patient recovered unexpectedly from gum infection while taking metronidazole for dysentery.

Mode of action. Metronidazole and tinidazole are very similar in action and act by interfering with bacterial DNA. Metronidazole is the more widely used but tinidazole has a longer duration of action. Their main use is in the treatment of deep-seated infections (such as abscesses).

Resistance. Rare.

GENERIC NAME	TRADE NAME	MAIN USES
METRONIDAZOLE	*ELYZOL (S)* *FLAGYL (TIS)* *FLAGYL COMPAK* *FLAGYL S (L)* *METROLYL (TIS)* *METRONIDAZOLE (T)* *NIDAZOL (T)* *ZADSTAT (TIS)*	Vaginal infections, pelvic infections, peritonitis, septicaemia, wound infections, osteomyelitis and abscesses. Also inflammation of the gums, colitis, dysentery and Guinea worm infestations.
TINIDAZOLE	*FLASIGYN (T)*	Similar to metronidazole. Longer action.

7 LINCOSAMIDES

Historical. Lincomycin is a natural antibiotic derived from a soil organism. Clindamycin is produced by chemical modification of lincomycin.

Common features. The two drugs that make up this group have similar properties. Their use is limited because of the serious adverse effects they may cause.

Mode of action. Lincosamides inhibit protein synthesis in bacterial cells, but not, apparently, human cells. They are bacteriostatic (stop bacterial growth) in low concentrations but can be bactericidal (kill bacteria) in high doses.

Resistance. Cross resistance may occur with macrolides. Staphylococci may develop resistance during treatment.

GENERIC NAME	TRADE NAME	MAIN USES
CLINDAMYCIN	*DALACIN C (CLI)*	Staphylococcal bone and joint infections, peritonitis, and infections of the female genital tract. May also be used to treat susceptible strains of *Staph. aureus* in people allergic to penicillins and/or cephalosporins.
LINCOMYCIN	*LINCOCIN (CLI)*	Lincomycin is no longer generally available. It has been replaced by clindamycin, which is more active and better absorbed.

8 MACROLIDES

Historical. Only erythromycin is now actually used in the UK. It was introduced in 1952 with the hope that it would solve the problem of resistant betalactamase producing bacteria. However, it was soon found that organisms (mainly *Staph. aureus*) could develop resistance during long courses of treatment.

Common features. Similar to tetracyclines. Bacteriostatic in low concentrations but can be bactericidal in high doses.

Mode of action. Erythromycin inhibits protein synthesis in bacterial cells but not, apparently, human cells. It has a similar spectrum of activity to benzylpenicillin.

Resistance. Resistance is rare during short-term treatment, but may occur during prolonged treatment.

GENERIC NAME	TRADE NAME	MAIN USES
AZITHROMYCIN	*Erythromycin (TL)* *Zithromax (C)*	As alternative to penicillin, particularly in penicillin-allergic people.
CLARITHROMYCIN	*Arpimycin (L)* *Klaricid (T)*	Used as drug of first choice in respiratory infections in children,
ERYTHROMYCIN	*Erycen (TL)* *Erymax (C)* *Erythrocin (TI)* *Erythrolar (L)* *Erythromid (T)* *Erythroped (TI)* *Ilosone (TCL)*	whooping-cough prevention, Legionnaires' disease, campylobacter, enteritis and chronic prostatitis.

9 PENICILLINS

Historical. Penicillin is produced by the fungus *Penicillium notatum* and was first described by Fleming in 1928. It was purified and adapted for therapeutic use by Florey and Chain in 1941. The first semi-synthetic penicillins were produced in 1957. Penicillins can be divided into the following groups:

Natural penicillins. **Betalactamase sensitive.** (Betalactamase is an enzyme made by certain bacteria which makes them resistant to betalactam antibiotics. See betalactams.)

Semisynthetic. **1 Betalactamase resistant:** Betalactamase resistant penicillins are used for serious infections (lung abscess, acute osteomyelitis, etc) caused by penicillinase producing staphylococci. 90 per cent of hospital acquired staphylococcal infections are caused by betalactamase (penicillinase) producing strains. Betalactamase resistant penicillins are effective against betalactamase-producing staphylococci, but these penicillins are far less effective against other bacterial species than benzyl penicillin.
2 Broad spectrum: These are subdivided into *aminopenicillins, ureidopenicillins, aminopenicillins (mecillinams) and antipseudomonal penicillins (*also known as *carboxypenicillins).*

Mode of action. The penicillins are bactericidal and act by interfering with bacterial cell wall synthesis. They are excreted in the urine. The drug Probenecid can be taken at the same time to achieve a higher concentration of penicillin in the body.

Non-human use. Penicillins are used extensively on farm animals to prevent and treat disease.

Resistance. Most staphylococci are now resistant to benzyl penicillin. *Staph. aureus* strains resistant to methicillin and cloxacillin (commonly called MRSAs) are a major problem in some hospitals; luckily these organisms so far remain sensitive to vancomycin. All the broad spectrum penicillins are inactivated by betalactamase producing bacteria. Cloxacillin and flucloxacillin are not completely resistant to staphylococcal betalactamases, and, for serious infection, they are used in combination with other antibiotics, such as gentamicin, fusidic acid or erythromycin.

BETALACTAMASE SENSITIVE (natural) PENICILLINS

GENERIC NAME	TRADE NAME	MAIN USES
BENZYL PENICILLIN (Penicillin G)	*Crystapen (I)*	Infections of skin, soft tissue, respiratory tract, ear, nose and throat.
BENETHAMINE* (Penicillin G)	*Triplopen (I)*	Also gonorrhoea and syphilis, bacterial endocarditis, meningitis,
BENZATHINE* (Penicillin G)	*Penidural (L)*	anthrax, gas gangrene, tetanus, leptospirosis and actinomycosis.
PHENETHICILLIN* (Penicillin V)	*Broxil (CL)*	Occasionally used for congenital syphilis in babies.
PHENOXYMETHYL PENICILLIN (Penicillin V)	*Apsin VK (CL)* *Distaquaine V-K (TL)* *Phenoxymethyl (C)* *Stabillin V-K (TL)* *V-Cil-K (TCL)*	Similar to benzylpenicillin, but less active. Mainly used for respiratory tract infections in children, middle ear infections, erysipelas, tonsillitis and for protection against infection following rheumatic fever.
PROCAINE PENICILLIN	*Bicillin (I)*	Useful against syphilis in early stages. Long acting intra-muscular injections are used to treat syphilis and gonorrhoea.

* Historically important, but no longer available.

BETALACTAMASE RESISTANT PENICILLINS

GENERIC NAME	TRADE NAME	MAIN USES
CLOXACILLIN	*CLOXACILLIN (C)* *ORBENIN (CLI)*	Infections due to betalactamase-producing staphylococci.
FLUCLOXACILLIN	*FLOXAPEN (CLI)* *FLUCLOXACILLIN (CL)* *LADROPEN (CI)* *MAGNAPEN (CLI)* *STAFOXIL (C)*	Similar to Cloxacillin but usually more effective.
TEMOCILLIN	*TEMOPEN (I)*	Infections due to penicillinase-producing bacteria.

AMINOPENICILLINS

GENERIC NAME	TRADE NAME	MAIN USES
AMOXYCILLIN	*ALMODAN (I)* *AMIX (C)* *AMORAM (C)* *AMOXIL (TCLI)* *AMOXYCILLIN (CL)* *AMOXYMED (C)* *AMRIT (C)* *GALENAMOX (C)* *RIMOXALLIN (C)*	Serious respiratory and urinary tract infections, gonorrhoea, ear, nose, throat and soft tissue infections.
AMPICILLIN	*AMFIPEN (L)* *AMPICILLIN (CL)* *PENBRITIN (CLI)* *RIMACILLIN (L)* *VIDOPEN (I)*	As above.

GENERIC NAME	TRADE NAME	MAIN USES
	Ampiclox (I) *Ampiclox Neonatal (L)*	Ear, nose, throat, respiratory and soft tissue infections. Urinary tract infections and gonorrhoea. Also before surgery.
with flucloxacillin	*Flu-Amp (C)* *Magnapen (CLI)*	
BACAMPICILLIN HYDROCHLORIDE	*Ambaxin (T)*	As above. Used in treatment of gonorrhoea.
CO-FLUAMPICIL	*Co-fluampicil (CLI)* *Flu-Amp (C)* *Magnapen (CLI)*	For infections involving betalactamase-producing staphylococci.
PIVAMPICILLIN	*Pondocillin (TCL)*	Infections of the respiratory tract, ear, nose and throat infections, skin, soft tissue, urinary tract infections and gonorrhoea.
with pivmecillinam	*Miraxid (TL)*	As for ampicillin and pivampicillin, also glandular fever.

BROAD SPECTRUM PENICILLINS COMBINED WITH BETALACTAMASE INHIBITORS

GENERIC NAME	TRADE NAME	MAIN USES
CO-AMOXICLAV	*Augmentin (TLI)*	Effective against most strains of penicillin/ amoxycillin resistant organisms. Mainly used for respiratory and urinary tract infections. Also used in typhoid and before dental surgery.

GENERIC NAME	TRADE NAME	MAIN USES
AMPICILLIN with sulbactam	*Dicapen (I)* *Unasyn (TI)*	For infections involving betalactamase producing bacteria. Also before surgery.

UREIDOPENICILLIN

GENERIC NAME	TRADE NAME	MAIN USES
MEZLOCILLIN	*Baypen (I)*	Used for infections following abdominal or gynaecological surgery.

CARBOXYPENICILLINS (antipseudomonal penicillins)

GENERIC NAME	TRADE NAME	MAIN USES
AZLOCILLIN	*Securopen (I)*	Systemic and local infections, especially of the respiratory and urinary tracts. Also post surgical infections, infected wounds and burns.
CARBENICILLIN	*Pyopen (I)*	
PIPERACILLIN with tazobactam	*Pipril (I)* *Tazocin (I)*	As azlocillin.
TICARCILLIN	*Ticar (I)*	As azlocillin.
with clavulanic acid	*Timentin (I)*	Severe infections in hospitalised patients with impaired or suppressed immune system.

AMIDINOPENICILLIN (Mecillinams)

GENERIC NAME	TRADE NAME	MAIN USES
MECILLINAM	*SELEXIDIN (I)*	Severe bowel infections. Urinary tract infections.
PIVMECILLINAM	*SELEXID (TL)*	Acute cystitis. Chronic or recurrent bacteria in the urine. Salmonella infection.
with pivampicillin	*PONDOCILLIN (T)* *MIRAXID (T)*	See pivampicillin.

10 POLYMYXINS

Historical. A family of antibiotics produced by a bacterium *(Bacillus polymyxa).*

Common features. Polymyxins are comparatively toxic and have been largely superseded by other antibiotics, like aminoglycosides and quinolones. They are not absorbed from the gut and are thus used mainly in topical preparations, for bladder irrigation and for bowel sterilisation. They are rarely used to treat systemic infections.

Mode of action. Disrupt cell membranes.

GENERIC NAME	TRADE NAME	MAIN USES
COLISTIN	*COLOMYCIN (TSI)*	See above.
POLYMYXIN B SULPHATE	*AEROSPORIN (I)* *POLYBACTRIN (L)*	See above. For bladder irrigation.

11 QUINOLONES

Historical. Nalidixic acid (discovered 1962) was the first quinolone to be synthesised. Its clinical use is limited by its narrow spectrum of activity and poor distribution in the body, other than in urine. The newer members of the group are called 4-quinolones.

Common features. Synthetic. Bactericidal. Used for the treatment of urinary tract infections and gut infections, notably dysentery. Should only be used for the treatment of infections caused by organisms resistant to standard drugs. The 4-quinolones need oxygen in order to kill bacteria. When oxygen is absent, they merely stop the growth of bacterial colonies.

Mode of action. Quinolones act on bacterial DNA.

Resistance. Quinolones have already been excessively used, and bacterial resistance is already a problem. Resistance has developed rapidly in patients suffering from infection with pseudomonas, citrobacter or campylobacter (causing wound, gut and bone infection). Resistance to one 4-quinolone seems to confer at least some resistance to the other members of the group.

GENERIC NAME	TRADE NAME	MAIN USES
ACROSOXACIN	*ERADACIN (C)*	Gonorrhoea.
CINOXACIN	*CINOBAC (C)*	Urinary tract infections.
CIPROFLOXACIN	*CIPROXIN (TI)*	Infections of the respiratory gastro-intestinal and urinary tracts. Also gonorrhoea and septicaemia.
ENOXACIN	*COMPRECIN (T)*	Urinary tract and skin infections. Also gonorrhoea and dysentery.

GENERIC NAME	TRADE NAME	MAIN USES
NALIDIXIC ACID	*NALIDIXIC ACID (T)* *MICTRAL (L)* *NEGRAM (TL)* *URIBEN (L)*	Urinary tract infections.
NORFLOXACIN	*UTINOR (T)*	Urinary tract infections.
OFLOXACIN	*TARIVID (TI)*	Urinary tract infections, lung infections, gonorrhoea, urethritis and cervicitis.

12 SULPHONAMIDES

Historical. Discovered in 1935. The first preparations were derived from dyes, but it was soon discovered that sulphonamides had antibacterial effects that did not depend on the presence of dye molecules. They made a dramatic impact on the hospital treatment of infections. Following the introduction of sulphonamide therapy, the mortality rate from streptococcal infections fell from 23 per cent in January 1938 to 4.7 per cent eight months later. In 1938, sulphapyridine (M&B 693) was introduced and a wide range of different preparations followed.

Common features. Broad spectrum. Synthetic. Old fashioned. Comparatively toxic. They all have a similar spectrum of activity. Rapidly absorbed from the gut. Excreted via the kidneys into the urine. Currently the main use is in the treatment of uncomplicated urinary tract infections and in the prophylaxis of recurrent urinary infections. Sulphapyridine in low doses over long periods may be used to control dermatitis herpetiformis. Sulphonamides are also used for the treatment of meningococcal meningitis (like sulpadiazine which enters the cerebrospinal fluid (CSF) more readily than the others).

Mode of action. Bacteria need folic acid for their growth. Sulphonamides 'look like' folic acid and fool the bacteria into absorbing them. The bacteria thus become deprived of folic acid and cease to multiply. Sulphonamides are thus 'bacteriostatic'.

Resistance. Now very common. Sulphonamides have increasingly been replaced by more active and less toxic antibiotics, apart from co-trimoxazole.

GENERIC NAME	TRADE NAME	MAIN USES
CO-TRIMOXAZOLE	*BACTRIM (TCLI)* *CHEMOTRIM (L)* *COMIXCO (L)* *COMOX (T)* *CO-TRIMOXAZOLE (TL)* *FECTRIM (T)* *FECTRIM FORTE (T)* *LARATRIM (L)* *SEPTRIN (TI)*	Widely used, particularly for urinary and respiratory tract infections. Also used for middle ear infection, sinusitis, typhoid, paratyphoid, cholera, shigellosis, skin and wound infections, acute and chronic osteomyelitis, brucellosis, and for gonorrhoea in penicillin sensitive patients.
SULFA-METOPYRAZINE	*KELFIZINE W (T)*	Urinary tract infections. Chronic bronchitis.
SULPHADIAZINE	*SULPHADIAZINE (TI)*	Meningitis.
SULPHADIMIDINE	*SULPHADIMIDINE (T)*	Urinary tract infections.
DAPSONE	*DAPSONE (T)* *MALOPRIM (T)*	Leprosy, dermatitis, herpetiformis, malaria.

13 TETRACYCLINES

Historical. The first broad spectrum bacteriostatic antibiotic to be discovered (1948). All tetracyclines are structurally related and have a similar spectrum of action.

Common features. Used in the treatment of acne, bronchitis, non specific urethritis, atypical pneumonia, typhus, brucellosis, lymphogranuloma venereum, Q fever, conjunctivitis, cholera, chlamydial infections and tropical sprue. However, bacterial resistance is increasing in an unpredictable manner and thus tetracyclines are rarely first choice drugs in the treatment of hospital infections.

Mode of action. Tetracyclines inhibit protein synthesis in bacteria and also affect protein metabolism in animal cells.

Non-human use. Oxytetracycline is used extensively on farm animals to prevent and treat disease. Cattle (beef and dairy), pigs and poultry are all treated routinely with tetracyclines. Tetracyclines are also used as antibiotics in horticulture and to promote growth on fruit trees.

Resistance. When tetracyclines were in widespread use for the treatment of common infections, unpredictable and increasing resistance was a major problem. However, the use of tetracyclines in Britain has declined in the last ten years and resistance has decreased accordingly. Resistance to one tetracycline automatically transfers to all the others.

GENERIC NAME	TRADE NAME	MAIN USES
TETRACYCLINE	*Achromycin (TCLI)* *Achromycin V (C)* *Deteclo (T)* *Sustamycin (C)* *Tetrabid (C)* *Tetrachel (TC)* *Tetracycline (T)* *Tetrex (C)*	Ear, nose and throat infections, lung infections, urinary tract infections, gut infections (e.g. cholera, dysentery), venereal diseases (e.g. gonorrhoea and syphilis), acne and soft tissue infections.
plus nystatin	*Mysteclin (T)*	
CHLORTETRACYCLINE	*Aureomycin (C)*	As tetracycline.
CLOMOCYCLINE SODIUM	*Megaclor (C)*	As tetracycline.
DEMECLOCYCLINE HYDROCHLORIDE	*Ledermycin (TC)*	As tetracycline.
DOXYCYCLINE	*Cyclodox (C)* *Demix (C)* *Doxycycline (C)* *Doxylar (C)* *Nordox (C)* *Ramysis (C)* *Vibramycin (CL)*	As tetracycline.
	Vibramycin-D (T)	Also prostatitis and sinusitis.
LYMECYCLINE	*Tetralysal 300 (C)*	As tetracycline.
MINOCYCLINE	*Aknemin (C)* *Blemix (T)* *Minocin (T)*	As tetracycline.
OXYTETRACYCLINE	*Berkmycen (T)* *Oxymycin (T)* *Oxytetracycline (TC)* *Oxytetramix (T)* *Terramycin (TC)*	As tetracycline.

14 TRIMETHOPRIM

Historical. For many years, trimethoprim was only available in combination with the sulphonamide sulphamethoxazole in a preparation called co-trimoxazole (see sulphonamides). This combination produces more adverse reactions than trimethoprim on its own.

Mode of action. Trimethoprim is a synthetic antibiotic. It is bacteriostatic (stops bacterial growth) and effective against a wide spectrum of bacteria. Acts by interfering with bacterial DNA. Theoretical risk of damage to human DNA. It is more active than the sulphonamides against most strains. It is used mainly for urinary infections.

Resistance. Uncommon.

GENERIC NAME	TRADE NAME	MAIN USES
TRIMETHOPRIM	*TRIMETHOPRIM (T)* *IPRAL (T)* *MONOTRIM (TLI)* *SYRAPRIM (TI)* *TRIMOGAL (T)* *TRIMOPAN (T)*	Urinary and respiratory tract infections. Malaria.

15 ANTIBIOTICS RESERVED FOR SPECIFIC INFECTIONS

Certain antibacterials are reserved for the treatment of specific infections. This is because some drugs are very toxic and only life threatening diseases can justify their use, and also because bacterial resistance increases with increased use of antibiotics. In order to deal with this problem some antibiotics are used only for specific conditions.

LEPROSY (Hansen's Disease)

Leprosy is still very common worldwide, especially in the tropics, subtropics and the Middle East. There are three major types, each requiring a different treatment regimen. Dapsone was the drug of first choice for many years, but resistance is becoming an increasing problem and the World Health Organisation is now advising a more varied treatment programme. The treatment is always long term, often lasting five years or more.

In the treatment of 'multibacillary leprosy' all three drugs are used together. For 'paucibacillary leprosy' rifampicin and dapsone are used together.

GENERIC NAME	TRADE NAME
CLOFAZIMINE	*LAMPRENE*
DAPSONE	*DAPSONE TABLETS*
RIFAMPICIN	*see under tuberculosis*

PENICILLIN RESISTANT STAPHYLOCOCCI

Sodium fusidate is a narrow spectrum steroid antibiotic reserved for severe infections caused by penicillin-resistant staphylococci. It is used as an alternative for patients allergic to penicillin and in the treatment of osteomyelitis. Resistance develops quickly so sodium fusidate is usually prescribed together with another antibiotic.

GENERIC NAME	TRADE NAME
SODIUM FUSIDATE	*FUCIDIN (TLI)*

TUBERCULOSIS

Some drugs are used solely for the treatment of tuberculosis. The treatment of TB has two phases, 'initial' and 'continuation'. The initial phase of treatment lasts eight weeks and aims to reduce the population of TB bacteria as quickly as possible. It involves the use of at least three drugs used simultaneously, such as isoniazid, rifampicin and pyrazinamide (ethambutol or streptomycin are added in cases of resistance). The continuation phase involves treatment with isoniazid, rifampicin, pyrazinamide or ethambutol and may last up to 9 months.

GENERIC NAME	TRADE NAME
CAPREOMYCIN	*CAPASTAT (I)*
CYCLOSERINE	*CYCLOSERINE (C)*
ETHAMBUTOL HYDROCHLORIDE	*MYAMBUTOL (T)* *MYNAH (T)*
ISONIAZID	*ISONIAZID (TL)* *RIMIFON (I)*
PYRAZINAMIDE	*ZINAMIDE (T)*
RIFABUTIN	*MYCOBUTIN (C)*
RIFAMPICIN combinations	*RIFADIN (CLI)* *RIFATER (T)* *RIFINAH 150 (T)* *RIFINAH 300 (T)* *RIMACTANE (CLI)* *RIMACTAZID 150 (T)* *RIMACTAZID 300 (T)*
STREPTOMYCIN	*STREPTOMYCIN SULPHATE (I)*

URINARY TRACT INFECTIONS

Many antibiotics are used for the treatment of urinary tract infections and can be found under their specific chemical groups elsewhere in the appendix. The antibiotics mentioned below do not fit in with any of those groups and are reserved for use against urinary tract infections only.

Urinary tract infections are much more common in women than in men. They tend to be chronic and recurrent. Before starting antibiotic therapy, a specimen of urine should be collected for tests. Bacterial resistance is an increasing problem in the management of urinary tract infections, but not (yet) to nitrofurantoin (below).

GENERIC NAME	TRADE NAME
NITROFURANTOIN	*FURADANTIN (TL)*
	MACROBID (C)
	MACRODANTIN (C)
	NITROFURANTOIN (T)
HEXAMINE HIPPURATE (Methanamine hippurate)	*HIPREX (T)*

16 ANTIFUNGAL DRUGS

Fungal cells are quite similar to animal cells and contain sophisticated intracellular structures which are not found in bacterial cells. While the differences between bacteria and animal cells enable antibacterial drugs to act selectively, the similarity between fungal and animal cells makes antifungal drugs generally more toxic than antibacterial drugs. Moreover, resistance often develops during antifungal treatment making fungal infections very hard to eradicate.

Some antifungals used to treat systemic infections have to be given by injection since they cannot be absorbed through the gut. However, oral preparations can be used to treat fungal infections in the mouth, oesophagus (gullet), stomach or intestine.

Fungal infections of the genitalia are commoner in women and can be treated with antifungal pessaries, capsules, tablets or cream inserted into the vagina (see Topical Preparations). Recurrence is common if the woman is pregnant, suffering from diabetes or is taking oral antibiotics or oral contraceptives. The risk of re-infection is high if there are fungal infections in other sites such as finger nails, umbilicus, gut or bladder. Sexual partners should be treated simultaneously. Treatment with oral antifungals is sometimes advised in cases of resistant or recurrent infections.

GENERIC NAME	TRADE NAME	MAIN USES
AMPHOTERICIN B	*AmBisome (I)* *Amphoul (I)* *Fungilin (TL)* *Fungizone (I)*	Given by injection to treat systemic fungal infections. Broad spectrum.
FLUCONAZOLE	*Diflucan (CI)*	Used orally for systemic fungal infections such as candidiasis, cryptococcal infections (e.g. meningitis in AIDS sufferers).
FLUCYTOSINE	*Alcobon (TI)*	Systemic fungal infections. Narrow spectrum.

GENERIC NAME	TRADE NAME	MAIN USES
GRISEOFULVIN	*FULCIN (TL)* *GRISOVIN (T)*	Fungal infections of skin, scalp, hair and nails. Skin infections need at least 6 weeks treatment and nail infections may take up to 12 months to eradicate.
ITRACONAZOLE	*SPORANOX (C)*	Fungal infections of skin and vagina.
KETOCONAZOLE	*NIZORAL (TL)*	Serious systemic thrush.
MICONAZOLE	*DAKTARIN (TLI)* *DIFLUCAN (C)*	Oral, vaginal and intestinal fungal infections, systemic candidiasis and ringworm.
NYSTATIN	*NYSTAN (TL)* *NYSTATIN (L)* *NYSTATIN-DOME (L)*	Mainly used for treatment of candida infection of skin and mucous membranes (as in gut and vagina). Too toxic to use by injection.
TERBINAFINE	*LAMISIL (T)*	Fungal skin infections.

17 TOPICAL (EXTERNAL) PREPARATIONS

Superficial infections of the skin, eyes, ears, nose, and genitalia can be caused by many different organisms and there are many topical preparations available containing antibiotics. Most doctors avoid using topical antibiotic preparations for skin infections, preferring instead to use simple disinfectants (except in the case of fungal skin infections where some antibiotic creams and ointments are of proven value).

GENERIC NAME	TRADE NAME	MAIN USES
AMOROLFINE	*Loceryl cream*	Skin
	Loceryl nail lacquer	Nails
CHLORAMPHENICOL	*Actinac*	Acne
	Chloramphenicol	Eye
	Chloramphenicol ear drops	Ear
	Chloromycetin-Hydrocortisone	Eye
	Chloromycetin-Sno Phenicol	Eye
	Minims-Chloramphenicol	Eye
	Opulets-Chloramphenicol	Eye
	Tanderil	Eye
CHLORTETRACYCLINE	*Aureomycin*	Eye/skin
CLINDAMYCIN	*Dalacin T*	Acne
CLIOQUINOL	*Barquinol HC*	Skin
	Betnovate-C	Skin
	Haelan-C	Skin
	Locorten-Vioform	Skin
	Vioform-Hydrocortisone	Skin
ERYTHROMYCIN	*Stiermycin*	Acne
FRAMYCETIN	*Framycetin-Sulphate*	Ear/eye/skin
	Framycort	Ear/eye/skin
	Framygen Soframycin	Ear/eye/skin

GENERIC NAME	TRADE NAME	MAIN USES
FUSIDIC ACID	*FUCIBET*	Skin
	FUCIDIN	Skin
	FUCIDIN H	Skin
	FUCIDIN INTERTULLE	Skin
	FUCITHALMIC	Eye
GENTAMICIN	*CIDOMYCIN*	Ear/eye
	CIDOMYCIN-TOPICAL	Skin
	GARAMYCIN	Ear/eye
	GENTICIN	Ear/eye/skin
	GENTICIN HC	Skin
	GENTISONE HC	Ear
	MINIMS-GENTAMICIN	Eye
METRONIDAZOLE	*METROGEL*	Acne
	METROTOP	Skin
MUPIROCIN (Pseudomonic Acid)	*BACTROBAN*	Nose/skin
NEOMYCIN	*AUDICORT*	Ear
	BETNESOL-N	Ear/eye/nose
	BETNOVATE-N	Skin
	CITATRIN	Skin
	DERMOVATE-NN	Skin
	EUMOVATE-N	Eye
	FML-NEO	Eye
	GRANEODIN	Eye
	GREGODERM	Skin
	MINIMS NEOMYCIN-SULPHATE	Eye
	NASEPTRIM	Nose
	NEO-CORTEF	Ear/eye
	NEOMYCIN	Eye
	NEOMYCIN CREAM	Skin
	NEOSPORIN	Eye
	OTOMIZE	Ear
	PREDSOL-N	Ear/eye
	STIEDEX-LPN	Skin

GENERIC NAME	TRADE NAME	MAIN USES
	Vibrosil	Nose
	Vista-Methasone N	Ear/eye/nose
NORFLOXACIN	*Noroxin opthalmic solution*	Eyes
OXYTETRACYCLINE	*Terra-Cortril*	Skin
POLYMYXIN	*Polyfax*	Eye/skin
	Polytrim	Eye
PROPAMIDINE ISETHIONATE	*Brolene*	Eye
SILVER SULPHADIAZINE	*Flamazine*	Skin/gums
SULPHACETAMIDE SODIUM	*Albucid*	Eye
	Minims Sulphacetamide Sodium	Eye
TETRACYCLINE	*Achromycin*	Ear/skin
	Aureocort	Skin
	Propaderm-A	Skin
	Tetracycline - Mixture	Mouthwash
	Topicycline	Acne
TOBRAMYCIN	*Tobralex*	Eye
NEOMYCIN/POLYMYXIN	*Maxitrol*	Eye
	Otosporin	Ear
	Polybactrin	Skin
	Tribiotic	Skin
FRAMYCETIN / GRAMICIDIN	*Sofradex*	Ear
	Soframycin	Ear
OXYTETRACYCLINE / POLYMYXIN	*Tetra-Cortril*	Ear
GRAMICIN/NEOMYCIN	*Adcortyl with Graneodin*	Skin
	Graneodin	Skin

GENERIC NAME	TRADE NAME	MAIN USES
GRAMICIDIN/NEOMYCIN/ NYSTATIN	*TRI-ADCORTYL*	Skin
	TRI-ADCORTYL OTIC	Ear
NYSTATIN/ OXYTETRACYCLINE	*TERRA-CORTRIL*	Ear
	TERRA-CORTRIL-NYSTATIN	Skin
	TRIMOVATE	Skin

18 TOPICAL PREPARATIONS FOR FUNGAL INFECTIONS

GENERIC NAME	TRADE NAME	MAIN USES
AMPHOTERICIN B	*FUNGILIN*	Genitalia Mouth/skin
BENZOIC ACID	*BENZOIC ACID - OINTMENT*	Ringworm
BENZOYL PEROXIDE	*QUINOPED*	Skin
CLOTRIMAZOLE	*CANESTEN*	Genitalia/skin/ ear
	CANESTEN HC	Skin
	LOTRIDERM	Skin
	MASNODERM	Skin
ECONAZOLE	*ECONACORT*	Genitalia/skin
	ECOSTATIN	Genitalia/skin
	ECOSTATIN-1	Genitalia
	GYNO-PEVARYL	Genitalia
	GYNO-PEVARYL-1	Genitalia/skin
	PEVARYL	Genitalia/skin
	PEVARYL TC	Skin
ISOCONAZOLE	*TRAVOGYN*	Genitalia
KETOCONAZOLE	*NIZORAL*	Genitalia/skin
MICONAZOLE	*DAKTACORT*	Skin
	DAKTARIN	Mouth/skin
	DUMICOAT	Nails
	GYNO-DAKTARIN	Genitalia
	GYNO-DAKTARIN 1	Genitalia
	MONISTAT	Genitalia
NATAMYCIN	*PIMAFUCIN*	Genitalia/skin/ mouth

GENERIC NAME	TRADE NAME	MAIN USES
NYSTATIN	*MULTILIND*	Skin
	NYSTADERMAL	Skin
	NYSTAFORM	Skin
	NYSTAN	Genitalia/ mouth/skin
	NYSTATIN	Mouth
	NYSTATIN-DOME	Mouth
	NYSTAVESCENT	Genitalia
	TIMODINE	Skin
	TINADERM-M	Skin
NYSTATIN/ METRONIDAZOLE	*FLAGYL COMPAK*	Genitalia/ mouth/skin
SALICYLIC ACID	*PHYTEX*	Nails
	PHYTOCIL	Ringworm
SULCONAZOLE	*EXELDERM*	Skin
TERBINAFINE	*LAMISIL*	Skin
TIOCONAZOLE	*TROSYL*	Nails
UNDECENOATES	*MONPHYTOL*	Skin/nails
	MYCOTA	
	PHYTOCIL	

Notes

Part One: **Blind Faith**

1. A comprehensive source of information about the uses and risks of drugs, including antibiotics, is *Martindale: the Extra Pharmacopeia*, the pharmacists' bible, published by the Pharmaceutical Press in London.

2. A reliable and well-written guide to drugs for the general reader is *Medical Treatments: the Benefits and Risks* (London: Penguin, 1991) by Dr Peter Parish. However, help is immediately at hand. The appendix to this book, 'The A–Z of Antibiotics', includes an easy-to-follow guide to all antibiotics now available on prescription for human use in the UK.

3. Berkow, R. (ed), *The Merck Manual* (Rahway, New Jersey: Merck, 1987). Updated every five years or so. This handy book of over 2500 pages, available in specialist bookshops, is a meticulous guide to diseases and their symptoms and treatments.

4. Halliday, J. (ed), *Antibiotics: the Comprehensive Guide* (London: Bloomsbury, 1990).

5. Kunin, C., 'Problems in antibiotic usage' in Mandell, G., Gordon Douglas, R., Bennett, J. (eds), *Principles and Practice of Infectious Diseases* (Edinburgh: Churchill Livingstone, 1985). You might suppose that physicians are familiar with the latest information on antibiotics. Usually, wrong: most general practitioners and hospital doctors and surgeons are far too busy to read textbooks.

6. Bochner, B., Lichtenstein, L., 'Anaphylaxis' (*N Eng J Med*, 1991; 324(25): 1785–90).

7. Wainwright, M., *Miracle Cure: the Story of Antibiotics* (Oxford: Blackwell, 1990).

8. Bennet, G., *The Wound and the Doctor. Healing, Power and Technology in Modern Medicine* (London: Secker and Warburg, 1987). Also see Anon, 'Burnished or burnt out: the delights and dangers of working in health' (*Lancet*, 1994: 344: 1583–4). On a similar theme, a book on the power of the medical profession over the media is Karpf, A., *Doctoring the Media* (London: Routledge, 1988).

9. In this book's conclusion and afterword, there is a guide for you and your doctor to help you make the best use of antibiotics.

10. Professor Parish's *Medicines: A Guide for Everybody* (London: Penguin, 1992) is also a valuable reference book.

11. The case that antibiotics are by their nature liable to be immunosuppressive, is made in Part 4, 'Apocalypse Now'.

12. Some antibiotics cause more ill-effects than others. Co-trimoxazole is a controversial drug. Because it is and has for years been used extensively by physicians for urinary tract, respiratory and other bacterial infections, reports of its toxicity are liable to be relatively frequent. However, it is relatively toxic, because it is partly made up of the sulphonamide sulphamethoxazole, and has the ill-effects of any sulphonamide. Critics point out that its benefits can be gained by use solely of its other ingredient, trimethoprim. The medical microbiologist Professor Richard Lacey believes that co-trimoxazole should be used rarely if at all, and said as much in his inaugural lecture. See the afterword of this book, and also Lacey, R., 'Do sulphonamide-trimethoprim combinations select less resistance in trimethoprim than trimethoprim alone?' (*J Med Microbiol*, 1982; 15: 403–27). A *Sunday Times* investigation noted that 113 deaths directly caused by co-trimoxazole have been reported to the UK Committee on Safety of Medicines, and also quoted the UK Medicines Control Agency as saying: 'Co-trimoxazole is an effective antibiotic that has been used in the UK and worldwide for many years. Its safety profile is well-known and documented.' See Deer, B., 'The pill that killed' (*The Sunday Times*, 20 March 1994).

13. The Association of British Pharmaceutical Industry (ABPI), the trade organisation for the drug industry, issues general practitioners with data sheets on drugs, including details of adverse effects. These are bound into an annual book, the *ABPI Data Sheet Compendium*. Doctors who prefer independent information can use the relatively brief British National Formulary, issued by the British Medical Association and The Royal Pharmaceutical Society.

14. Mathisen, G., 'Antibiotic pharmacology. Erythromycin, parts 1 and 2' (*The APUA Newsletter*, 1989; 7/1 and 2).

15. WHO Scientific Working Group, 'Antimicrobial resistance' (*Bull WHO*, 1983; 61(3): 383–94).

16. This and the next example are cited in: Medawar, C., *The Wrong Kind of Medicine?* (London: Hodder and Stoughton, 1984). Charles Medawar, founder and director of the drug watchdog Social Audit, has done as much as anybody in Britain to alert citizens to the problems of prescription drugs.

17. Antibiotics work against bacteria and other micro-organisms such as fungi. Antibacterial is a more specific name for antibiotics that work against bacteria. Antimicrobial is a more general name. But antibiotics do not work against viral infections, with a few exceptions. Viral infections range from the common cold to AIDS. Many common infections, for example of the throat, may be viral or bacterial, and thus tempt the physician to try an antibiotic 'just in case'.

18. Swindell, P., Reeves, D., Bullock, D. et al., 'Audits of antibiotic prescribing in a Bristol hospital' (*Br Med J* 1983; 286: 118–21).

19. Anon, 'Surveys of antibiotic prescribing' (*Lancet*, 1983; I: 1084–5).

20. Anon, 'Antibiotic audit' (*Lancet*, 1981; I: 310–11).

21. Moss, F., McNicol, M., McSwiggan, D., Miller, D., 'Survey of antibiotic prescribing in a district general hospital' (*Lancet*, 1981; II: 349–52, 407–9, 461–2).

22. Kunin, C., 'Evidence of inappropriate use of antimicrobial agents', in Mandell, G., Gordon Douglas, R., Bennett, J. (eds), *Principles and Practice of Infectious Diseases* (Edinburgh: Churchill Livingstone, 1985).

23. Silverman, M., Lee, P., *Pills, Profits, and Politics* (Berkeley: University of California Press, 1974).

24. Greenwood, D. (ed), *Antimicrobial Therapy* (Oxford: University Press, 1989).

25. National Institutes of Health Study on Antibiotic Use and Antibiotic Resistance Worldwide, 'Reports of Task Force 1 and Task Force 6' (*Rev Infect Dis*, 1987; 9(3): S232–S243, S297–S312).

26. Kim, J., Gallis, H., 'Observations on spiralling empiricism: its causes, allure and perils, with particular reference to antibiotic therapy' (*Am J Med*, 1989; 87: 201–6).

27. Lacey, R., 'General use of antibiotics' (*Update*, 1 March 1988: 1811–17). Also, Lacey, R., 'A rational approach to antibiotics' (*Br J Sex Med*, 1988; March: 106–10). And see the afterword to this book.

28. 'Complete the course' has an additional rationale: that an incomplete course is more likely to breed drug-resistant bacteria in the body. But microbiologists take the opposite view, pointing out that the longer any course of antibiotics, the greater the risk of resistance. The phenomenon of drug resistance is dealt with in Part 5, 'Superbug'.

29. In the foreword and afterword to this book Professor Lacey proposes that antibiotic use should be reduced to one tenth or less of current rate. And see Lacey, R., 'Have antibiotics killed microbiology?' (*University of Leeds Review*, 1985–6; 28: 213–26).

30. Campbell, E., Scadding, J., Roberts, R., 'The concept of disease' (*Br Med J*, 1979; 2: 757–62).

31. Department of Health and Social Security, *Prevention and Health: Everybody's Business* (London: HMSO, 1976).

32. McKeown, T., *The Role of Medicine. Dream, Mirage or Nemesis?* (Oxford: Blackwell, 1979). This great book proves that drug therapy, while it may be effective in the treatment of individual patients, has not had much effect on the general incidence of disease. His thesis has not been contradicted with any authority; but, since its publication, drugs have continued to dominate modern medicine.

33. Two books written by Dubos relied upon here (and in Part 3, 'Bug Wars') are *The White Plague* (reissued by Rutgers University Press in 1987) and *Mirage of Health* (Allen and Unwin, 1960). An excellent profile of Dubos was published in the May 1991 issue of *Scientific American.*

34. The rate of infectious disease in any community is mainly determined by the state of public and personal health. Well-nourished people are thereby protected against infection. See Scrimshaw, N., Taylor, C., Gordon, J., *Interactions of Nutrition and Infection* (Geneva: World Health Organisation, 1968). *See also* Part 5 of this book.

35. World Health Organisation, 'World tuberculosis toll is rising' (Geneva: *WHO* (Features, no. 148), October 1990).

36. Murray, C., Styblo, K., Rouillon, A., 'Tuberculosis in developing countries: Burden, intervention and cost' (*Bull Int Union Against TB and Lung Disease*, 1990; 65 (1): 2–20).

37. Anon, 'The global challenge of tuberculosis' (*Lancet*, 1994; 344: 277–9).

38. Bloom, B., Murray, C., 'Tuberculosis: commentary on a re-emergent killer' (*Science*, 1992; 257: 1055–64).

39. Watson, J., Tuberculosis in Britain today (*Br Med J*, 1993; 306: 221–2).

40. O'Neill, S., 'TB menace rises again among the homeless' (*Independent on Sunday*, 31 March 1991).

41. Culliton, B., 'Drug-resistant TB may bring epidemic' (*Nature*, 1992; 356: 473).

42. Weman, M., 'Treatment of multi drug-resistant tuberculosis' (*N Eng J Med*, 1993; 329(ii): 784–91).

43. Royal College of Physicians and Royal College of Pathologists, *Training in infectious diseases* (Report and press release, May 1990).

44. Fletcher, D., 'New infections defy drugs war on diseases' (*The Daily Telegraph*, 31 May 1990).

45. Parliamentary Office of Science and Technology, *Diseases fighting back. The growing resistance of TB and other bacterial diseases* (London: POST, 1994).

Part Two: **On the Treadmill**

1. A useful textbook if you want to know more is: Ketchum, P., *Microbiology* (New York: John Wiley, 1984).

2. Conventionally, all living things are classified into five categories: animals (including humans), plants, fungi, protista (such as algae), and the single-cell prokaryotic bacteria. New thinking based on DNA analysis is that all living things should be classified into three groups, of which two are bacteria. See: Margulis, L., Guerrero, R., 'Kingdoms in turmoil' (*New Scientist*, 23 March 1991). Either way, bacteria are fundamental in evolution.

3. So adaptable that some biologists are beginning to believe that Darwin's theory of evolution by random mutation applies only to higher forms of life, and that Lamarck's theory that species change in response to environmental forces applies to bacteria. See: Lewin, R., 'Can bacteria direct their own evolution?' (*New Scientist*, 15 September 1990). Also: Symonds, N., 'A fitter theory of evolution.' (*New Scientist*, 21 September 1991). And see Part 5.

4. Bacteria are categorised in other ways. All bacteria are either 'Gram-positive' or 'Gram-negative', depending on whether or not they can be permanently stained using a method devised by the Danish microbiologist Hans Christian Gram. This distinction is not merely cosmetic; the staining procedure reveals differences in cell-wall structure which is useful information for medical microbiologists. Bacteria are also categorised according to whether they are aerobic (requiring oxygen) or anaerobic (viable without oxygen). See Part 3, 'Bug Wars' for an explanation of the relevance of this distinction.

5. Sources used for the account of bacteria in this section include: Sleigh, D., Timbury, M., *Notes on Medical Bacteriology* (Edinburgh: Churchill Livingstone, 1986), as well as numerous reviews and research papers, notably by Dr Peter Borriello, Dr B. S. Drasar and Professor Sydney Finegold.

6. Thomas, L., *The Wonderful Mistake* (Oxford: University Press, 1988).

7. 'Antibiotic' is a general term now usually applied to drugs used to treat bacterial, fungal and other infections. An alternative term, is antimicrobial. More precise terms are antibacterial, antifungal, anti-protozoal, and anti-helminthic (used against worms). Surface infections may be treated with antibiotics or alternatively by antiseptics which are chemicals generally not classified as drugs, such as chlorine, phenols and hydrogen peroxide, that have a detergent effect and don't work internally, or else are too toxic for internal use. Antiseptics are sometimes called germicides, and may be used in soap, toothpaste and gargles. Disinfectants such as household bleaches are also germicidal.

8. Bacteria may be classified according to their bacteriophage content. Thus, the modern epidemic of food-borne salmonella infection in Britain is carried by *Salmonella enteritidis* phage 4.

9. 'The A–Z of Antibiotics', the appendix to this book, lists all antibiotics prescribed in Britain for human use. In it antibiotics are arranged by group or 'family', with information about how they work and what infections they are normally used for. See also the afterword by Professor Richard Lacey.

10. Sources used for this section include: Pratt, W., Fekety, R., *The Antimicrobial Drugs* (Oxford: University Press, 1986). Laurence, D., Bennett, P., *Clinical Pharmacology* (Edinburgh: Churchill Livingstone, 1992).

11. Part 1, notes 2, 10.

12. Harris, R., *The Real Voice* (New York: Macmillan, 1964). Also Inglis, B., *Drugs, Doctors and Disease* (London: André Deutsch, 1965).

13. Lappé, M., *When Antibiotics Fail. Restoring the Ecology of the Body* (Berkeley, California: North Atlantic Books, 1986).

14. Van den Bosch, R., *The Pesticide Conspiracy* (New York: Doubleday, 1978).

15. Metcalf, R., 'Insect resistance to insecticides' (*Pestic Sci*, 1989: 26: 333–58).

16. Royal Commission on Environmental Pollution, *Seventh report: Agriculture and Pollution* (London: HMSO, 1979).

17. Anti-protozoal drugs are a type of antibiotic, but are not listed in 'The A–Z of Antibiotics', the appendix to this book.

18. Wilkie, T., 'Monster bugs thrive as chemical arsenal fails' (*Independent*, 20 February 1989).

19. See Part 5 for a fuller account.

20. Koshland, D., 'The microbial wars' (*Science* 1992; 257: 1021).

21. Kunin, C., 'The responsibility of the infectious disease community for the optimum use of antimicrobial agents' (*J Infect Dis*, 1985; 151(3): 388–97). Also: Kunin, C., 'Rational use of antibiotics' (*WHO Drug Information*, 1990; 4(1): 4–7).

22. Begley, S., 'The end of antibiotics' (*Newsweek*, 28 March 1994).

23. As in the USA and the UK the rise of the German pharmaceutical industry after World War II was principally due to the phenomenal success of antibiotics.

24. Sources used for the accounts of antibiotics in this section include: Goodman-Gilman, A., Rowe, T., Nies, A., Taylor, P. (eds), *Pharmacological Basis of Therapeutics* (Oxford, Pergamon, 1990). National Institutes of Health Study on Antibiotic Use and Antibiotic Resistance Worldwide. 'Report of Task Force 2' (*Rev Infect Dis*, 1987; 9(3): S244–S260). Greenwood, D. (ed), *Antimicrobial Therapy* (Part 1, note 24). *Martindale: the Extra Pharmacopoeia* (Part 1, note 1). *The Merck Manual* (Part 1, note 3). Milton Wainwright's *Miracle Cure* (Part 1, note 7).

25. Cowe, R., 'One could argue with this kind of neat theory. Top 10 European drug companies' (*Guardian*, 14 December 1989). Also Elliott L., Cowe R. 'Drug companies struggle to get fit' (*Guardian*, 7 May 1994).

26. Part 1, note 1. As already mentioned, co-trimoxazole as a sulphonamide combination also has these ill-effects.

27. Gross R., Rowe, B., Cheasty, T., Thomas, L., 'Increase in drug resistance among *Shigella dysenteriae, Sh. flexneri*, and *Sh. boydii*' (*Br. Med J* 1981; 283: 575–6).

28. *See also* Part 5, 'Superbug'.

29. Finch, R., 'The penicillins today' (*Br Med J*, 1990; 300: 1289–90).

30. Archer, A., 'Alliances offer a model' (*Financial Times Pharmaceutical Survey*, 23 July 1991).

31. Aral, S., Holmes, K., 'Sexually transmitted diseases in the AIDS era' (*Scientific American*, 1991; 264(2): 18–25).

32. Ison, C., Branley, N., Kirtland, K., Easmon, C., 'Surveillance of antibiotic resistance in clinical isolates of *Neisseria gonorrhoeae*' (*Br Med J*, 1991; 303: 1307).

33. Yeung, K., Dillon, J., 'Norfloxacin resistant *Neisseria gonorrhoeae* in North America' (*Lancet*, 1991; 336: 759).

34. Part 1, note 25.

35. Pratt, R., Dufrenoy, J., *Antibiotics* (Philadelphia: Lippincott, 1949).

36. Part 1, note 7.

37. Melrose, D., *Bitter Pills. Medicines and the Third World Poor* (Oxford: Oxfam, 1982).

38. Burns, I., Hodgman, J., Cass, A., 'Fatal circulatory collapse in premature infants receiving chloramphenicol' (*N Eng J Med*, 1959; 261: 1318–21). Anon, 'Danger of chloramphenicol' (*Br Med J*, 1952; 19 July: 136–8). Anon. 'Mortality from chloramphenicol' (*Br Med J*, 1961; 8 April: 1019–20).

39. Part 1, note 13.

40. Geneva: WHO Programme for Control of Diarrhoeal Diseases 1988.

41. Yergin, D., *The Prize* (New York: Simon and Schuster, 1991).

42. Braithwaite, J., *Corporate Crime in the Pharmaceutical Industry* (London: Routledge and Kegan Paul, 1984). This contains a fuller account of the tetracycline industry in the 1950s; and also of the postwar German pharmaceutical industry.

43. Hooper, D., Wolfson, J., 'Fluoroquinolone antimicrobial agents' (*New Eng J Med*, 1991; 324(6): 384–94).

44. Hunt, L., 'Withdrawn drug "introduced rapidly"' (*Independent*, 15 June 1992).

45. Pinn, S., 'Quinolone to conquer resistance of bacteria' (*Hospital Doctor*, 12 September 1991).

46. Abbott Laboratories. Temafloxacin (Teflox/Teflox 400) – worldwide withdrawal. Letter to doctors, 6 June 1992.

47. Lacey, R., 'Are better drugs on the way?' (*MIMS* magazine, 1 September 1986).

48. Midtvedt, T., 'Quinolones and the environment' (*Lancet*, 1989; ii: 1040).

49. Maskell, R., '4-fluoroquinolones and *Lactobacilli* spp as emerging pathogens' (*Lancet*, 1992; 399(i): 929).

50. As for example: Dukes, M., Aronson, J. (eds), *Side Effects of Drugs Annual 15* (Amsterdam: Elsevier, 1991).

51. Liss, R., Batchelor, F., 'Economic evaluations of antibiotic use and resistance – a perspective, Report of Task Force 6 of the NIH Study on Antibiotic Use and Antibiotic Resistance Worldwide' (*Rev Infect Dis*, 1987; 9 (3): S297–S311). These figures were also cited by an expert group convened by the World Health Organisation in 1988. See Kunin, C., Johansen, K. et al., 'Report on a symposium on use and abuse of antibiotics worldwide' (*Rev Infect Dis*, 1990; 12(1): 12–19).

52. Col, N., O'Connor, R., 'Estimating worldwide current antibiotic usage. Report of Task Force 1 of the NIH Study on Antibiotic Use and Antibiotic Resistance Worldwide' (*Rev Infect Dis*, 1987; 9(3): S232–S243).

53. Lowe, D., 'Manufacture of penicillin' in Queener, S. et al. (eds), *Beta-lactam antibiotics for clinical use* (New York: Marcel Dekker, 1986).

54. British Society for Antimicrobial Chemotherapy, General Practice Working Group, 1994, *Report to the Council of the BSAC by the General Practice Group on Community Antibiotics Usage in England and Scotland from 1980–93* (BSAC, 1995).

55. Iglehart, J., 'The Food and Drug Administration and its problems' (*N Eng J Med 1991*; 325(3): 217–20).

56. Mihill, C., 'A very British drugs ailment' (*Guardian*, 15 June 1990).

57. This impressive sum includes all the costs of developing as well as researching a successful drug. It also includes the costs of research and development of unsuccessful drugs, and the costs of drugs that are expensive to develop are passed on to the customer, which in Britain is usually the National Health Service. And see Muller, M., *The Health of Nations* (London: Faber, 1982).

58. Commission of the European Communities, *The Community's Pharmaceutical Industry* (Luxembourg: CEC, 1985).

59. Cowe, R., 'The ultimate drug deal' (*Guardian*, 24 January 1995).

60. Anon, 'Private policing' (*The Economist*, 20 April 1991).

61. As quoted in Dr Joe Collier's book *The Health Conspiracy*, published in the UK by Century in 1989.

62. Anon, 'The doctors' dilemma' (*The Economist*, 27 January 1990).

63. Illich, I., 'Body history' (*Lancet*, 1986; ii: 1325–6).

Part Three: **Bug Wars**

1. This chapter owes much to the thinking of Professor Lewis Thomas, as well as to Professor René Dubos, already cited in Part 1. 'Germs' by Lewis Thomas is from his book *The Wonderful Mistake* published by Oxford University Press in 1988.

2. Lacey, R., *Safe Shopping, Safe Cooking, Safe Eating* (London: Penguin, 1989).

3. Susan Sontag's *Illness as Metaphor* (Allen Lane, 1979) is an illuminating account of how the language we use shapes our attitude to disease and ourselves. Her own focus is tuberculosis and cancer. She points out that 'the military metaphor in medicine first came into wide use in the 1880s, with the identification of bacteria as agents of disease'.

4. Hodgkin, K. (ed), *Family Medical Adviser* (London: Reader's Digest, 1983).

5. Vaccination is a subject worth a book in itself. As with antibiotics, vaccination has played only a small part in the decline of epidemic infections. Homoeopathic doctors believe that vaccination lowers the body's natural resistance to disease.

6. I have drawn from Bernard Dixon's excellent book *Beyond the Magic Bullet*, published by Allen and Unwin in 1978, for this passage.

7. The overpowering influence of Pasteur is delineated in Professor Bruno Latour's remarkable book *The Pasteurisation of France*, published by Harvard University Press in 1988.

8. Trélat, E., 'La salubrité' (*Revue Scientifique*, 1895; 10/8: 163–70).

9. World Health Organisation, 'Declaration of Alma Ata' (*Lancet*, 1978; ii: 1040–1).

10. Dunlop, D., *World Medicine*, 18 October 1972.

11. Sources used for the account of gut flora in this section include the following. Hentges, D. (ed), *Human Intestinal Flora in Health and Disease* (New York: Academic Press, 1983). Grubb, R., Midtvedt, T., Norin, E. (eds), *The Regulatory and Protective Role of the Normal Microflora* (New York: Macmillan, 1989).

12. Gurr, M., 'The nutrition of microbes and man' (Editorial, *Br J Nutr*, 1990; 63: 5–6).

13. Booth, C., 'Introduction to Conference on Intestinal Flora in Health and Disease' (*Ann Ist Super Sanita*, 1986; 22/3: 727–8).

14. Sir Arbuthnot Lane, now generally seen as a butcher, may have had a point. Diets heavy in meat in which cereal, vegetables and fruit were almost absent, were fashionable at the time; such diets can cause intense constipation and even a seizing up of the colon. This problem is not caused by bacteria. In extreme cases it can be solved only by surgery. Lane himself was a dietary reformer whose ideas on a healthy diet are similar to those generally accepted today.

15. Hill, M., Hudson, M., Borriello, P., 'Factors controlling the intestinal flora' (*Eur J Chemotherap and Antibiotics*, 1982; 2: 51–6).

16. Gorbach, S., 'Biochemical methods and experimental models for studying the intestinal flora' (*Ann Ist Super Sanita*, 1986; 22/3: 739–48).

17. Midtvedt, T., 'The normal microflora, intestinal motility and influence of antibiotics. An overview', in Grubb, R., Midtvedt, T., Norin, E. (eds), *The Regulatory and Protective Role of the Normal Microflora* (New York: Macmillan, 1989).

18. van der Waaij, D., de Vries-Hospers, H., 'Colonisation resistance of the digestive tract; mechanism and clinical consequences' *Ann Ist Super Sanita*, 1986; 22/3: 875–82.

19. van der Waaij, D., de Vries, J., Lekkerkerk van der Wees, J., 'Colonisation resistance of the digestive tract in conventional and antibiotic-treated mice' (*J Hyg*, 1971; 69: 405–11).

20. So what this means, is that antibiotics are liable to damage the body's outer immune defences, and to expose its inner immune defences. The consequent ill-effects are discussed in detail in Part 4, 'Apocalypse Now'.

21. Sources used for this section include Lehninger, A., *Biochemistry* (New York: Worth, 1975).

22. Schell, O., *Modern Meat* (New York: Random House, 1984).

23. Part 1, note 7.

24. The pharmacological as distinct from nutritional qualities of food and drink is now a subject of great scientific interest. An excellent recent popular book is Jean Carper's *Food Pharmacy*, published by Simon and Schuster in 1989. Other references are as follows. Beuchat, L., Brackett, R., 'Inhibitory effects of raw carrots on *Listeria monocytogenes*' (*Appl & Environ Microbiol*, 1990; 56(6): 1734–42). Baumgartner, B., Erdelmeier, C., Wright, A. et al., 'An antimicrobial alkaloid from *Ficus septica*' (*Phytochemistry*, 1990;

29(10): 3237–330). Haffejee, I., Moosa, A., 'Honey in the treatment of infantile gastroenteritis' (*Br Med J*, 1985; 290: 1866–7). Anon, 'Olive yields antibiotic' (*GP*, 9 March 1990). Diker, K., Akan, M., Hascelik, G. et al. 'The bacteriocidal activity of tea against *Campylobacter jejuni* and *Campylobacter coli*' (Letters in *Appl Microbiology*, 1991; 12: 34–5). Mihill, C., 'Garlic fights food bugs' (*Guardian*, 15 July 1993).

Part Four: **Apocalypse Now**

1. Brumfitt, W., 'Progress in understanding urinary infection' (*J Antimicrob Chemotherap*, 1991; 27: 9–22).

2. Part 1, note 3.

3. Sources used for the accounts of the ill-effects of antibiotics in this chapter include microbiological and pharmacological textbooks already referred to, and also the following: Hugo, W., Russell, A. (eds), *Pharmacological Microbiology* (Oxford: Blackwell, 1991). Pratt, W., Fekety, R., *The Antimicrobial Drugs* (Oxford: University Press, 1986).

4. Reid, G., Bruce, A., Cook, R., Llano, M., 'Effect on urogenital flora of antibiotic therapy for urinary tract infection' (*Scand Infect Dis*, 1990; 22: 43–7). Also, Reid, G., Bruce, A., Beheshti, M., 'Effect of antibiotic treatment on receptivity of uroepithelial cells to uropathogens' (*Can J Microbiol*, 1988; 34: 327–31). See also Maskell, R., 'Antibacterial agents and urinary tract infection: a paradox' (*Br J Gen Pract* April 1992: 138–9).

5. Sources used for this section include the following. Balmer, S., Wharton, B., 'Diet and faecal flora in the newborn: breast milk and infant formula' (*Arch Dis Child*, 1989; 64: 1672–7). Bennet, R., Eriksson, M., Nord, C. et al., 'Faecal bacterial microflora of newborn infants during intensive care management and treatment with five antibiotic regimes' (*Ped Infect Dis*, 1986; 5: 533–9). Bennet, R., Nord, C., 'The intestinal microflora during the first weeks of life: normal development and changes induced by caesarian section, pre-term birth and antimicrobial treatment' in

Grubb, R., Midtvedt, T., Norin, E. (eds), *The Regulatory and Protective Role of the Normal Microflora* (New York: Macmillan, 1989). Hall, M., Cole, C., Smith, S. et al., 'Factors influencing the presence of faecal lactobacilli in early infancy' (*Arch Dis Child*, 1990; 65: 185–8). Raibaud, P., 'Factors controlling the bacterial colonisation of the neonatal intestine', in Hanson, L. (ed), *Biology of Human Milk* (New York: Raven Press, 1988).

6. Anybody who needs reminding of the vital importance of breastmilk should read Gabrielle Palmer's book *The Politics of Breastfeeding*, published in 1988 by Pandora Books.

7. This is true both in the developed world and in developing countries and is of special importance in the latter.

8. Sources used for this section include the following. Anon, 'The management of acute otitis media' (*Drugs and Therapy Bull*, 1984; 22(14): 53–5). Mills, R., 'Policies on antibiotics of south-east London general practitioners for managing acute otitis media in children' (*Br Med J*, 1984; 288: 1199–1202). Browning, G., 'Childhood otalgia: acute otitis media. Antibiotics not necessary in most cases' (*Br Med J*, 1990; 300: 1005–6). Placito, M., 'Antibiotics "slow rate of otitis recovery"' (*Doctor*, 8 March 1990). Skinner, D., Pritchard, A., Narula, A., 'Acute otitis media' (*Br Med J*, 1990; 300: 1524). Van Buchem, F., Peeters, M., Van't Hof, M., 'Acute otitis media: a new treatment strategy' (*Br Med J*, 1985; 290: 1033–7).

9. Rheumatic fever, causing swelling in the joints and sometimes damage to the heart, is indeed now very rare in Britain, but new strains of *S. pyogenes* are an increasing cause of serious infections, including rheumatic fever, in the USA. Antibiotics are certainly indicated if a patient not only has an acute sore throat but also swelling in the joints (polyarthritis); but not just for simple sore throats. There is also an ethical issue involved here. Physicians who prescribe antibiotics not to treat a disease but to prevent a complication should always make this clear.

10. The classic account of the dangers of pesticides, including superpests, is Rachel Carson's book *Silent Spring*, first published in 1962, and now available from Penguin.

11. Hentges, D., 'Role of the intestinal microflora in host defence against infection', in Hentges, D. (ed), *Human Intestinal Microflora in Health and Disease* (New York: Academic Press, 1983).

12. Freter, R., 'Experimental enteric shigella and vibrio infections in mice and guinea pigs' (*J Exp Med* 1956; 104: 411–18).

13. Miller, C., 'Protective action of the normal microflora against enteric infection: an experimental study in the mouse' (*Univ Mich Med Bull*, 1959; 25: 272–9).

14. Finegold, S., 'Intestinal microbial changes and disease as a result of antimicrobial use' (*Ped Infect Dis*, 1986; 5(1): S88–S90).

15. This work goes back to Huppert, M., Cazin, J., Smith, H., 'Pathogenesis of *Candida albicans* infection following antibiotic therapy' (*J Bacteriol*, 1955; 70: 440–7). Professor Hentges (note 11, above) provides other references and there are more later in this chapter.

16. For example, Fekety, R., Kim, K., Batts, D. et al., 'Studies on the epidemiology of antibiotic-associated *Clostridium difficile* colitis' (*Am J Clin Nutr*, 1980; 33: 2527–32).

17. Infants are vulnerable to botulism. And see note 11, above.

18. Hentges, D., Stein, A., Casey, S., Que, J., 'Protective role of intestinal flora against infection with *Pseudomonas aeruginosa* in mice: influence of antibiotics with colonisation resistance' (*Infect and Immun*, 1985; 47(1): 118–22).

19. Guiliano, M., Barza, M., Jacobus, N., Gorbach, S., 'Effect of broad-spectrum parenteral antibiotics on composition of intestinal microflora of humans' (*Antimicrob Agents and Chemotherap*, 1987; 31(2): 202–6. Also, 32(5): 723–7).

20. van Saene, H., Stoutenbeek, C., Geitz, J. et al., 'Effect of amoxycillin on colonisation resistance in human volunteers' (*Microb Ecol in Health and Dis*, 1986; 1: 169–77).

21. Sources for this section include the following: George, W., Sutter, V., Finegold, S., 'Antimicrobial agent-induced diarrhoea – a bacterial disease' (*J Infect Dis*, 1977; 136(6): 822–8). Anon, 'Antibiotic-associated colitis – the continuing saga' (*Br Med J*, 1981; 282: 1913–14). George, W., Finegold, S., 'Clostridia in the human gastrointestinal flora' in Borriello, P. (ed), *Clostridia in Gastrointestinal Disease* (Boca Raton, Florida: CRC Press, 1985). Lyerly, D., Krivan, H., Wilkins, T., '*Clostridium difficile*: its diseases and toxins' (*Clin Microbiol Rev*, 1988; 1(1): 1–18).

22. Kelly, C., Pothoulakis, C., LaMont, J., '*Clostridium difficile* colitis' (*N Eng J Med*, 1994; 330(4): 257–62).

23. Brazier, J., Duerden, B., et al., 'Clostridium difficile – progress report' (*PHLS Microbiology Digest*, 1994; 10(2): 76–90).

24. Sources for this section include the following: Anon, 'An irritable mind or an irritable bowel?' (Editorial, *Lancet*, 1984; ii: 1249–50). Welch, G., Hillman, I., Pomare, E., 'Psychoneurotic symptomatology in the irritable bowel syndrome: a study of reporters and non-reporters' (*Br Med J*, 1985; 291: 1382–4).

25. Sources for this and the next sections include the following: Anon, 'Crohn's Disease: 40 years on' (Editorial, *Br Med J*, 1978; 1106–7). Anon, 'Management of Crohn's disease: time for audit?' (Editorial, *Br Med J*, 1980; 281: 893–4). Gazzard, B., Price, H., Libby, G., Dawson, A., 'The social toll of Crohn's disease' (*Br Med J*, 1978; 1117–19). Heaton, K., 'Crohn's disease and ulcerative colitis' in Trowell, H., Burkitt, D., Heaton, K. (eds), *Fibre, Fibre-Depleted Foods and Disease* (London: Academic Press, 1985). Hunt, L., 'Number of children with serious bowel disorder triples' (*Independent*, 11 November 1989).

26. Mallett, S., Lennard-Jones, J., Bingley, J., Gilon, E., 'Colitis' (*Lancet*, 1978; ii: 619–21).

27. Bayliss, C., Bradley, H., Alun Jones, V., Hunter, J., 'Some aspects of colonic microbial activity in irritable bowel syndrome associated with food intolerance' (*Ann Ist Super Sanita*, 1986; 22(3): 959–64). Hunter, J., Alun Jones, V., 'Studies on the pathogenesis

of irritable bowel syndrome produced by food intolerance' in Read, N. (ed), *Irritable Bowel Syndrome* (New York: Grune and Stratton, 1985). Hunter, J., 'Irritable bowel syndrome' (*Proc Nut Soc*, 1985; 44: 141–3).

28. Dickinson, R., 'Enteric infection and ulcerative colitis' (thesis, 1982, unpublished).

29. Part 3, note 18.

30. Taylor-Robinson, S., Miles, R., Whitehead, A., Dickinson, R., 'Salmonella infection and ulcerative colitis' (*Lancet*, 1989; i: 1145).

31. Seneca, H., Henderson, E., 'Normal intestinal bacteria in ulcerative colitis' (*Gastroenterol*, 1950; 15: 34–9). Shorter, R., Huizenga, K., Spencer, R., 'A working hypothesis for the aetiology and pathogenesis of non-specific inflammatory bowel disease' (*Digestive Dis*, 1972; 17: 1024–32). Tabaqchali, S., Tanaka, K., Wilks, M., 'Bacterial flora and intestinal chronic disease' (*Ann Ist Super Sanita*, 1986; 22(3): 921–32). Hudson, M., Hill, M., Lennard-Jones, J., 'Bacteria associated with the colo-rectal mucosa in patients with inflammatory bowel disease' (*Microecol and Therapy*, 1984; 14: 287–8).

32. van Saene, H., *Pathogenesis of Inflammatory Bowel Diseases* (Holland: Lannoo Tielt-Bussum, 1982).

33. Dr Hunter has co-written a self-help book for people who suffer from irritable bowel syndrome and from food allergy. The reference is: Workman, E., Hunter, J., Alun Jones, V., *The Allergy Diet* (London: Martin Dunitz, 1984).

34. Brostoff, J., Gamlin, L., *The Complete Guide to Food Allergy and Intolerance* (London: Bloomsbury, 1989). This is also an excellent manual and self-help guide.

35. Hunter, J., 'Food allergy – or enterometabolic disorder?' (*Lancet*, 1991; 338: 495–6).

36. Ebringer, A., 'The relationship between klebsiella infection and ankylosing spondylitis' (*Ballière's Clinical Rheumatology*, 1989; 3(2): 321–88). Ebringer, A., Ptasyznska, T., Corbett, T. et al., 'Antibodies to proteus in rheumatoid arthritis' (*Lancet*, 1985; ii: 305–7). Ebringer, A., Khalafpour, S., Wilson, C., 'Rheumatoid arthritis and proteus: a possible aetiological association' (*Rheumatol Int*, 1989; 9: 223–8). Linehan, L., 'How potatoes and pasta can damage the bones' (*Independent*, 8 November 1988).

37. Fryden, A., Bengtsson, A., Foberg, U. et al., 'Early antibiotic treatment of reactive arthritis associated with enteric infections: clinical and serological study' (*Br Med J*, 1990; 301: 1299–1302).

38. Cannon, W., *The Wisdom of the Body* (New York: Norton, 1963).

39. The standard textbook is: Odds, F., *Candida and Candidosis* (London: Ballière Tindall, 1988).

40. Part 1, note 24.

41. See the appendix for an account of all the anti-fungal drugs now available in Britain.

42. Abrahams, P., 'OTC sales prove addictive' (*Financial Times*, 21 August 1992).

43. The 'candida missionaries' who believe there is an epidemic of candida superinfection in our midst, are Dr C. Orian Truss and Dr William Crook. See Truss, C., *The Missing Diagnosis* (PO Box 26508, Birmingham, Alabama 35226, USA) and Crook, W., *The Yeast Connection* (Professional Books, PO Box 3494, Jackson, Tennessee 38301, USA). The claims made in these books are generally felt to be over-enthusiastic. A useful self-help book is Jacobs, G., *Candida albicans* (London: Optima, 1990).

44. Blonz, E., 'Is there an epidemic of chronic candida in our midst?' (*JAMA*, 1986; 256: 3138–9).

45. Seelig, M., 'Mechanisms by which antibiotics increase the incidence and severity of candidiasis and alter the immunological defences' (*Bacteriol Rev*, 1966; 30: 442–59).

46. Witkin, S., 'Defective immune responses in patients with recurrent candidiasis' (*Infect in Med*, 1985; May/June: 129–32).

47. See also Galland, L., Bueno, H., 'Mucosal inhibition of candida growth as a possible marker of candida hypersensitivity' (paper presented at Candida Update conference, Memphis, 16–18 September 1988).

48. Bennett, 'Searching for the yeast connection' (*N Eng J Med*, 1990; 323(25): 1766–7). This leading article commented on the results of a trial showing that anti-fungal drugs (like nystatin) by themselves are not effective treatment for candidiasis. The reference for this study is: Dismukes, W., Scott Wade, J., Lee, J. et al., 'A randomised, double-blind trial of nystatin therapy for the candidiasis hypersensitivity syndrome' (*N Eng J Med*, 1990; 323(25): 1717–23). Also: Edwards, J., 'Invasive candida infections. Evolution of a fungal pathogen' (N Eng J Med, 1991: 1060-2).

49. Sources used for this section include the following: Jenkins, R., Mowbray, J. (eds), *Post-Viral Fatigue Syndrome* (New York: Wiley, 1991). Goudsmit, E., 'Myalgic encephalomyelitis: a review of the literature' (unpublished).

50. Mihill, C., 'ME "in everyone" says specialists' (*Guardian*, 1 September 1990).

51. Yousef, G., Mann, G., Smith, D. et al., 'Chronic enterovirus infection in patients with postviral fatigue syndrome' (*Lancet*, 1988; i: 146–50).

52. Jessop, C., 'Chronic fatigue syndrome' (presentation for conference, San Francisco, 15 April 1989, unpublished).

53. Weir, D., *Immunology* (Edinburgh: Churchill Livingstone, 1983).

54. Anon, 'Antibiotics as biological response modifiers' (*Lancet*, 1991; 337: 400–1).

55. Raeburn, J., 'Antibiotics and immunodeficiency' (*Lancet*, 1972; ii: 954–6).

56. Hauser, W., Remington, J., 'Effect of antimicrobial agents on the immune response' in Ristuccia, A. (ed), *Antimicrobial Therapy* (New York: Raven Press, 1984).

57. Hall, C., 'Sexual diseases hit epidemic levels' (*Independent*, 28 December 1990).

58. Fisher, J., *The Plague Makers* (New York: Simon and Schuster, 1994).

59. Rutherford, G., 'Long term survival in HIV-1 infection' (*Br Med J*, 1994; 309: 283–4).

60. Note 25, above. Also: Willett, W., 'The search for the causes of breast and colon cancer' (*Nature*, 1989; 338: 389–94).

61. Hill, M., 'Bile, bacteria and colon cancer' (*Gut*, 1983; 24: 871–5).

Part Five: **Superbug**

1. Part 2, note 5.

2. Neu, H., 'The crisis in antibiotic resistance' (*Science*, 1992; 257: 1064–72).

3. Cooper, T., 'Infectious diseases: no cause for complacency' (*J Infect Dis*, 1976; 134: 510–12). Tomasz, A., 'Multiple-antibiotic-resistant pathogenic bacteria' (*New Eng J Med*, 1994; 330(17): 1247–51).

4. Hunt, L., 'Children's ward is closed after two babies die' (*Independent*, 5 August 1992).

5. Rogers, L. '1 in 5 patients picks up an infection in hospital' (*Evening Standard*, 6 August 1992).

6. World Health Organisation, *Antimicrobial resistance. Report of scientific working group* (Geneva: WHO, 1982).

7. Mayon-White, R., Ducel, G., Kereselidze, T., Tikomirov, E., 'An international survey of the prevalence of hospital-acquired infection' (*J Hosp Infect*, 1988; 11(A): 43–8).

8. Anon, 'Are hospitals the worst places to get well?' (*Which? Way to Health*, April 1990).

9. de Bruxelles, S., Ferriman, A., 'Deadly "super bug" spreads through wards' (*Observer*, 31 August 1986).

10. Hill, G., Prentice, T., Wright, P., Stuttaford, T., 'Under siege from a super-bug' (*The Times*, 3 March 1987).

11. Part 2, note 1.

12. Part 2, note 5.

13. Staphylococci have always been a pest. Boils were one of the ten plagues visited on biblical Egypt. In the nineteenth century post-operative staph infection was generally epidemic; it's said that the operating theatre at the University of Aberdeen had the text 'Prepare to meet thy God' hung on the wall.

14. Brumfitt, W., Hamilton-Miller, J., 'Methicillin-resistant *Staphylococcus aureus*' (*N Eng J Med*, 1989; 320(18): 1188–96).

15. Sanderson, P., 'Staying one jump ahead of resistant *Staphylococcus aureus*' (*Br Med J*, 1986; 293: 573–4).

16. Part 2, note 24.

17. Hall, C., 'Fears raised by superbug secrecy' (*Independent*, 6 April 1989).

18. Maycock, J., Personal communication. Also see Maycock, J., 'An isolating experience' (*Nursing Times*, 1989; 85(13): 75).

19. Hopper, P., Turner, A., Law, M., Gill, M., 'Control of MRSA' (confidential interim report, 8 August 1986, unpublished).

20. Duckworth, G., Lothian, J., Williams, J., 'Methicillin-resistant *Staphylococcus aureus*: report of an outbreak at a London teaching hospital' (*J Hosp Infect*, 1988; 11: 1–15).

21. Quoted in: Hill, G., Prentice, T., Wright, P., Stuttaford, T., 'From wonder drug to bitter pill' (*The Times*, 2 March 1987).

22. Nash, M., 'Attack of the Superbugs' (*Time*, 31 August 1992).

23. Cohen, M., 'Epidemiology of drug resistance: implications for a post-antimicrobial era' (*Science*, 1992; 257: 1050–5).

24. Austrian, R., 'Some observations on the pneumococcus and on the current status of pneumococcal disease and its prevention' (*Rev Infect Dis*, 1981; 3(S1): (S1–17).

25. And also see Kunin, C., 'Resistance to antimicrobial drugs – a worldwide calamity' (*Ann Intern Med* 1993; 118: 557–61).

26. Moellering, R., 'The enterococcus: a classic example of the impact of antimocrobial therapy on therapeutic options' (The Garrod Lecture, *J Antimicrob Therap*, 1991; 28: 1–12).

27. Shiaes, D., Al-Obeid, A., Gutman, L., 'Enterococcal resistance to vancomycin and teicoplanin' (APUA newsletter 1989; 7(4): 1, 4).

28. French, G., Abdulla, Y., Heathcock, R., et al., 'Vancomycin resistance in south London' (*Lancet*, 1992; 338: 28 March). Friedan, T., Munsiff, S., Low, D. et al., 'Emergence of vancomycin-resistant enterococci in New York City' (*Lancet*, 1993; 342: 76–9).

29. Fraimow, H., Jungkind, D., Lander, D. et al., 'Urinary tract infection with an *Enterococcus faecalis* isolate that requires vancomycin for growth' (*Ann Int Med*, 1994; 121(1): 23–6).

30. Woodford, N., Johnson, A., Morrison, D. et al., 'Vancomycin-dependent enterococci in the United Kingdom' (*J Antimicrob Chemother*, 1994; 33: 1066).

31. Florey, H., 'Clinical use of penicillin' (*Br Med J*, 1944; 2: 9–13).

32. Monod, J., *Chance and Necessity* (London: Collins, 1972). I have altered some of the words but not the sense of the English translation.

33. It may be that mammoths were more adaptable than commonly thought. In 1993 Russian scientists announced the discovery of remains of a miniature variety on an Arctic island, which may have survived until a few thousand years ago.

34. Sometimes drug resistance can be overcome by giving relatively massive doses of antibiotics.

35. Bacillary dysentery is uncommon in Europe, America, and other temperate zones, in which the species of shigella bacilli that cause dysentery are less severe in their effect.

36. Watanabe, T., 'Infective heredity of multiple drug resistance in bacteria' (*Bacteriol Rev*, 1963; 27: 87–103).

37. Akiba, T., Koyama, K., Isiki, Y., et al., 'On the mechanism of the development of multiple-drug-resistant clones of shigella' (*Jap J Microb*, 1960; 4: 219).

38. Ochai, K., Yamanaka, T., Kimura, K., Sawada, O., 'Inheritance of drug resistance (and its transfer) between shigella strains and between shigella strains and *E. coli* strains' (*Nhonji-shimpo*, 1959; 1861: 34–6).

39. Sometimes plasmids are called 'R factors', the 'R' standing for 'resistance'. To be precise, the term 'R factor' applies only to that part of the plasmid's genetic structure that confers and transfers drug resistance.

40. A lucid account of plasmids is: Novick, R., 'Plasmids' (*Scientific American*, 1980; 243(6): 102–7).

41. In an interview with the American farmer and writer Orville Schell, first published in the *New Yorker*, and then in Schell's excellent and provocative book, *Modern Meat* (Part 3, note 22).

42. Dr Watanabe's work became well known in the scientific world a decade after his first findings were published in specialist journals, with publication of this warning. The reference is: Watanabe, T., 'Infectious Drug Resistance' (*Scientific American*, 1967; 217: 19–27).

43. Studies in which plasmids have been found in remote 'pre-antibiotic' communities are cited by Professor Stanley Falkow of Stanford University, in a pioneering book. The reference is: Falkow, S., *Infectious Multiple Drug Resistance* (London: Methuen (distributors), 1975).

44. The classic study made by Dr Naomi Datta of Hammersmith Hospital in London, of bacteria collected early this century, also found plasmids. See for example: Datta, N., Hughes, V., 'Plasmids of the same Inc groups in enterobacteria before and after the medical use of antibiotics' (*Nature*, 1983; 306: 616).

45. Resistance genes were found in remote communities studied in modern times (note 43, above) but hardly at all in pre-antibiotic bacteria (note 44, above). Perhaps bacteria made resistant by antibiotics managed somehow to travel and infect remote native peoples, perhaps carried by animals, traders, or research scientists.

46. See Part 2.

47. Levy, S., Marshall, B., Schleuderberg, S. et al., 'High frequency of antimicrobial resistance in human faecal flora' (*Antimicrob Agents Chemotherap*, 1988; 32: 1801–6).

48. Dr O'Brien is here describing recent medical practice in the USA. Third-generation cephalosporins are indeed very expensive, and in other developed countries such as the UK are therefore used uncommonly, for obstinate infections in hospital patients. Such 'luxury' drugs are available only for the rich in developing countries.

49. Dr O'Brien has proposed that 'a low level of carriage of resistant strains [of bacteria] should become a public health goal, as have normal blood pressure and lower serum cholesterol levels'. See

Lester, S., Pilar Pla, M., Wang, F. et al., 'The carriage of *Escherichia coli* resistant to antimicrobial agents by healthy children in Boston, in Caracas, Venezuela, and in Qin Pu, China' (*N Eng J Med*, 1990; 323(5): 285–9).

50. Part 2, note 37.

51. National Institutes of Health Study on Antibiotic Use and Antibiotic Resistance Worldwide, 'Report of Task Force 4' (*Rev Infect Dis*, 1987; 9(3): S270–S285).

52. Just how virulent an organism is, critically depends on the immune strength of the infected person. Micro-organisms may be particularly virulent because they secrete most toxin, multiply most rapidly, or because they are especially adhesive and/or invasive.

53. Much of the information in this section is taken from reports prepared by Health Action International, the leading global public interest group concerned with drugs. The reports include the following. *Antibiotics: the wrong drugs for diarrhoea. Problem Drugs: Antidiarrhoeals* (Antidiarr 1A). *Antidiarrhoeals containing antibiotics* (Antidiarr 1B). *Hydroxyquinolines* (Antidiarr 1C). HAI has gained the respect of the drug industry and of regulatory authorities; its reports are meticulous. Its address in Europe is J. van Lennepkade 334-T, 1053 NJ Amsterdam, the Netherlands.

54. Information correct in 1988–9.

55. World Health Organisation, *Programme for the Control of Diarrhoeal Diseases. A manual for the treatment of diarrhoea* (Geneva: WHO, 1990).

56. World Health Organisation, *Diarrhoeal Disease Control Programme* (Geneva: WHO, 1988).

57. Anon, 'Porter v Ohmae' (*The Economist*, 4 August 1990).

58. Christie, D., 'Third World in Action' (*The Listener*, 12 October 1989).

59. World Health Organisation, *The rational use of drugs in the management of acute diarrhoea in children* (Geneva: WHO, 1991).

60. Gorbach, S., Edelman, R., 'Travelers' diarrhea' (National Institutes of Health Consensus Development Conference, *Rev Infect Dis*, 1986; 8: suppl 2: S109–S233).

61. Hyams, K., Bourgeois, A., Merrell, B. et al., 'Diarrhoeal disease during Operation Desert Shield' (*N Eng J Med*, 1991; 325: 1423–8).

62. Scotland, S., 'The occurrence of plasmids carrying genes for both enterotoxin production and drug resistance in *E. coli*.' (*J Hyg (Cambridge)*, 1979; 83: 531–7).

63. Nandan, G., 'Troops battle to contain India's outbreak of plague' (*Br Med J*, 1994; 309: 827).

64. Olarte, J., 'Chloramphenicol-resistant typhoid fever in Mexico: update since 1972' (The Alliance for the Prudent Use of Antibiotics (APUA) newsletter 1984; 2/4).

65. Lee, P., Statement before the US Senate Sub-Committee on Monopoly, 26 May 1976 (personal communication from Professor Lee).

66. Wallace, M., Yousif, A., Mahroos, G. et al, 'Ciprofloxacin versus ceftriaxone in the treatment of multiresistant typhoid fever' (*Eur J Clin Microbiol Infect Dis,* 1993; 12(12): 907–10).

67. Mandal, B., '*Salmonella typhi* and other salmonellas' (*Gut*, 1994; 35: 726–8).

68. Threlfall, E., Rowe, B., Ward, L., 'Occurrence and treatment of multi-resistant *Salmonella typhi* in the UK' (*PHLS Microbiology Digest*, 1991; 8/2). Also Rowe, B., Ward, R., Threlfall, E., 'Treatment of multi-resistant typhoid fever' (*Lancet*, 1991; I: 1422).

69. Threlfall, E., Said, B., Rowe, B. et al., 'Emergence of multiple drug resistance in Vibrio cholerae 01 El Tor from Ecuador' (*Lancet*, 1993; 342: 1173).

70. Cholera Working Group, 'Large epidemic of cholera-like diseases in Bangladesh caused by *Vibrio cholerae* 0139 synonym Bengal' (*Lancet*, 1993; 342: 387–90).

71. World Health Organisation, *The rational use of drugs. Report of the conference of experts, Nairobi, 25–29 November 1985* (Geneva: WHO, 1987).

72. Fabricant, N., Hirschhorn, N., 'Deranged distribution, perverse prescription, unprotected use: the irrationality of pharmaceuticals in the developing world' (*Health Pol and Plan*, 1987; 2(3): 204–13).

73. World Health Organisation, *The world drug situation* (Geneva: WHO, 1988).

74. Pradervand, P., *Tetracycline lemonade. Report prepared for HAI International* (The Hague: HAI, 1984).

75. Tan, M., *Dying for Drugs. Pill power and politics in the Philippines* (Quezon City, Philippines: HAI, 1986).

76. Consumers' Association of Penang, *Drugs and the Third World. Tetracyclines – urgent control needed on sale and use* (Penang: CAP, 1989).

77. Management Services for Health, *Where does the tetracycline go? Health center prescribing and child survival in East Java and Kalimantan* (Boston: MSH, 1988).

78. Obaseiki-Ebor, E., Ebea, P., 'A survey of antibiotic outpatient prescribing and antibiotic self-medication'. Also another multi-authored paper (*J Antimicrob Chemotherap*, 1987, 1989; 759–63, 641–51).

79. Ferraz, E., 'Changing antibiotic usage in Brazil' (The APUA Newsletter 1989; 7/1).

80. Holmberg, S., Solomon, S., Blake, P., 'Health and economic aspects of antibiotic resistance' (*Rev Infect Dis*, 1987; 9(6): 1065–78).

81. The chemical industry, grown enormous because of the Second World War, was redesigned to produce agrichemicals after the war. Pre-chemical farming, well within the memories of people born in the 1920s or before, is evoked notably in John Stewart Collis's book *The Worm Forgives the Plough*' (London: Barrie and Jenkins, 1988).

82. In the UK, use of antibiotics on animals is officially restricted, following government's acceptance of recommendations made by an expert committee chaired by Professor Michael Swann in 1969. In particular, antibiotics used for growth promotion should not be those used as human medicine. This has not prevented the spread of drug-resistant infection from animals to people, however. See: Joint Committee on the Use of Antibiotics in Animal Husbandry and Veterinary Medicine (London: HMSO, 1969). Also: Anon, 'Why has Swann failed?' (*Br Med J*, 1980; 6225: 1195–6).

83. The use of drugs to treat and prevent infection in animals should be supervised by veterinary surgeons. Whether or not this is so in practice depends on the country (some are better regulated than others) and on the farmer (some are more scrupulous than others). Given the scale of meat and dairy production in developing countries, vets cannot systematically control or monitor the use of drugs on animals, especially when black markets flourish.

84. See Part 2.

85. Arguments between farmers who use modern (chemical) methods, and those who use traditional ('organic') methods of animal husbandry, can be bitter. The accusation that antibiotics and other drugs are used as a substitute for good farming practice, is often made by those who oppose intensive agricultural methods. Certainly, regular use of antibiotics on animals makes meat cheaper.

86. Novick, R., 'Antibiotics: wonder drugs or chicken feed?' (*The Sciences*, July–August 1979; 14–17).

87. British Veterinary Association, *Animal use of antibiotics* (issued by the BVA Medicines Committee, May 1989).

88. In the United States, an example of hostility to the use of antibiotics on animals being contained within a general ideological framework is, Jeremy Rifkin's book *Beyond Beef* (New York: Penguin, 1992). In Britain, as one example, the animal rights' group Chickens' Lib from time to time emphasises the dangers of antibiotics as used in the intensive rearing of poultry.

89. Ministry of Agriculture, Fisheries and Food, *Anabolic, antihelminthic and antimicrobial agents. The twenty-second report of the Steering Group on Food Surveillance. The Working Party on Veterinary Residues in Animal Products* (London: HMSO, 1987).

90. World Health Organisation, *Evaluation of certain veterinary drug residues in food. Thirty-fourth report of the joint FAO/WHO expert committee on food additives. Technical report series 788* (Geneva: WHO, 1989).

91. Ministry of Agriculture, Fisheries and Food, *Veterinary residues in animal products 1986 to 1990. The Government's response to the advice of its advisory committees* (London: MAFF, June 1992).

92. Wray, C., Furniss, S., Benham, C., 'Feeding antibiotic-contaminated waste milk to calves – effects on physical performance and antibiotic sensitivity of gut flora' (*Br Vet J*, 1990; 146: 80–7).

93. A balanced summary account, 'The use of antibiotics in food production' has been published in the UK by the Consumers Europe Group in May 1990. It is obtainable from CEG at 24 Tufton Street, London SW1P 3RB.

94. As reported in Erlichman, J., 'Cover-up that may help the superbugs' (*Guardian*, 7 April 1987).

95. Most but not all antibiotic residues are found in meat, meat products, and other food of animal origin. Antibiotics are also sometimes used in effect as pesticides against bacterial infections of fruit.

96. Lacey, R., *Unfit for Human Consumption* (London: Souvenir Press, 1991).

97. Levy, S., 'Playing antibiotic pool: time to tally the score' (*New Eng J Med*, 1984; 311(10): 663–4). This editorial was written to accompany a remarkable study by Dr Scott Holmberg of the US Centers for Disease Control and colleagues. See 'Drug resistant salmonella from animals fed antibiotics' (*N Eng J Med*, 1984; 311 (19): 617–22) tracing an outbreak of multiple drug-resistant salmonella infection back to its origins in a beef herd fed tetracyclines for growth promotion.

98. Institute of Medicine of the National Academy of Sciences, *Human health risks with the subtherapeutic use of penicillin or tetracyclines in animal feed* (Washington: National Academy Press, 1988).

99. World Health Organisation, *Salmonellosis control: the role of animal and product hygiene. Technical report series 774* (Geneva: WHO, 1988).

100. Cohen, M., Tauxe, R., 'Drug-resistant salmonella in the United States: an epidemiologic perspective' (*Science*, 1986; 234: 964–9).

101. Bingham, S., 'Agricultural chemicals in the food chain' (*J Roy Soc Med*, 1989; 82: 311–12).

102. Rampling, A., Upson, R., Brown, D., 'Nitrofurantoin resistance in isolates of *Salmonella enteritidis* phage type 4 from poultry and humans' (*J Antimicrob Therap*, 1990; 25: 285–90).

103. Holmberg, S., Wells, J., Cohen, M., 'Animal-to-man transmission of antimicrobial-resistant salmonella: investigations of US outbreaks, 1971–1983' (*Science*, 1984; 225: 833–5).

104. Novick, R., 'The development and spread of antibiotic-resistant bacteria as a consequence of feeding antibiotics to livestock' (1981: Annals of the New York Academy of Sciences, 23–59).

105. Page, W., Huyer, G., Huyer, M., Worobec, E., 'Characterisation of the porins of *Campylobacter jejuni* and *Campylobacter coli* and implications for antibiotic susceptibility' (*Antimicrob Agents and Chemotherap*, 1989; 33(3): 297–303).

106. Poyart-Salmeron, C., Carlier, C., Trieu-Cuot P. et al., 'Transferable plasmid-mediated antibiotic resistance in *Listeria monocytogenes*' (*Lancet*, 1990; 335: 1422–6).

107. Wray, C., 'Some aspects of the occurrence of resistant bacteria in the normal animal flora' (*J Antimicrob Therap*, 1986; 18 (C): 141–7).

108. Williams Smith, H., Lovell, M., '*Escherichia coli* resistant to tetracyclines and to other antibiotics in the faeces of UK chickens and pigs in 1980' (*J Hyg Camb*, 1981; 87: 477–83).

109. Levy, S., FitzGerald, G., Macone, A., 'Changes in intestinal flora after introduction of a tetraycline-supplemented feed on a farm' (*New Eng J Med*, 1976; 295: 583–8).

110. Linton, A., Howe, K., Bennett, P., Richmond, M. (*J Appl Bacteriol*, 1977; 43: 465–9).

CONCLUSION

1. DuPont, H., Ericsson, C., 'Prevention and treatment of traveler's diarrhea' (*New Eng J Med*, 1993; 328(25): 1821–7). The judgements cited derive from a consensus conference on the use of drugs to prevent traveller's diarrhoea held at the US National Institutes of Health in January 1985: see *Rev Infect Dis*, 1986; 8: Suppl 2: S109–S233.

2. Public opinion polls taken in the USA, the UK, and elsewhere in Europe, consistently show that personal and family health is the issue that above all concerns us – more than work and the prospect of unemployment, more than love, more than fear of war. After all, without health, what is worth having?

3. World Health Organisation, *The selection of essential drugs. Technical report series 615* (Geneva: WHO, 1977).

4. In 1977 the list of essential antibiotics published by WHO included five penicillins (benzyl penicillin, benethamine benzyl penicillin, phenoxymethyl penicillin, cloxacillin, ampicillin), three sulphonamides (salazosulphapyridine, sulphadimidine, and the trimethoprim cocktail co-trimoxazole), together with an aminoglycoside (gentamicin), chloramphenicol, the macrolide erythromycin, and tetracycline. The toxicity of chloramphenicol was noted. The complementary list was an aminoglycoside (amikacin) for drug-resistance infection, a penicillin (procaine penicillin) whose toxicity was noted, a sulphonamide (sulphadiazine), and a tetracycline (doxycycline). An updated list, or a list suitable for the UK and other developed countries now, would be somewhat different: see Professor Richard Lacey's afterword to this book.

5. Published regularly by the British Medical Association and the Royal Pharmacological Society of Great Britain, the BNF is a reliable but brief source of information about drugs.

6. As for example the 'Antibiotics Guidelines' for hospital practice and the 'Antibiotic Prescribing Guidelines for Common Infections in General Practice' issued by the Health Authority in Leeds. Prepared by an expert committee chaired by Professor Lacey, these have been adapted by him in his afterword to this book.

7. WHONET was begun and is kept going by Professor Thomas O'Brien in Boston. The address is Laboratory of Microbiology, Brigham and Women's Hospital, 75 Francis Street, Boston, Mass. 02115, USA.

8. Anon, 'Over-the-counter drugs' (*Lancet*, 1994; 343: 1374–75).

9. See, for example, *Bad Medicine* by Milton Silverman, Mia Lydecker and Philip Lee (Stanford University Press, 1982). In Britain Charles Medawar of Social Audit has co-written and published *Drug Dependency*. The address of Social Audit is PO Box 111, London NW1 8XG.

10. The address of the Consumers' Association of Penang is: No. 87, Jalan Cantonment, 10250 Pulau Penang, Malaysia.

11. The address of the Alliance for the Prudent Use of Antibiotics is PO Box 1372, Boston, Mass. 02117, USA. APUA was begun and is kept going above all by Professor Levy.

12. The address of the International Organisation of Consumer Unions in Europe is Emmastraat 9, 2595 The Hague, The Netherlands.

13. Until the 1980s and 1990s few nutritionists would dare say that wholefoods protect against infection as well as against non-infectious diseases. But although research remains patchy, it is likely that a great range of raw and lightly cooked foods of vegetable origin are protective.